The essays in this thought-provoking volume provide a critical perspective on women's responses to biomedical and other technologies affecting reproduction and health in general. A theoretical introduction, which argues for a rethinking of the concepts of biopower, medicalization, agency, and resistance, challenges the assumption that women are passive recipients of technological innovations. Thirteen case studies show that it is usually pragmatism that motivates women's behavior, explaining why their reactions to technology may range from acceptance to rejection or indifference, depending on whether its use fits with their own priorities and values. Essay topics include infertility in east Africa, prenatal diagnostic screening in America, AIDS in Africa, reproductive technologies in China and Japan, the emergence of the breast cancer movement, and health and environmental issues in Egypt and First Nations communities in Canada. Challenging conventional assumptions about the relationship between women and technology, this book is indispensible reading for anthropologists, sociologists, and gender studies scholars.

Pragmatic women and body politics

Cambridge Studies in Medical Anthropology 5

Editors
Ronald Frankenberg, *Centre for Medical Social Anthropology, University of Keele*
Byron Good, *Department of Social Medicine, Harvard Medical School*
Alan Harwood, *Department of Anthropology, University of Massachusetts, Boston*
Gilbert Lewis, *Department of Social Anthropology, University of Cambridge*
Roland Littlewood, *Department of Anthropology, University College London*
Margaret Lock, *Department of Social Studies of Medicine, McGill University*
Nancy Scheper-Hughes, *Department of Anthropology, University of California, Berkeley*

Medical anthropology is the fastest growing specialist area within anthropology, both in North America and in Europe. Beginning as an applied field serving public health specialists, medical anthropology now provides a significant forum for many of the most urgent debates in anthropology and the humanities.

Medical anthropology includes the study of medical institutions and health care in a variety of rich and poor societies, the investigation of the cultural construction of illness, and the analysis of ideas about the body, birth, maturation, ageing, and death.

This new series includes theoretically innovative monographs, state-of-the-art collections of essays on current issues, and short books introducing the main themes in the subdiscipline.

1 Lynn M. Morgan, *Community participation in health: the politics of primary care in Costa Rica*
2 Thomas J. Csordos, *Embodiment and experience: The existential ground of culture and self*
3 Paul Brodwin, *Medicine and morality in Haiti: the contest for healing power*
4 Susan Reynolds Whyte, *Questioning misfortune: the pragmatics of uncertainty in eastern Uganda*

Pragmatic women
and body politics

Edited by

Margaret Lock
McGill University

Patricia A. Kaufert
University of Manitoba

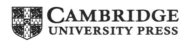
CAMBRIDGE
UNIVERSITY PRESS

CAMBRIDGE UNIVERSITY PRESS
Cambridge, New York, Melbourne, Madrid, Cape Town, Singapore, São Paulo

Cambridge University Press
The Edinburgh Building, Cambridge CB2 2RU, UK

Published in the United States of America by Cambridge University Press, New York

www.cambridge.org
Information on this title: www.cambridge.org/9780521620994

First published 1998

A catalogue record for this publication is available from the British Library

Library of Congress Cataloguing in Publication data

Pragmatic women and body politics/ edited by Margaret Lock, Patricia A.
Kaufert.
    p.   cm. – (Cambridge studies in medical anthropology 2)
Includes index.
ISBN 0 521 62099 6 – ISBN 0 521 62929 2 (pbk)
1. Women – Health and hygiene. 2. Women – Medical care. 3. Women – Social
conditions. 4. Medical technology – Social aspects. 5. Human reproductive
technology – Social aspects. 6. Medical anthropology. I. Lock, Margaret II.
Kaufert, Patricia A. (Patricia Alice) III. Series.
RA564.85.P73 1997
362.1'082–dc21   97–10263 CIP

ISBN-13 978-0-521-62099-4 hardback
ISBN-10 0-521-62099-6 hardback

ISBN-13 978-0-521-62929-4 paperback
ISBN-10 0-521-62929-2 paperback

Transferred to digital printing 2006

Contents

Contributors

EMILY K. ABEL Emily Abel, Professor of Health Services and Women's Studies, UCLA, is the author of *Who Cares for the Elderly? Public Policy and the Experience of Adult Daughters* (Temple, 1991) and co-editor with Margaret K. Nelson of *Circles of Care: Work and Identity in Women's Lives* (SUNY Press, 1990). She is writing a history of women's care for sick and disabled family members in the United States from 1850–1940.

JANICE BODDY Janice Boddy is Professor of Anthropology at the University of Toronto. She is the author of *Wombs and Alien Spirits: Women, Men and the Zar Cult in Northern Sudan* (1989), articles on spirit possession, feminism, female circumcision, and popular anthropology, and co-author of *Aman: The Story of a Somali Girl* (1994; translated into fourteen languages). She is currently doing archival research for a book on attempts by the British colonial administration to reform women's bodies and Sudanese society in the first half of this century.

CAROLE H. BROWNER Carole Browner is a Professor in the Department of Psychiatry and Biobehavioral Sciences, and in the Department of Anthropology at UCLA. She is a social anthropologist whose research interests lie at the intersection of gender, health, and development. She has published extensively on field studies in urban Columbia, rural Mexico, and the US.

BRENDA D. ELIAS Brenda Elias is a Ph.D. student and research associate in Community Health Sciences. Her interests are in cultural risk assessment, management, and communication. She has presented and co-published papers and reports concerning the social and cultural construction of risk perceptions in the Canadian North. She has worked collaboratively with First Nation peoples, currently with a First Nation University Research Team on a national–regional health survey in Manitoba First Nation communities (Canada).

ELLEN GRUENBAUM Ellen Gruenbaum is Professor of Anthropology at California State University, San Bernardino, where she also served as the Director of Women's Studies for six years. She lived in Sudan for five years, during which time she taught at the University of Khartoum and conducted ethnographic research. She is currently writing a book using an anthropological perspective on the "female circumcision" controversy.

LISA HANDWERKER Lisa Handwerker, a medical anthropologist, is currently an Associate Professor at the California Institute of Integral Studies and research affiliate at the Institute for Research on Women and Gender at Stanford University. She was recently elected to the board of the National Women's Health Network and chairs the reproductive health committee. She is also chair of the Council on Anthropology and Reproduction of the Society of Medical Anthropology, American Anthropological Association.

PATRICIA A. KAUFERT Patricia Kaufert has done research and published on a number of topics related to women's health including menopause, childbirth, and screening for breast cancer. She has been a member of numerous provincial and national committees in Canada concerned with women's health. She is at present working with Margaret Lock on a project looking at the communication of risk in relation to hormone therapy.

KARINA KIELMANN Karina Kielmann is currently working towards her doctorate from the Johns Hopkins School of Public Health. Drawing on a combined background of medical anthropology and international health, her work juxtaposes medical and public health discourses on reproductive health with women's interpretations and experiences of health and illness. She has lived and worked in Kenya, Tanzania, and most recently India.

ELLEN LEWIN Ellen Lewin is the author of *Lesbian Mothers: Accounts of Gender in American Culture*. Her most recent book is *Recognizing Ourselves: Rituals of Lesbian and Gay Commitment in America* to be published by Columbia University Press. She is currently an Affiliated Scholar at the Institute for Research on Women and Gender at Stanford University.

MARGARET LOCK Margaret Lock is Professor in the Department of Social Studies of Medicine and the Department of Anthropology at McGill University. She is the author of *East Asian medicine in Urban Japan: Varieties of Medical Experience* (California: 1980), and the prize-winning *Encounters with Aging: Mythologies of Menopause in Japan and North America* (California: 1993). Lock has edited four other books and written over 100 scholarly articles. She is part president of the Society for Medical Anthropology, American Anthropological Association, and a member of the Royal Society of Canada and the Canadian Institute for Advanced Research (CIAR). She is currently writing a book on biomedical technologies and changing conceptions of life and death.

IRIS LOPEZ Iris Lopez is an anthropologist and the Director of the Women's Studies Program at City College (CCNY). She has taught in the department of Latin American and Caribbean Studies at the City College of New York since 1985 and has also been a visiting professor at the University of California in Los Angeles. She spent one year doing a postdoctorate at the University of Hawaii at Manoa. Currently, she is writing a book on sterilization and Puerto Rican women in New York City.

SOHEIR A. MORSY Soheir Morsy is Associate Professor of Anthropology and Director of Women's Studies at Tufts University. Her work with the United Nations in parts of Asia and Africa has dealt with issues of development, particularly in terms of gender, health, education, and agrarian schemes.

MARK NICHTER Mark Nichter is a Professor of Anthropology at the University of Arizona, Tucson, who specializes in the study of the anthropology of the body, medical anthropology, and ethnomedicine. In addition to anthropology, Mark has postgraduate training in international health and psychiatry and has a joint appointment in the department of family and community medicine. He is the author of over thirty articles and two books in the field of medical anthropology and is actively engaged in research in North America, as well as in South and South-East Asia.

JOHN D. O'NEIL John O'Neil is a medical anthropologist who has worked with Aboriginal people in Canada, Australia, and Siberia over the past twenty years on a variety of issues related to community health. The focus of this work has been to establish a critique of the colonizing effects of Western health care practices on Aboriginal understandings of health and healing. Significant publications include several book chapters (co-authored with Patricia Kaufert) examining the impact of obstetric practices in Inuit communities, and a series of "definitive" papers examining Aboriginal health policy issues in Canada published in conjunction with the various reports of the Royal Commission on Aboriginal Peoples (1993–7).

BROOKE GRUNDFEST SCHOEPF Brooke Grundfest Schoepf, an economic and medical anthropologist, obtained her doctorate from Columbia University in 1969. She has conducted field research in England, France, the US, and ten countries in Africa, most recently in Rwanda. Currently, Schoepf is on faculty at the Institute for Health and Social Justice, the Department of Social Medicine of Harvard University Medical School (Boston), and the National University of Rwanda (Butare).

ANNALEE YASSI Annalee Yassi is the Director of Environmental and Occupational Medicine at the University of Manitoba. She has published extensively in the areas of environmental health surveillance, occupational health for health care workers, and cross-cultural environmental and occupational epidemiology. Yassi is currently working on a book and an international training program in basic environmental health through the World Health Organization. She is also working on several environmental health projects in Latin America.

1 Introduction

Margaret Lock and Patricia A. Kaufert

Living in the twentieth century, women have experienced an increasing appropriation of their bodies as a site for medical practice, particularly in connection with pregnancy, childbirth, and the end of menstruation. This phenomenon forms one of the cornerstones of "the medicalization of life" (Illich 1992:230), a process which is likely to become more intrusive with the laboratory manipulation of human conception and the routinization of mass screening programs for genetic disease. Medicalization has been characterized as the making of a "body pliant to power" (Grosz 1993:199), but the authors who have contributed to this book (thirteen anthropologists, together with two epidemiologists and an historian as co-authors on two of the essays) start out from the position that medicalization and power are ideas which must be grounded historically and culturally, as must resistance, agency, and autonomy. However, although we believe that the creation of nuanced relativistic explanations is essential, these accounts are not our final objective. Situated accounts should stimulate self-reflection – an exercise which, if successful, encourages analysts of social and political events to pay attention to the way in which "our own common sense is structured" (Zito and Barlow 1994, see also Rabinow 1977). It is only on the basis of this semiotic turn, in which certain truth claims are decentered, including those originating with the medical sciences, that attempts can be made to generalize about body politics.

In concluding this introduction, given the rapid spread of knowledge and technologies, we will call for yet another move, a "semiotic return" to local sites of research in order to understand better how globalization affects body politics.

In putting this book together, our primary concern was with the "microphysics of power" (in Foucault's idiom) and its operation in everyday life. We set out to provide a series of accounts of women's knowledge about and responses to body technologies of various kinds, but we wanted also to situate the subjectivity and agency of women in the context of their lived experience. We have tried to make clear the extent to which biomedical technologies are not autonomous, but are themselves the products of the same historical, cultural, and political contexts to which women are responding. Finally, we sought to elaborate further on social science theory in connection with body politics, and to this end we build on several books written by feminist anthropologists and historians (see, for example, Atkinson and Errington 1990; Ginsburg and Rapp 1995; Strathern 1992; Yanagisako and Delaney 1995; Zito and Barlow 1994).

Practices and discourse which have particular implications for women and their health are central in all the essays in this book. Their common aim is to illustrate the complexity of women's responses to the process of medicalization, responses which may range from selective resistance to selective compliance, although women may also be indifferent. However, these essays suggest that ambivalence coupled with pragmatism may be the dominant mode of response to medicalization by women.

Focusing, therefore, on the complexity of women's relationship with technology, these essays take a quite different position from those discussions which start from the assumption that women are passive vessels, simply acting in culturally determined ways with little possibility for reflection on their own condition. Neither do the authors set off from the opposite premise which defines women as inherently suspicious of and resistant to technological interventions. Rather, the contributors propose that women's relationships with technology are usually grounded in existing habits of pragmatism. For by force of the circumstances of their lives, women have always had to learn how they may best use what is available to them. If the *apparent* benefits outweigh the costs to themselves, and if technology serves their own ends, then most women will avail themselves of what is offered.

To the extent that any thinking about women and the body must confront issues of reproduction, we have included a number of essays in this collection which deal with different aspects of the reproductive body. Lisa Handwerker and Karina Kielmann explore the meaning of infertility for women living in countries – China and Tanzania – in which the state and the medical system construe women's bodies in terms of fertility to be controlled. Iris Lopez explores the decisions made by Puerto Rican women in curtailing their fertility. Ellen Lewin discusses the ways of becoming fertile chosen by lesbian women. Emily Abel and Carole Browner focus on the relationship between experimental knowledge of the pregnant body and the quasi-scientific knowledge of the prenatal advice literature. Janice Boddy reflects on her experience as a witness to childbirth in Canada and the Sudan, creating a compelling account of the different forms that the "colonization of consciousness" with respect to childbirth takes in these two cultural settings. Ellen Gruenbaum situates the fertility and childbirth of Sudanese women as one important element in the wider context of their overall health.

Yet, we also wanted to steer the book away from the current tendency (encouraged, perhaps, by our fascination with the new reproductive technologies) to portray women's lives as though consumed by reproduction. By privileging for analysis problems relating to reproduction, of outstanding importance though they be, the danger is that one of the most intransigent stereotypes – woman equals reproduction – simply slips by unexamined. Hence other essays in the book have been deliberately selected because they deal with quite different dimensions of women's experience. Emily Abel and Carole Browner explore the experience of being a daughter to aging parents; Margaret Lock describes being mother to a child with Down syndrome in Japan. Soheir Morsy and John O'Neil and colleagues focus on women who question not only the impact of science and technology, but also the role of the state in the protection of public health. Brooke Grundfest Schoepf discusses women and AIDS in Zaire, while Patricia Kaufert reviews the history of the breast cancer movement in the United States.

Although diverse in topic, these essays share some commonalities of approach, such as a mutual commitment to the long overdue but growing recognition that it is inappropriate to conceptualize a "one culture/one gender system" when representing women. While some feminist anthropologists have chosen to minimize differences in economic and power relations between women, we have tried to avoid that particular trap, believing that the behavior and subjectivity of individual women cannot be explicated on the basis of gender alone, even when appropriately contextualized. As many of these essays show, gender is cross-cut by other categories of class, religion, language, and ethnicity, whether at the local level (as in the village communities described by Gruenbaum) or at the level of international politics (as in the conferences described by Morsy).

By their use of the ethnographic method in which due attention is paid to both local practices and local knowledge, these essays run counter to the critique of resistance studies recently made by Ortner, namely that they are "ethnographically thin" (1995:190). Considered as a whole, this book displays a wide array of anthropological techniques, although most authors make use of the "ethnographic stance" (Ortner 1995:173) in which they present empirically rich, contextualized case studies. The essays by Janice Boddy, Ellen Gruenbaum, and Brooke

Grundfest Schoepf, for example, are based on years of ethnographic fieldwork in the same villages and with the same people. Ellen Lewin, Iris Lopez and Margaret Lock adopt the technique of allowing women to present their own stories, but then situate these accounts in the larger context of dominant ideologies about reproduction, fertility, and infertility. Soheir Morsy and Patricia Kaufert draw on official records, documentary evidence, government reports, the scientific literatures, using these materials to reconstruct the history of particular protest movements. Despite these differences in materials and methods of research, the essays are linked by a common preoccupation with medicalization, the politics of the body and the responses of women to biopower in its many different forms.

Contesting the common sense of culture

Before specifically considering the medicalization of female bodies, it may be helpful to outline our position on the central concepts of culture, ideology, and hegemony, concepts which are used explicitly in many chapters, and implicitly in the others.

There are several reasons why the idea of hegemony has appeal for cultural anthropologists. As the Comaroffs note, it appears to offer a ready *rapprochement* between practice and theory, action and thought, and ideology and power – dualities which many cultural anthropologists work hard to paste over (Comaroff and Comaroff 1991). For Antonio Gramsci, the creator of the concept, "nothing is anchored to . . . master narratives, to stable (positive) identities, to fixed and certain meanings: all social and semantic relations are contestable, hence mutable" (Hebdige 1988:206). Thus hegemony is not a given, nor simply a product of oppressive forces or class difference, but is realized only through negotiation among competing forces.

Gramsci, and later Raymond Williams (1977), both emphasized that the ideas of hegemony, culture, and ideology should be kept distinct, arguing that they cannot be reduced to, or subsumed by, one another. Taking this lead, the Comaroffs define culture as:

[T]he space of signifying practice, the semantic ground on which human beings seek to construct and represent themselves and others – and, hence, society and history. As this suggests [culture] is not simply a pot of messages, a repertoire of signs to be flashed across a neutral mental screen. It has form as well as content; is born in action as well as thought; is a product of human creativity as well as mimesis; and, above all, is empowered. But it is not all empowered in the same way, all of the time.

This is where hegemony and ideology become salient . . . They are the two dominant forms in which power enters – or, more accurately, is entailed in culture. (Comaroff and Comaroff 1991:22)

The majority of anthropologists do not think of culture as a stable entity, as something which coincides with a nation, society, ethnic group, or professional organization. Instead they think in terms of landscapes of group identity – "ethnoscapes" – in which groups are no longer conceptualized as tightly territorialized, spatially bounded, historically unselfconscious, or culturally homogenous units (Apparudai 1991:192). Few populations have lived in total and permanent isolation from others, although relatively large portions of the world's population have lived for long periods of time within clearly defined boundaries. Today virtually no people remain untouched by the transnational networks of communication in which we all participate.

This insight does not dispose of culture as a salient concept around which meanings are mobilized; it does, however, alert one to the way in which the dialectics of domination and resistance take place in a cultural field which is fluid and continually open to contestation (see, for example, Nordstrom and Martin 1992). Globalization has ensured that the majority of the world's people are aware, as never before, that other ways of being exist beyond the boundaries of their respective communities. This experience encourages reflection, heightens the possibility of resistance to local social arrangements, or alternatively may lead to a reaffirmation of tradition. More frequently, the consequence is an unstable mix of ongoing contestation. As a result of globalization, hegemonic power, "that order of signs and practices, relations and distinctions, images and epistemologies – drawn from a historically situated cultural field – that come to be taken-for-granted as the natural and received shape of the world and everything that inhabits it" (Comaroff and Comaroff 1991:23), is a shrinking domain. In other words, common sense – the unspoken authority of everyday life – becomes increasingly subject to disputation. Orthodoxy – that which is "naturalized," hegemonic, and taken as self-evident – is brought into consciousness and made recognizable as ideology, and is therefore laid bare for criticism.

It is at this disjunction, where tacit culturally shaped knowledge lies exposed, that the assertion of power and associated ideological truth claims become most evident. Evidence that individuals who challenge institutionalized power bases can be perceived as a serious threat is to be found at times in brutal acts of violence, whether it be the murder of gynecologists who assist women in obtaining an abortion, or the slaughter of Algerian women who choose not to conform to Islamic fundamentalism. Individuals who dispute either physical violence or "symbolic violence" – the institutionalized violence of everyday life (Bourdieu 1977:190) – are considered dangerous to a conservative moral order, which is itself undergoing a renewed vitalization with the resurgence of various forms of global fundamentalism and the elaboration in North America of the New Right.

Biopower and subjectivity

In this book we are concerned primarily with taken-for-granted knowledge as it manifests itself in the practices of medicine and public health. The claims of medical knowledge to a privileged status depend on the belief, shared by medical professionals and the public alike, that scientific knowledge, being factual, cannot be subject to epistemological scrutiny. Together with a gathering number of other dissidents, we reject this view of science, and start out from the assumption that science and technological practices are historically and culturally produced. Thus biomedicine and its associated technologies, like all other cultural domains, are subject to discursive negotiation.

In *Discipline and Punish* (1979), Foucault made a distinction between two types of power, one in which authoritative control is exerted directly over others (which is how medicalization is usually thought to be enacted), and a second, more insidious form which "proliferates outside the realm of institutional politics, saturating such things as aesthetics and ethics, built form and bodily representation, medical knowledge and mundane usage" (see Comaroff and Comaroff 1991:22). We believe that this division is too stark, for although the practice of biomedicine can be described as paternalistic and exerting authoritative control, characterizing it by the first type of power would be a gross oversimplification. Our concern here is particularly with the second kind of hegemonic power, for we argue that tacit knowledge not only shapes the behavior of practitioners, but accounts for the mixed and ambivalent reception of medicalization on the part of women.

We do not conceptualize power, therefore, simply as negativity, oppression, and constraint imposed from the top down. Rather we draw on Foucault's notion of biopower which, following Nietzsche's lead, emphasizes localized, routinized bodily practices in families, communities, and institutions. This type of body politics, which Foucault argued emerged in Euro-America from the beginning of the nineteenth century, construes the body as a corporeal entity, the boundaries of which are clearly demarcated anatomically. This physical entity has become the systematic target for disciplinary measures implemented by experts of various kinds. Biopower is conceptualized by Foucault as having two poles: that of "anatomo-politics" focused on the manipulation of individual bodies and, at the other pole, the manipulation and control of populations, systematized from the mid-nineteenth century onwards through "techniques of the survey," which ensured the possibility for regulation of both public and private life (Armstrong 1983; Foucault 1979). One of Foucault's most pertinent insights was his assertion that biopower, in creating a domain of expertise, constitutes its own objects of analysis to which it then responds. In other words, bodily states are labeled by experts as diseases; certain behaviors are defined as deviant, unnatural, immoral, opening up the way for systematic and legitimized attempts at medicalization of both body and behavior. Nowhere is this more apparent than in the lives of those women who do not fit within normalized categories, such as the infertile women in China (Handwerker) or Tanzania (Kielmann), Japanese women who produce "deficient" children (Lock), the fertile lesbian women in California (Lewin). Such women become ready-made targets of the medical gaze.

Our position here is not simply one of social constructivism, however; for while we recognize with Foucault that the classification of illness and deviancy is a discursive exercise, we would also argue that the labeling and diagnosis of physical states often serves its denoted purpose, namely, as an opening to obtaining a therapeutic regimen for the relief of pain and misery and as a barrier against death. Hence for women with breast cancer, it is their dependency on medicine for therapy and relief of suffering that defines the central core of the relationship with biomedical research and technology (see Kaufert, this volume).

At the site of the individual body, therefore, biopower may be experienced as enabling, or as providing a resource which can be used as a defense against other forms of power. At the centre of many of the essays in this book stands a pragmatic woman willing to use whatever biomedicine can provide in pursuit of her own goals or the protection of her independence. This type of pragmatism explains why infertile women in Zanzibar went to see a gynecologist (see Kielmann, this volume) or a lesbian woman in California went to her local medical clinic when she wanted to become pregnant (see Lewin, this volume). Both groups of women were willing to use a biomedical solution if it would ensure their fertility. Similarly, Japanese women will embrace reproductive technologies if seen as a valid means to achieve their social and culturally defined priorities, namely a family in which biological and social parentage are one and the same (see Lock, this volume). The realities of being a Puerto Rican woman, trying to survive and raise children in New York, set boundaries beyond the control of the individual woman. Continuing life as a fertile woman almost ceases to be a meaningful choice, as Iris Lopez shows. Yet, given the wider system of economic and social oppression, being sterilized may also be interpreted as a source of freedom, providing women with some minimal control over their bodies relative to other forms and conditions of either contraception or childbearing. Tubal ligation, known familiarly as *la operacion*, becomes accepted practice, its necessity recognized, but resented.

Foucault himself argued that subjects of biopower are not passive recipients; on the contrary the body becomes the center of a "dialectical force relation" in which it stands as a "metaphor for the anatomical focus and embodiment of power; a materiality that acts as a source and target of power, whether expressed politically, sexually, juridically or in discourse. It is not assigned a binary value as either active or passive, as the perpetrator or recipient of power" (Hewitt 1991:231). Although subjects do not control the direction of history writ large, Foucault insisted that people have the ability to choose among available discourse and practices, to use them creatively, and to reflect on them. Thus the subject is "neither entirely autonomous nor enslaved, neither the originator of the discourses and practices that constitute its experiences, nor determined by them" (Sawicki 1991:104).

Foucault's theory of biopower is clearly insightful, but feminist critics are uncomfortable with the way in which subjects, although not rendered passive, remain marginalized. Many argue that power relations make competing demands on people, and that the complex responses of individuals to both coercive and more subtle "common-sense" hierarchies and oppression are underestimated by Foucault. For this reason alone research should privilege the standpoint of those who are the usual targets for normalizing discourse and practices, and feminists who live and work outside the Euro-American tradition have been particularly active in developing important critiques of much of the research on subjectivity and agency.

Kumar (1994), for example, takes exception to the idea of subjugated (marginalized) knowledge as conceptualized by Foucault, because women and other disenfranchised people are inevitably understood in this scheme as fully constituted by and reacting only to those at the center of powerful institutions. Limiting analysis to relationships of domination directed from the top down, even when the subject is made active, fails to decenter the loci of power it is assigned. In a Foucauldian analysis, these hubs of hegemonic engagement remain as the dominant "other" in terms of which women everywhere are produced and produce themselves as irrevocably different – usually as inferior or wanting in some way.

Radical feminists point out that it is necessary to locate "new idioms of alterity" (Suleri 1992:1), to seek out the often subtle ways in which those who do not apparently control their own lives actually constitute different local worlds for themselves, worlds from which they can reflect upon the ironies of their situation, both locally and globally. Joan, the woman at the centre of Mark Nichter's contribution to this book, observes both herself and the medical care system, seeking always to subvert its accustomed order, relishing her successes, conscious all the time of the battle engaged.

In a different but related vein it has been argued by feminists that a widely shared female subjectivity cannot exist, largely because forms of patriarchy, tacit knowledge, and power relations are not universal. Kumar criticizes the tendency in many feminist analyses to dehistoricize and essentialize the subject, whether it be "women, peasants, or tribals" (1994:7). She stresses the importance of understanding the power ploy involved in the constitution of "woman as subject" with its emphasis on the "inborn" qualities of women defined as femininity, virtue, purity, nurturance, and so on. She goes on to argue that the implementation of such concepts varies through time and space and, therefore, contextualization is imperative.

Without historical contextualization these papers could be in danger of being dismissed as anthropological trivia – culturally relative, but with little significance outside the societies in question. Historically grounded ethnography permits perceptive comparisons, highlights the resilience of culturally constructed value systems, and above all forces an engagement with body politics within and between societies. The women around whom these essays are constructed all exist in the context of a densely described historical past. In Mark Nichter's chapter, this past is a single life history, but in the other contributions the relevant past includes the history of colonial policy in the Sudan (Boddy; Gruenbaum), the more recent impact of the World Bank and international development and population policies in Egypt (Morsy), China's population policies and its culturally constructed history of infertility (Handwerker), the centuries-long history of the planned family in Japan, together with the cultural history of reproduction there, with its focus on the production of children who are wanted by society (Lock), and the remarkable history of *la operacion* in Puerto Rico (Lopez).

Similarly, the essays all locate the development and implementation of technologies of the body not only with respect to the lives of individual women, but also in larger social, political, and global contexts. However, when discussing situated local practices, levels of analysis shift between a focus on the single woman (Nichter), one or two women with a single gynecologist (Kielmann), or families of women functioning within the context of their village community (Gruenbaum). By using the comparative method to examine case studies of individual women in Canada and the Sudan, Janice Boddy provides a compelling re-creation of the lived experiences of these women, but also reveals significant differences in the form and functioning of the family in the two settings. In her conclusion, Boddy draws on a careful review of the causes of maternal deaths to make a powerful statement for improved public health and better distribution of global resources rather than the increasing medicalization of the birth process. Similarly, other essays move from micro- to macrolevels to reveal contradictions between the everyday lives of women and dominant discourses and policy making, as in Morsy's analysis of the impact on women of relationships between the Egyptian state and international capitalism, and in Handwerker's exposé of the management of reproduction by the Chinese government. Childless women remain subject in China to harassment and discrimination, rather than being lauded for their contribution to the nationally recognized problem of "overpopulation." Women have now been provided with access to IVF technologies as the means of overcoming the "deficiency" of their infertility.

As several of the essays show, women may react against local hegemonies which pit women against women, but they may also collaborate or remain silent. Schoepf, for example, writes about a woman telling how she was driven from her home after the death of her husband by his sisters, who, falsely accusing her of having given him AIDS, seized all his wealth and property. Janice Boddy explores the different reasons for a young woman's death, including the reluctance of her mother-in-law to offend the family of the local midwife by seeking care from a more competent practitioner in a neighboring village. Greed in the first case, respect for convention in the other, took precedence over solidarity among women.

Personal gain, class interests, or adherence to tradition are powerful forces capable of withstanding efforts to overcome exploitation by "consciousness raising" and appeals to female solidarity (Lock 1993; hooks 1990). Appeals to some universal form of feminist solidarity are themselves suspect. Many of the European and North American delegates attending the International Conference on Population and Development in Cairo in 1994 or the United Nations Fourth World Conference on Women in Beijing in 1995 wanted to transcend their respective cultures and join together with women from a wide range of societies. Yet writing about these meetings, Soheir Morsy describes a reaction against Western feminist dreams of creating an international consciousness of oppression, arguing that other women saw the Euro-American tradition in academic and feminist writing as another form of imperialism. While interested in the creation of a shared discourse, many delegates wanted to emphasize local problems and local needs as defined by local women. Aware of the problems which this split had caused in Cairo, some participants in the Beijing conference tried to bridge the gap and achieve a mix of sensitivity to the particularities of local context (thus avoiding the trap of essentialism) while at the same time speaking out on issues which had universal relevance for women, including issues of power and women's potential for resistance.

Playing with power

Many of the authors are concerned with the very notion of resistance, involving as it does the question of consciousness of the motives for one's own behavior on the part of the women studied, and also the assumption that resistance is the only form of active (as opposed to passive) behaviour available to women (Abel and Browner; Handwerker; Kielmann; Lock). Few of the women portrayed in these essays are passive, although the constraints under which many must resist, or make their choices, are often narrow. Women in the two villages studied by Gruenbaum maneuver within the changing patterns of constraints on their lives, trying always to maximize their control over their own lives and the lives of their children. Their resistance is for essentially pragmatic rather than ideological ends, but it is in direct response to male power.

Foucault's famous assertion: "Where there is power, there is resistance" has been too often cited out of context, in order to force an assessment of power as entirely authoritarian. For Foucault, although networks of power facilitate surveillance, they also produce pleasure, knowledge, goods, and technologies, and they are, therefore, seductive, not only to those who instigate them but to potential recipients who may choose to comply. Foucault also recognized a "plurality of resistances" to power networks, but asserted that resistance is never exterior to power, nor is it necessarily designed to overthrow any given regime or institution.

James Scott, when doing research in Malaysia, described everyday activities such as gossip, slander, foot-dragging, and pilfering as the "weapons of the weak" (1985:29). He understood these activities as one of the few forms of resistance available to those with little room to maneuver in their daily lives. As seen by Scheper-Hughes, the many different forms of "foot-dragging" used by women are calculated responses designed to annoy in situations of repression and orthodoxy (1992). Other anthropologists have focused on the sites where poetry, laments, trance, dance, and other cultural forms are made use of to express dissent, often in an effort to bring to light the "resilience and creativity of the human spirit in its refusal to be dominated" (Abu-Lughod 1990:42; see also Boddy 1989; Seremetakis 1991; Trawick 1988).

Ellen Lewin (in this volume), however, suggests that: "'resistance' is rapidly becoming a word that covers anything, defines itself, and may be said to exist because we insist that it do so" (p. 164). In her view, feminists have been overeager to accept "the discovery of evidence of even indirect or unconscious resistance." She warns us that those forms of resistance which particularly delight anthropologists, because of their subtlety and their symbolic overlay, are particularly amenable to misinterpretation.

Like Lewin, Abu-Lughod has criticized other anthropologists for their romantic portrayals of resistance. She sees this as the result of an overeagerness to show that subordinated peoples are not unreflecting automatons, but find ways to respond critically, even if elliptically, to their respective situations. Recognizing the force of Foucault's insight, Abu-Lughod has strategically inverted his statement to read, "where there is resistance, there is power" (1990:42). From this vantage point, the behavior and responses of individuals to their lived experiences can be read at times as resistance, but simultaneously as commentaries on the workings of networks of power.

How then is resistance to be defined? Karina Kielmann takes a relatively extreme position in her essay, suggesting that "we can only start to attribute meanings of resistance when women themselves envisage and express the possibility of options diverging from orthodox frameworks of meaning surrounding the body" (p. 136). This position is similar to that of Fegan, who argued several years earlier that the question of intention is important, and that without conscious intention an act cannot be interpreted as one of resistance (1986). Like Fegan, Keilmann has chosen to set aside the Freudian notion of repression, a move with which not all readers may agree.

If Lewin's, Abu-Lughod's, and Kielmann's positions are accepted, then it is questionable whether a whole range of subtle forms of culturally instituted behaviors, many of which are not fully accessible to consciousness, constitute resistance. If one accepts that it is only when "common sense" is liberated from hegemonic discourse into the realm of ideology that the possibility for resistance is made fully conscious and available to clear articulation, then it may well be appropriate to confine use of the word resistance to self-consciously calculated responses to situations of domination. The breast cancer movement would be one example of this (see Kaufert, this volume). Yet, the vast array of culturally shaped resistance-like behaviors, responses on the part of individuals to inchoate feelings of a lack of justice, distress, exploitation, and so on, nevertheless remain as crucial activities for the attention of social scientists and feminists alike.

In addition to the question of consciousness, Kielmann is rightly concerned, as are other authors in this book, with apparent contradictions in the ways in which people selectively pursue strategies of consent and dissent within the constraints set out by society. She notes that practices which women carry out as individuals may negate the dominant ideologies to which they claim their behavior conforms. Private and public domains are frequently not well articulated with one another and ambiguities are clearly evident. This is where research into the lived experience and pragmatics of behaviors by those who ostensibly lack power is essential, if the subtleties of compliance and resistance are to be exposed.

Marx cautioned many years ago that intention evolves through practice. Moreover, as Scott has pointed out, even when public representations for change in the dominant system are actively demanded by subordinated groups, such representations nearly always have a strategic or dialogic dimension to the form that they take (1990:92). Thus, outright demands for complete reform and potentially revolutionary activities are unusual. Resistance, as both Kielmann and Lock argue in their chapters, is shaped by the existing moral order, even while simultaneously undertaking a reimagining and challenging of that order.

What appears to be political resistance may at times be driven by delusions and madness, or by anger at purely personal events, as might be argued in relation to Joan, the woman portrayed in Nichter's essay. Alternatively, resistance may be dreamt about, but ultimately discarded as an unrealistic hope. Under conditions of extreme violence, open resistance becomes effectively impossible except for those willing to become martyrs. Millions of women work with determination behind the scenes, often clandestinely in both the public and private domains to bring about justice and change in their lives and societies. Anthropologists, journalists, and other outsiders are not privy to the bulk of this activity which is therefore unlikely to be publicly articulated except when forcibly routed out and exposed by those in power. This patient, resilient form of resistance nevertheless constitutes vital and constructive political activity in local settings. Finally, resistance may also exist in the form of an organized, structured movement or protest, as in the case of environmentalists protesting to the government in Egypt (Morsy) or Canada (O'Neil and colleagues), or women with breast cancer working the lobbies on Capitol Hill.

The body as a site for resistance

Medical anthropologists have long argued that the human body, being the prime target for surveillance and control in societies everywhere, inevitably becomes a contested domain, a quintessential site where power is enacted, leading to somatic responses which are most often interpreted as illness. Such bodily response has been designated as "idioms of distress" (Nichter 1981). The very existence of such tropes tends to focus attention on somatic states, thus muting an exploration of possible social relations complicit in the onset of distress. Similarly, medicalization and more recently geneticization (the process whereby diseases are labeled as genetic in origin, Lippman 1993) individualize illness and deflect attention away from social relations. Recently, for example, professional literature and the media have given extensive coverage to the discovery of two of the genes implicated in breast cancer. These findings are usually presented without the crucial caveat, namely that nutritional, toxic, and environmental factors alone are believed to be implicated in up to 85 percent of breast cancers and that, even where inherited susceptibility plays a role, cancer does not manifest itself unless triggered by some extraneous event (Lock in press). A displacement occurs from social and political issues to the body, for the maintenance of good health in which individuals can be held responsible.

In contrast to most medical and even much epidemiological literature, analytical emphasis on bodily praxis tends to foreground the sickening social order, while simultaneously paying attention to body semiosis and individual distress (Lock and Scheper-Hughes 1990). So, for example, Ong interpreted attacks of spirit possession on the shop floor of multinational factories in Malaysia as part of a complex negotiation in which young women respond to violations of their gendered sense of self, difficult work conditions, and the process of modernization (1988). Similarly, the refusal of certain Japanese adolescents to go to school can be understood as a muted form of resistance to manipulation by families, peers, and teachers. In addition it can be interpreted as an expression of the malaise widely experienced by many Japanese as a result of the competitive and debilitating learning and working conditions in their society, which is in turn linked to modernization (Lock 1991). The Kleinmans have analyzed narratives about chronic pain in China to show an association between chaotic political change at the national level, collective and personal delegitimation in local worlds, and the subjective experience of physical malaise (1991).

Based on her work in a Brazilian shantytown, Scheper-Hughes describes an "epidemic of *nervoso*" which she interprets as having multiple meanings. At times, it is the refusal of men to continue demeaning and debilitating labor: at other times, the response of women to violent shock or tragedy, and also in part to the ongoing state of emergency in everyday life. The epidemic signals a nervous agitation, "a state of disequilibrium" – one of the few means of expressing dissent in a very repressive society. Individuals may well be conscious of the injustice of their situation, but at the same time exhibit ambivalence and describe their own bodies as "worthless" or "used up" (1992:187). Scheper-Hughes concludes that the semi-willingness of people to participate in the medicalization of their bodies is the result of participating in the same moral world as their oppressors.

Regardless of how people account for the origins of their sickness, they often seek out medical help. For although most people will do what they can to relieve their physical suffering, this does not necessitate their giving up political explanations for their distress. One does not have to share the same explanatory system as the medical professional to procure medicine. Moreover, some medical professionals are acutely aware of the political origins of sickness. Susan Love, a physician but also a fierce opponent of the "cancer establishment," is a rare but powerful example (see Kaufert, this volume).

Yet, political explanations for the origins of sickness are relatively rare among physicians, or even within the general population of the suffering. As a good number of medical anthropologists have shown, most people who seek out help for malaise of all kinds understand their problem primarily or exclusively as somatic – an interpretation which is, of course, reinforced by the majority of biomedical practitioners and also by local explanations for distress when they focus exclusively on physical discomfort (Good and Good 1988). Young has shown, moreover, that psychiatric treatment for post-traumatic stress disorder is expressly designed to encourage the patient to participate in the moral world of the physician (1993). Mark Nichter, however, presents us with Joan, a woman impressive in her ability to impose her script on the medical care system and deny physicians their customary right of orchestrating their medical encounters with patients. In a reversal of the usual patient-as-object of the clinical gaze, physicians are the object of Joan's gaze and the victims of her mission to reform medicine in accordance with her own vision of its proper practice.

Yet, it is inappropriate to think of biomedicine as a monolithic enterprise. Biomedical knowledge is complex, often not standardized, and always open to contestation from both within the profession and outside. Enormous variation exists both within and among the biomedicines institutionalized around the world today, and tacit knowledge embedded in the cultures of biomedicine makes translation among them exceedingly difficult.

Several important lessons can be gleaned from years of research in medical anthropology, among them that the body in sickness is a polysemic system, subject to numerous interpretations which are shaped, but not determined, by culture. Attitudes towards medicalization can be positive, negative, or ambivalent, and in any case are not stable. The response of women to medicalization is often mixed. They rarely react to the specific technology, or simply to the manipulation of their bodies, but rather on the basis of their perceptions as to how medical surveillance and interventions might enhance or worsen their daily lives. Indeed, for some women in some situations, such as being diagnosed with breast cancer, medical technology may hold out their only hope of survival. Through their demands that funding be increased and dedicated to research on breast cancer, women challenged the usual relationship of the scientific establishment with the state (Kaufert). Seen from this perspective, the breast cancer movement provides an opportunity to explore patterns of resistance which are not contingent upon withdrawal outside of medical control, but attack that control from within the system. Rather than decrying medical knowledge – as in the case of feminist critiques of childbirth – these women demand that the resources of medical science should be refocused, concentrated on discovering the causes and cures of breast cancer.

One strength of anthropological analyses is the elicitation of subjective accounts as told by informants which can then be juxtaposed with other versions of reality. The networks of the microphysics of power remain as abstract constructs of the imagination unless they are fleshed out with narratives produced by those on whom power is practiced. Mark Nichter presents Joan also as a woman constantly engaged in the process of creating and recreating the story of her body and its suffering. Janice Boddy uses her essay partly as an elegy to Amal, a woman who risked the survival of her body against her deeper commitment to maintaining its privacy and its impermeability to the gaze of male outsiders. Both Joan and Amal, and many of the other women who figure in these essays, are remarkable in their capacity to impose their presence even through the words of the observing/listening anthropologist. Mbeya, a Zairian woman, talks about her husband, who died of AIDS but refused to use condoms despite the risk to her. Driven out by his family, probably herself now dead, Mbeya's resistance is partly through the telling of her story (Schoepf). Yamada-san is the mother of a child, and both of them have been devalued and rendered almost invisible in their society of Japan because the child has Down syndrome. Yamada-san's invitation for the anthropologist to come to her home can be interpreted as resistance on her part, as she strove to make her intolerable situation public (Lock). Demands for visibility and voice were central elements in the resistance of women with breast cancer, and a motivating force in the emergence of the breast cancer movement (Kaufert).

Earlier we cited the Comaroffs' definition of hegemony as that part of the dominant world view that has come "to be taken-for-granted as the natural and received shape of the world and everything that inhabits it." The women in these essays challenged the taken-for-granted social and political ordering of their world. Resistance may be a single woman's rejection of medical advice on the placement of an aging parent (Abel and Browner), or the Tanzanian women who can be seen as rejecting the usual construction of the barren body in their society by seeking a cure for their infertility in biomedical clinics (Kielmann). Women in the breast cancer movement, and in the movements described by Soheir Morsy and John O'Neil *et al.*, saw themselves as acting in defense of their bodies and those of other women.

Medicalization revisited

The majority of feminists writing about "body politics" seek to alert readers to the dangers inherent in the transformation of the female body into a site for technological intervention (Katz Rothman 1989; Basen *et al.* 1993), but sociologists (more than other social scientists) have for some time now tried to contextualize the process of medicalization, at least in terms of institutional arrangements.

Conrad (1992), following Zola, argues that for medicalization to take place, specific behaviors and conditions must first be conceptualized as medical or biological "problems" (in other words, they must be "naturalized" as disease), secondly, recognition by medical institutions and policy making committees is essential so that appropriate services can be created, and thirdly, they must be diagnosed and interpreted in medical settings as diseases or abnormalities. If these requirements are met, then the health care professions are in a position to claim these conditions as coming under their jurisdiction, making medicine an institution of social control (Zola 1972). We would suggest that it could be equally well argued that recognition of diseases comes from changes in medical knowledge which is then disseminated to society at large (see, for example, Lock 1993; Young 1995), but the end result may well be the same.

Several authors have argued that analyses of the social construction of diseases and the institutionalization of associated medical practices provide too narrow a lens with which to account for medicalization. The discussion in the preceding section suggests that an account limited to the interests of the medical profession and of the state is inadequate, because medicalization cannot proceed unless a cooperative population of patients exists on whom techniques can be performed (Conrad 1992). However, Reissman reminds us once again, this time specifically in connection with medicalization, that women are "not simply passive victims of medical ascendancy. To cast them solely in a passive role is to perpetuate the very kinds of assumptions about women that feminists have been trying to challenge" (1983:3). Thus, as we have been arguing throughout this introduction, while bodies inevitably mediate all reflection and action on the world, and can be read as culturally produced (Lock and Scheper-Hughes 1990), individual behavior and responses are not determined by dominant ideologies. Although the conflation of knowledge/power postulated by Foucault serves to legitimize biomedical knowledge as scientific and rational, and thus to "naturalize" it, an uncritical reception of its truth claims by either individuals, populations at large, or medical professionals cannot be assumed.

Actual medical practitioners are absent or shadowy figures in all but Mark Nichter's paper and that of Janice Boddy, where the Sudanese midwives play major roles. In the others essays, physicians appear briefly as advice givers to women who are pregnant or caring for an aging parent (Abel and Browner), sources of assistance with methods of insemination (Lewin), having the power to diagnose and possibly treat infertility (Handwerker; Kielmann), counselors on genetic risk (Lock), tellers of bad news to women with breast cancer (Kaufert). Alternatively, physicians may not appear at all, even when female sterilization is the subject for discussion (Lopez).

While biomedicine is configured mainly in terms of its diverse relationships with the reproductive body, many of these essays come from a different perspective. Kaufert, for example, looks at the complex relationship between women and biomedicine, when the presence of cancer precludes resistance by withdrawal from treatment. Lock looks at genetic disease as expressed in the lives of a mother and her son and in terms of their social relationships, rather than their relationship with biomedicine. Both Gruenbaum and Morsy raise issues in the area of public or community health, being concerned with the impact on health of agricultural development policies, either the direct effect of pesticides and polluted water sources, or the indirect implications of social and economic changes for women's health and well-being. Soheir Morsy discusses these issues at the level of state policy, whereas Gruenbaum focuses on the position of wives and mothers within a changing Islamic household, but the forces are similar.

Further, the essays in this book make it clear that women's lives are not preoccupied with medicine and that, for most women, reproduction does not occupy an undue proportion of their energy. Feminists writing in the Western intellectual tradition have often granted an importance to medicine approaching that which the medical establishment gives itself, but ethnographic accounts in which attention is paid to everyday life make it clear that it is more appropriate to understand women's responses in medical settings as reflecting their daily experiences as part of a domestic group, a community, or a society. Most of the literature on medicalization focuses on clinical settings, individual women, and the manipulation of their bodies. The contributions by Gruenbaum, Lopez, O'Neil et al., and Morsy all make clear in their different ways that women are concerned not simply with their own bodies, but with what might be glossed as public health issues – that is, with the bodies of others. Many of them are working for better conditions in their communities at large, activities which are sometimes peripheral or even removed from medicine, but which ultimately have profound effects on health.

Creating needs: technologies of naturalization

The concept of "nature" is, of course, culturally constructed, and the meanings attributed to it change through time and space. A scientific, post-Enlightenment account assumes nature to be subject to experimental manipulation and ultimately understandable as a set of universal laws. In theory, this approach visualizes nature as a domain entirely separate from the moral order. In practice, however, "nature" often continues to serve, as it did prior to the Enlightenment, as a moral touchstone, the effects of which are especially evident at the culturally constructed margins between "nature" and "culture" (Lock 1995).

Nature is usually drawn on as a moral arbitrator in one of three ways. People can be chastised if their behavior does not conform to what is understood as "natural" – in scientific parlance, certain behaviors are understood as biologically "determined" and therefore inevitable. Culturally constructed gendered and age-related behavioral norms, for example, are frequently legitimized as naturally determined: thus in many cultures women are believed to be "naturally" nurturant, while men are inevitably assertive. One logical extension of this type of argument is that women must conceive and reproduce in order to be "real" women. A woman who rejects fertility in China is defined as not "normal," while the "infertile" woman demonstrates her normality by seeking treatment (Handwerker, this volume). A second way in which nature is used as ideological commentary on the social order is by categorizing certain individuals and groups as "wild" or "uncultured," closer to nature, and as a consequence potentially dangerous (Douglas 1970; Yoshida 1967). Feminists writing about the management of women's bodies cite numerous nineteenth- and twentieth-century texts which reveal such an attitude toward women in Euro-America (Leys Stepan 1986; Jordanova 1989; Duden 1993). Nature is used in a third way to legitimize moral commentary in connection with manipulation of what is taken to be the natural order itself – attempts to intervene and destroy or transform nature in inappropriate ways may disrupt society (O'Neil *et al.* and Morsy, this volume).

How nature is demarcated from culture in local discourse gives considerable room for contestation and ideological manipulation. Although scientific accounts tend to dismiss this polysemy as so much cultural flotsam to be stripped away to reveal the "natural" facts inscribed in the universal physical body, it is at these "blurred boundaries," at the "intersection of discourses," that dissent, doubt, anxiety, hope, and challenges to structures of power can best be seen. As Balsamo has noted, "investigating the interaction between material bodies and new technologies illuminates the work of ideology-in-progress" (1996:10). This is what makes women's responses to medicalization so interesting and so difficult to interpret. The very act of medicalization naturalizes and hence legitimizes manipulation of the "abnormal" body as the source of distress. Attention is deflected away from hierarchical arrangements, the control of knowledge, and the making of the body docile, because medicalization is perceived as benevolent – a manifestation of our mastery of the vagaries of nature. Once understood this way, as a cultural improvement on nature, then compliance with and resistance to medicalization becomes all the more remarkable, and highly significant for what it can teach us about hegemony and power.

The history of medical knowledge and medical technologies has usually been transmitted as an heroic tale about the conquest of the enemy, whether it be human or nature – a narrative of progress, and of the betterment of humanity in general. This dominant ideology has, for the past 100 years at least, been accompanied by a counter-discourse replete with ambivalence and warnings about the consequences of technology gone wild. From Mary Wollstonecraft Shelley to Kurt Vonnegut, novels have been used to describe the havoc and misery which technology can create. The humanities and social sciences have also sounded regular warnings: Ellul claimed, for example, that "Technique has become *autonomous*; it has fashioned an omnivorous world which obeys its own laws and which has renounced all tradition" (1964, emphasis added). But, as Winner has pointed out, the very idea of an autonomous technology raises an "unsettling irony, for the expected relationship of subject and object is exactly reversed" (1977:16).

In this book we understand technology not simply as tools and machines, but, following Foucault, as also techniques of quantification, systematization, and routinization: in short, the gamut of human effort to manipulate and control what is available to it in order to produce an effect or an end-product perceived to be beneficial in some way to individuals and also society (see also Escobar 1995).

A common assumption is that the driving force behind the creation of technologies is to meet universal human needs. Both Marcuse and Habermas claim that there is little inherently questionable about technological developments provided that we go about them in the right way. Others, including Basalla (1988) and Sahlins (1976), take a more radical position. They stress that, aside from the fundamental requisites for sustaining life, it is culture and not nature which defines necessity. Necessity is not the mother of invention in any predetermined way: on the contrary, human technology is a "material manifestation of the various ways men and women throughout time have chosen to define and pursue existence" (Basalla 1988:14). Technology is thus an integral part of the history of human aspirations and simply to associate it with power and economic systems, as do Marcuse, Habermas, and others, is to leave tacit the dominant modernist ideology of progress as an inherently rational pursuit to which culture makes no contribution.

It is easy to presume that of all forms of technology, medical technologies exist to meet basic human needs, above all to reduce suffering and avoid premature death. Techniques that allow us to penetrate with increasing facility into the recesses of the body, together with those that prolong life, are surely for the good. But since the 1970s it has become increasingly clear that biomedical technology is by no means autonomous. Disputes with respect to biomedical technology in societies driven by technological development usually revolve today around questions of individual rights, autonomy, and justice. Activists have focused on abuse of individual patients by powerful elites. Very few commentators have stepped back to look at the larger picture and ask why, for example, infertility, menopause, and aging are conceptualized as diseases, or why we strive so hard to conquer death. Nor do we ask why manifestations of distress are given labels such as anorexia nervosa, attention deficit disorder, post-traumatic stress syndrome, or false memory syndrome. By defining them as behavioral problems, responsibility is located with the individual and the family, while the complex social and political origins of these conditions are made opaque.

The view from the margins

We have argued thus far for a decentering of certain important concepts which frequently go unexamined. Such an exercise permits a contextualization of knowledge production, including that of biomedicine, as well as a sensitivity to the ways in which subjectivity and agency are enacted in different sites. This exercise is a rather sophisticated extension of the original anthropological endeavor because, ideally, anthropologists have never been content simply with portrayals of other cultural formations, but use their findings to reflect on tacit knowledge embedded in their own belief systems. One major contribution of medical anthropology has been to introduce a critical approach to biomedical knowledge and practice, in part an extension of research into the cultural construction of medical systems in other parts of the world; the more sophisticated forms of this research succeed in highlighting the epistemological foundations of all types of medical practice (see, for example, Farquhar 1993).

Recent critiques of cultural anthropology claim that anthropologists remain insufficiently sensitive to the way in which their interpretations create an appearance of a cultural coherence in the societies which they study, a coherence which is in fact an artifact produced by the intellectual gaze from afar (Said 1978; Clifford and Marcus 1986). Tsing has argued that it is important to transgress "conventions of segregated 'internal' and 'external' cultural analysis" in order to reveal cultural heterogeneity and the "trans-communal links through which 'communities' are forged" (1993:9). We follow Ginsburg and Rapp in defining "local" as "any small-scale arena in which social meanings are informed and adjusted through negotiated face-to-face interaction" and transnational or global processes as "those through which specific arenas of knowledge and power escape the communities of their creation to be embraced by or imposed on people beyond those communities" (1995:8–9). When the flow of ideas and technology is perceived as being from "advanced" societies to the "developing" world, then an assumption is often made that recipient societies undergo a process of secularization and rationalization, an integral part of modernization. It is abundantly clear, however, that no such simple trajectory occurs, and that reversals and other unanticipated outcomes are common, in both "developed" and "developing" societies.

Given increasing globalization and its resultant complexities, a cultural critique which simply uses knowledge from afar to reflect intellectually on the condition of the so-called advanced societies does not go far enough. One must make yet another move – a semiotic return – to local sites of research for further reflection on the way in which competing truth claims and practices are contested as a result of the ceaseless appearance of new knowledge which in turn provides a continual challenge to common-sense knowledge. This semiotic return includes a consideration of body politics – individual and communal. Whatever their declared ethnicity and wherever their geographical location, the majority of women are responding today not simply to "tradition" and local hegemonies, but also to the effects that globally circulating knowledge and practices have on their lives. Moreover these responses have no close association with exposure to formal education.

The impact of circulating knowledge and technologies on the bodies of women may become immediately visible in the rapid adoption of contraceptive technologies to prevent fertility (Morsy, this volume) or the adoption of new techniques to overcome infertility (Handwerker, this volume). But Morsy looks also at the impact of agricultural pesticides on women's bodies, and breast cancer activists link their own tumors with an environment polluted by a cocktail of carcinogenic chemicals, the byproducts of technological development. Such technologies, whether embraced or decried by women, are rarely perceived as morally neutral, by the state or local governments, by women themselves, or by health care professionals, both local and outsiders.

New technologies inevitably suggest possibilities for increased freedom and innovative change, but they also frequently open the door to new forms of illness, domination, or neo-colonial expansion. Most often such technologies inspire ambivalence and cause debate to erupt about the perceived breakdown of moral order. It is in this analytic space that the contributions to this book are concentrated – a space which reverberates with the unresolvable tensions created for women by being marginalized, often in multiple ways, as they respond both to the power of "tradition" and the power of technological innovation, neither of which forces is stable nor situated unambiguously within or outside their communities.

Increasingly in the present global political climate, people find themselves marginalized through isolation or expulsion from community and often family. For example, young women in many Asian countries are sold by their families into servitude as poorly paid labor or as sex workers. In Central and South America and in China there are repeated reports of girls and young women being stolen from their families (Anagnost 1995). In North America, immigrant labor, frequently women working for the garment industry, are employed in illegal, hidden sweat shops for considerably less than minimum wage or else are forced into insecure piece work in their own domestic space, a practice which is on the increase because employers can thus avoid scrutiny. The possibilities for resistance or critical reflection in situations of extreme isolation where structural violence is at its most constraining, as Scott noted (1990), are minimal. When the evil conditions under which so many women live and work are taken into account, then the type of postmodern analysis which plays with the idea of multiplicity, with the possibilities for individual remaking of the world, and with the invention of "incalculable choreographies" (McDonald 1982) seems flagrantly irresponsible. Similarly, analyses which understand women above all as autonomous, rational actors negotiating reality in order to improve their lot are badly flawed. Serious political accounts must contextualize women's lives and pay close attention to their structural positions in various human groupings. As Lopez notes in her essay, one must ask exactly what concepts such as "choice" and "voluntary" mean in the context of women's lives. At the same time it is important to generalize across difference whenever possible, if the lived experiences of women as portrayed in ethnographic accounts are to break through the bonds of "common sense."

REFERENCES

Abu-Lughod, Lila 1990, "The romance of resistance: tracing transformations of power through Bedouin women," *American Ethnologist* 17:41–55.
Anagnost, Ann 1995, "A surfeit of bodies: population and the rationality of the state in post-Mao China," in Ginsburg and Rapp 1995, pp. 22–41.
Apparudai, Arjun 1991, "Global ethnoscapes: notes and queries for a transna-

tional anthropology," in R. G. Fox (ed.), *Recapturing Anthropology: Working in the Present*, Santa Fe, New Mexico: School of American Research Press, pp. 191–210.

Armstrong, David 1983, *Political Anatomy of the Body: Medical Knowledge in Britain in the Twentieth Century*, Cambridge: Cambridge University Press.

Atkinson, Jane Monnig and Errington, Shelly 1990, *Power and Difference*, Stanford: Stanford University Press.

Balsamo, Anne 1996, *Technologies of the Gendered Body*, Durham, NC: Duke University Press.

Basalla, George 1988, *The Evolution of Technology*, Cambridge: Cambridge University Press.

Basen, Gwynne, Eichler, Magrit and Lippman, Abby (eds.) 1993, *Misconceptions: The Social Construction of Choice and the New Reproductive and Genetic Technologies*, Hull, Quebec: Voyageur Publishing.

Boddy, Janice 1989, *Wombs and Alien Spirits: Women, Men and the Zar Cult in Northern Sudan*, Madison: University of Wisconsin Press.

Bourdieu, Pierre 1977, *Outline of a Theory of Practice*, Cambridge: Cambridge University Press.

Clifford, James and Marcus, George (eds.) 1986, *Writing Culture: The Poetics and Politics of Ethnography*, Berkeley: University of California Press.

Comaroff, J. and Comaroff, J. L. 1991, *Of Revelation and Revolution: Christianity, Colonialism and Consciousness in South Africa*, Vol. 1, Chicago: University of Chicago Press.

Conrad, Peter 1992, "Medicalization and social control," *Annual Review of Sociology* 18:209–32.

Douglas, Mary 1970, *Natural Symbols*, New York: Vintage.

Duden, Barbara 1993, *Disembodying Women: Perspectives on Pregnancy and the Unborn*, Cambridge: Harvard University Press.

Ellul, Jacques 1964, *The Technological Society*, trans. John Wilkinson, New York: Alfred A. Knopf.

Escobar, Arturo 1995, *Encountering Development: The Making and Unmaking of the Third World*, Princeton: Princeton University Press.

Farquhar, Judith 1993, *Knowing Practice: The Clinical Environment of Chinese Medicine*, Boulder, Colorado: Westview Press.

Fegan, Brian 1986, "Tenants' non-violent resistance to landowner claims in a central Luzon village," *Journal of Peasant Studies* 13:87–106.

Foucault, Michel 1979, *Discipline and Punish: The Birth of the Prison*, trans. Alan Sheridan, New York: Vintage.

Ginsburg, Faye and Rapp, Rayna (eds.) 1995, *Conceiving the New World Order: The Global Politics of Reproduction*, Berkeley: University of California Press.

Good Delvecchio, Mary-Jo and Good, Byron J. 1988, "Ritual, the state and the transformation of emotional discourse in Iranian society," *Culture, Medicine and Psychiatry* 12:43–63.

Grosz, Elizabeth 1993, "Bodies and knowledge: feminism and the crisis of reason," in L. Alcoff and E. Potter (eds.), *Feminist Epistemologies*, New York: Routledge, pp. 187–216.

Hebdige, Dick 1988, *Hiding in the Light: On Images and Things*, New York: Routledge.

Hewitt, Martin 1991, "Bio-politics and social policy: Foucault's account of welfare," in M. Featherstone, M. Hepworth and B. S. Turner (eds.), *The Body: Social Process and Cultural Theory*, London: Sage Publications, pp. 225–55.

hooks, Bell 1990, *Yearning: Race, Gender, and Cultural Politics*, Toronto: Between the Lines.

Illich, Ivan 1992, *In the Mirror of the Past: Lectures and Addresses 1978–1990*, New York: Marion Boyars.

Jordanova, Ludmilla 1989, *Sexual Visions: Images of Gender in Science and Medicine Between the Eighteenth and Twentieth Centuries*, Madison: University of Wisconsin Press.

Kleinman, Arthur and Kleinman, Joan 1991, "Suffering and its professional transformation: toward an ethnography of interpersonal experience," *Culture, Medicine and Psychiatry* 15(3):275–301.

Kumar, Nita (ed.) 1994, "Introduction," in *Women as Subjects: South Asian Histories*, Charlottesville: University of Virginia Press, pp. 1–25.

Leys Stepan, Nancy 1986, "Race and gender: the role of analogy in science," *Isis* 77:261–77.

Lippman, Abby 1993, "Worrying – and worrying about – the geneticization of reproduction and health," in Basen *et al.*, pp. 39–65.

Lock, Margaret 1991, "Flawed jewels and national dis/order: narratives on adolescent dissent in Japan," Festschrift for George DeVos, *Journal of Psychohistory* 18:507–31.

　1993, *Encounters With Aging: Mythologies of Menopause in Japan and North America*, Berkeley: University of California Press.

　1995, "Contesting the natural in Japan: moral dilemmas and technologies of dying," *Culture, Medicine and Psychiatry* 19:1–38.

　in press, "Social and cultural issues in connection with breast cancer testing and screening," in B. Koenig and H. Greely (eds.), *Genetic Testing for Breast Cancer Susceptibility: The Science, The Ethics, The Future*, Cambridge, Cambridge University Press.

Lock, Margaret and Scheper-Hughes, Nancy 1990, "A critical-interpretive approach in medical anthropology: rituals and routines of discipline and dissent," in T. Johnson and C. Sargent (eds.), *Medical Anthropology: A Handbook of Theory and Method*, New York: Greenwood Press, pp. 47–72.

McDonald, Christie 1982, "Choreographies: interview with Jacques Derrida," ed. and trans. C. McDonald, *Diacritics* 12:66–76.

Nichter, Mark 1981, "Idioms of distress," *Culture, Medicine and Psychiatry* 5:379–408.

Nordstrom, Carolyn and Martin, JoAnn (eds.) 1992, *The Paths to Domination, Resistance, and Terror*, Berkeley: University of California Press.

Ong, Aihwa 1988, "The production of possession: spirits and the multinational corporation in Malaysia," *American Ethnologist* 15:28–42.

Ortner, Sherry 1995, "Resistance and the problem of ethnographic refusal," *Comparative Studies of Society and History* 37:173–93.

Rabinow, Paul 1977, *Reflections on Fieldwork in Morocco*, Chicago: University of Chicago Press.

Reissman, C. K. 1983, "Women and medicalization: a new perspective," *Social Policy* 14:3–18.

Rothman, Barbara 1989, *Recreating Motherhood: Ideology and Technology in a Patriarchal Society*, New York: W.W. Norton and Co.

Sahlins, Marshall 1976, *Culture and Practical Reason*, Chicago: University of Chicago Press.

Said, Edward 1978, *Orientalism*, New York: Pantheon.

Sawicki, Jana 1991, *Disciplining Foucault: Feminism, Power, and the Body*, New York: Routledge.

Scheper-Hughes, Nancy 1992, *Death Without Weeping: The Violence of Everyday Life in Brazil*, Berkeley: University of California Press.

Scott, James 1985, *Weapons of the Weak: Everyday Forms of Peasant Resistance*, New Haven: Yale University Press.

1990, *Domination and the Arts of Resistance*, New Haven: Yale University Press.

Seremetakis, C. Nadia 1991, *The Last Word: Women, Death, and Divination in Inner Mani*, Chicago: University of Chicago Press.

Strathern, Marilyn 1992, *Reproducing the Future: Anthropology, Kinship and the New Reproductive Technologies*, New York: Routledge.

Suleri, Sara 1992, *The Rhetoric of English India*, Chicago: University of Chicago Press.

Trawick, Margaret 1988, "Spirits and voices in Tamil songs," *American Ethnologist* 15:193–215.

Tsing, Anna Lowenhaupt 1993, *In the Realm of the Diamond Queen*, Princeton: Princeton University Press.

Williams, Raymond 1977, *Marxism and Literature*, London: Oxford University Press.

Winner, Langdon 1977, *Autonomous Technology: Technics-out-of-Control as a Theme in Political Thought*, Cambridge: The MIT Press.

Yanagisako, Sylvia and Delaney, Carol (eds.) 1995, *Naturalizing Power: Essays in Feminist Cultural Analysis*, New York: Routledge.

Yoshida, Teigo 1967, "Mystical retribution, spirit possession, and social structure in a Japanese village," *Ethnology* 6:237–62.

Young, Allan 1993, "A description of how ideology shapes knowledge of a mental disorder (posttraumatic stress disorder)," in S. Lindenbaum and M. Lock (eds.) *Knowledge, Power and Practice: The Anthropology of Medicine and Everyday Life*, Berkeley: University of California Press.

1995, *The Harmony of Illusions: Inventing Posttraumatic Stress Disorder*, Princeton: Princeton University Press.

Zito, Angela and Barlow, Tani E. (eds.) 1994, *Body, Subject and Power in China*, Chicago: University of Chicago Press.

Zola, Irving K. 1972, "Medicine as an institution of social control," *Sociological Review* 20:487–504.

2   Remembering Amal: on birth and the British in northern Sudan

Janice Boddy

November 1994: The ochre light of dusk, birds clamoring in the ne'em tree, a muezzin's call to prayer. I open the familiar blue door and enter the courtyard without knocking. A sense of home engulfs me. Everything seems as it was: to my left, the breezeway sheltering water jars, its earth floor damp and cool; to my right, the gallery off the storeroom where we sat to pound spices, wash clothes, brew coffee, and talk. Ahead is the *saysaban* Salima planted all those years ago, alive still, miraculously grown, marking time. But the far verandah has been walled for rooms. There is a new garden with morning glories, sunflowers, and henna, gifts of piped water one hour a day.

Salima emerges from the goat pen at the back. She sets her milk bowl on the kitchen sill, embraces me without a word. At once she starts to tremble, weeping. She wails a rhythmic mourning phrase whose drawn out words I cannot catch. Now I am crying too, holding her shoulders as she holds mine.

Moments later we sit and dry our eyes in silence. Then, abruptly, she smiles. "You've been a long time away," she says. "Much has happened. Awad has two more daughters, both very young. Would you like to meet his new wife? Would you like to see Amal's little girl? She's ten years old now, and very smart, first in her class at school."

Awad and his wife appear, each with a freshly bathed toddler in arms. Amal's daughter, tall for her age, hangs back, hiding behind her father's legs. He places a hand on her shoulder and gently draws her forth. "Her name is Nura," he says. "We named her for our grandmother." The girl is a miniature of her mother, over half as old as she was at her death.

For several months in the mid-1980s, I lived with Salima, Awad, their parents, and Amal, Awad's bride, on the east bank of the Nile in an Arab Sudanese village I call Hofriyat. I had spent over a year there in the mid-1970s doing ethnographic research and had returned to continue the work. Amal was pregnant and understandably apprehensive. She had been ill with malaria, anemia, and a bladder infection.

The clinician had detected proteins in her urine; she seemed always to be in pain. Whole days she lay groaning on an *angareeb* (rope bed) in the gallery. Other days she insisted on doing her share of the work, hauling water home from the well, scrubbing Awad's clothes.

From the moment she knew she was expecting, Amal wore her wedding gold to thwart capricious spirits that might seize her womb and loosen its captive seed. Amal's body had become a protected domestic space, a figurative house wherein mingle the male and female contributions that shape and sustain human life (Boddy 1989). Her blood nurtured a kindred being who would remain an intimate part of herself even after birth.

Amal ate well when she could, "clean," expensive foods – eggs, grapefruit, guavas, tomatoes, meat, fava beans, lentils – that Awad supplied to help build her blood.[1] She went to the village clinic for weekly prenatal checks, but the government midwife was never there – out on call Amal was told. Only the male nurse's aide in charge of the tiny, woefully understocked dispensary had examined Amal – or so she said.

Later she revealed that he had not. She did not trust the man; he is not related to the people of Hofriyat. Worse, he's rumoured to be possessed by *zar* spirits that are known to play havoc with women's fertility. At his office he is regularly found listening to recordings of *zar* songs to appease his spirits. We suspect he is possessed by the European Doctor *zar*, Hakim-bi-Dor (Doctor by Turns), because both man and spirit are least discontent when patients are lined up waiting to see them. The clinician often roams the village in character: stethoscope slung round his neck, blood pressure cuff strapped to his arm. Neither implement is properly functional, as his watch lacks a second-hand. The spirit-possessed clinician is a parody of Western medicine, a stinging, if suitable, comment on its efficacy in impoverished postcolonial Sudan. Amal would not let him palpate her belly; she was too shy, she said, too ashamed. Besides, he was always trying to sell her more vitamins to "fix her body" and had once advised a lengthy course of tetracycline which Awad vetoed, aware of the harm it could cause the unborn child.

Awad and I begged her to see a proper doctor in Shendi, the closest town, 30 kilometers away. We offered countless times to accompany her there on the bus. I would approach the doctor, I said, and I would stay with her; she need not feel ashamed, pregnancy was natural, she was a married woman, it was important to take care of herself and the baby. Awad even ordered her to go, but she refused, and left to stay with her mother a few doors away.

Amal's stubbornness was not without reason; she confided that she could not bear the thought of being examined by strangers, all of them men. Hofriyati women conceal their pregnancies in public, something that modesty wraps and a preference for corpulent figures make it possible to do. Even close female kin refer to the condition euphemistically, for pregnancy is unmistakable evidence of sexual activity, and it is shameful for women to evince their sexuality. It is doubly improper to do so in front of men.[2]

So we sent for Miriam, the busy district midwife, who questioned Amal and examined her eyes and mouth but was not alarmed. When the pains returned I suggested we call for Sheffa, the midwife from a neighboring district, who had impressed me with her cool professionalism and kindly, no-nonsense approach. Sheffa was a qualified nurse's aide – well beyond Miriam's achievements. She had a confidence Miriam lacked, and a bedside manner that would, I was sure, convince Amal to seek the medical help she clearly required. But the family objected that Miriam would take offense, placing their good relations with her, hence the welfare of all its women, in jeopardy. Midwives are powerful people; their prompt response can mean life rather than death for mothers and infants alike.

I left Hofriyat shortly before Amal's baby was due. Hugging her good-bye on boarding the rickety bus for Khartoum, I feared I would not see her again. I think she knew that I would not.

I have since had the luxury to ponder Amal's response and my insistence, my undeterred faith in biomedical technology, a faith that increasingly resides with Hofriyati too. I am less certain now that Amal's death in childbirth was readily preventable, and less convinced that she died for the sake of shame, or if she did, that it was a meaningless or, for her, avoidable act. I have no answers, only half figured questions and a weight of accumulating ironies for consolation. This essay juggles and tries to make sense of these by exploring some politics of female reproductive experience.

A few months before leaving for Hofriyat in 1983, I played labor coach to my friend, Melanie, then in the last trimester of pregnancy with a husband stationed abroad. Together we attended prenatal classes, practised breathing, saw films of normal and cesarean births that made our blood run cold. Melanie had ceased being herself when she learned she was expecting: she stopped smoking, drank no alcohol, ate a diet rich in protein, calcium, iron, folic acid, all the things a fetus needs. Pregnancy consumed her. She consulted books to learn what her body was doing at every stage. She stoically eschewed medication:

nary an aspirin passed her lips the whole nine months. She came to regard herself as an incubator, nature's perfect instrument for growing human life, and was confirmed in her assessment when we at last saw her baby on the monitor of an ultrasound machine. The sonogram ratified the internal evidence of her body, offering objective corroboration that motherhood was imminent and real. Melanie's fetus now became a person, someone distinct from herself. And in her culture, persons are identified by the things that surround them, by what they possess.[3]

So Melanie devoted her prenatal work-leave to fixing up a nursery. She papered and painted in primary colors to stimulate the baby's mind; hung cheerful, clinky mobiles; put an array of stuffed animals on a bookshelf placed within sight of the crib. She bought tiny outfits, baby blankets, sheets, sleepers, vests, bibs, box upon box of disposable diapers. At the supermarket check-out she found a booklet called "Name Your Baby."

Friends and family threw a surprise shower replete with pink and blue balloons and a caffeine-free teddy-bear cake. They gave her a Jolly-Jumper, a highchair, cups with lids and perforated spouts, the requisite Beatrix Potter bowl.

I moved in for the final month. We cleaned her house from bottom to top, disinfected bathrooms and kitchen appliances, banished unsuspecting cats from upstairs rooms. Melanie drank milk and took vitamins every day. She listened to soothing music, walked in the evenings to keep in shape, began to see her obstetrician once a week. She was rhesus negative, thirty years old, and pregnant for the first time – not a "low risk" case.

Her due date arrived but the baby did not. The next check-up came, and the one after that. She was agitated driving back from her latest appointment, so we decided to stop at the mall; maybe window shopping would persuade the baby to be born.

When we got home there was a message on the answering machine. Melanie must return to hospital right away: she would deliver by cesarean section that afternoon.

In Canada maternal mortality rates are among the lowest in the world: four deaths per 100,000 live births in 1985. In Ontario the rate that year was seven.[4] But only about two-thirds of that province's births were normal vaginal deliveries and few of these took place at home. Fully one in five was a cesarean section and a further one in ten was operative, performed with forceps or vacuum extraction (Ontario Government 1987a:80–1).

In 1983 Ontario's perinatal (still birth plus early neonatal [within the first week of life]) mortality rate was 6.7 per thousand births (Ontario Government 1987b:118). The rate for early neonatal deaths alone was under five (*ibid.*:74).

For Sudan such finely calibrated statistics are impossible to get. Infant mortality (live births surviving less than a year) is estimated to be somewhere between 110 and 120 per thousand based on imperfect census reports from 1973 (Sudan Government 1982:7). The time of Amal's pregnancy (1983–4) was one of hardship; the north was on the brink of famine and even bread was scarce. Since nutrition plays a major role in determining pregnancy outcome, rates were likely higher then and continued so in the difficult years that ensued.[5] Figures from the 1920s, though of questionable reliability, hint at deteriorating conditions since the heyday of colonial rule: in the northern provinces in 1926, infant mortality was recorded at seventy-one per thousand. By 1929 that rate had dropped to sixty.[6]

To put this in perspective, the infant mortality rate in England and Wales between 1896 and 1900, when the British were engaged in conquering Sudan, was 156 per thousand. By the early 1930s, with improved hygiene and nutrition especially for the poor, it had fallen to sixty-two, on a par with figures for northern Sudan.[7]

Rates of maternal mortality in Sudan are comparatively high, with figures ranging from 655 to 2270 per 100,000 live births.[8] Because this figure is based on *live* births, it does not, of course, include women who died during pregnancy, as a complication of pregnancy following still birth, miscarriage, or induced abortion, or as a long-term consequence of childbearing. Since deaths are seldom reported at all (Sudan Government 1982:4), it is subject to gross distortion. Even so, it means that in Sudan, where the number of live births a woman can expect to experience averages seven,[9] a conservative estimate of her lifetime risk of dying as a result of pregnancy is one in twenty-one. A more realistic figure (assuming the underreporting of both maternal deaths[10] and pregnancies) could well be one in nine.[11] By contrast, the lifetime risk in developed regions is as low as one in 10,000 (Abou Zahr 1993). I would stress that these are actuarial figures, and do not convey risks to individual women. Several studies have shown that in the developing world maternal mortality rates for girls who become pregnant before age 15 are five to seven times higher than for those aged 20 or more; for those in their late teens, the rates are still two to three times as high (Abou Zahr and Royston 1991:6).

By 1983 a handful of Hofriyati had delivered in hospital, at least two by cesarean section.[12] And in 1994 there was widespread talk in the village about being able soon to "reserve" a hospital bed for childbirth, as is increasingly done in the city.

Life for women in Hofriyat is undeniably precarious and it is understandable that many seek to minimize childbearing risks by all available means. Most marry young and experience early and multiple pregnancies. All in prepubescence undergo infibulation, a form of "female circumcision" in which the midwife excises the girl's clitoris and inner labia, then pares her outer labia and stitches them together so as to "cover" or "veil" the vaginal meatus, leaving a pinhole opening for the elimination of urine and menstrual blood.[13] A girl's virginity thus becomes a revisable social assertion rather than one whose expression is natural and discrete (Hayes 1975). At marriage many infibulated women must be surgically opened in order to have sexual intercourse; in labor all require the presence of a midwife to perform one or more episiotomies before the baby can be born. After delivery a woman is resewn, and thereby regains a measure of virginal status.

While infibulation is designed to safeguard reproductive capacity (Boddy 1982; 1989), sadly, it often precipitates its distress. This frustrates the cultural imperative that married women demonstrate fecundity, and may lead to devastating loss of status and economic support through divorce or co-wifery. Infibulation is clearly hazardous to health. Most of its complications are long term, and derive from improper drainage of urine and menstrual blood.[14] Childbirth is problematic, as the inelastic scar may prolong the second stage of labor, the contraction phase when the baby is leaving the womb, and, even when a midwife is present to cut through the fibrous tissue, the outcome can be death or brain damage to the child. For the mother, lengthy delivery can cause fistulae (passages) to develop between the vagina and bladder or rectum, resulting in incontinence for which she may face ostracism and divorce (Toubia 1994:713; Dareer 1982:38). Dermoid cysts have been reported to develop in the line of the scar, and keloids sometimes form that complicate an anterior episiotomy (Abdalla 1982:23). Maternal death can result from blood loss and exhaustion or a revisitation of unsanitary conditions attending the original operation. In order to avoid traumatic delivery some women in their third trimester cut back on their food, resulting in low birth weights, a problematic start for the child, and slow recovery for the mother (cf. Mohamud 1991:208; van der Kwaak 1992:780). Still, whatever its risks to individuals, infibulation seems not to have had a negative effect on overall fertility levels in Sudan, where the annual rate of increase hovers around 3 percent (Sudan Government 1982:60–1, 7; Spencer

1994:123). Infibulation transforms a woman's natural fertility into a moral asset that defines her sense of self; despite growing awareness of its harmfulness, no Hofriyati woman I spoke to in the mid-1970s or early 1980s was willing to give up the practice.

Soon after arriving in Hofriyat in 1976, I was taken to witness a birth. The setting was an ordinary room in an ordinary mud-brick house, but on that day it was dank and unbearably hot, packed with women fingering worry-beads, chanting invocations to drown any cries from the mother-to-be. Windows giving onto the alley were shuttered for privacy, leaving the doorway and a window overlooking the courtyard as the only sources of light. The packed earth floor had been wetted down to offset the heat; flies were thick wherever some moisture remained.

The laboring woman lay flat on her back on an *angareeb* that had been spread with a mattress topped by an auspiciously "red" fibrous mat linked to demonstrations of female fertility. The lower end of the mattress was slightly elevated and covered with a waterproof sheet. This supported the woman's hips and heels. Her knees were raised in a local equivalent of the stirruped birthing posture customary in Western societies. To deliver, she would have to push the baby uphill. Stretched over her legs was a *towb*, the length of cloth that, worn circling the body and covering the head, is women's everyday modesty garb. A washbasin was placed on the floor at the foot of the bed and behind it sat Miriam, the midwife, on a low woven stool. A nearby table held her midwife's tin box, opened and ready, and a bowl of water containing her implements. Beneath the bed smoked a censer of fragrant bridal woods.

Periodically, Miriam thrust her head beneath the cloth while female kin held the *towb* tight lest it slip and expose the woman to view. When Miriam felt the head crowning, she injected the woman with anesthetic, took scissors from the bowl and cut. The room filled with joyous ululations. A baby girl was safely born inside the tent after a long and sonorous labor; the mother, though weak, was well.

The prone or "lithotomy" birthing posture was introduced to Sudan by British sisters, Mabel and Gertrude Wolff, who, in the 1920s and 1930s, established the Midwives Training School in Omdurman adjacent to Khartoum. British motives for initiating midwifery reform were (rhetorically, at least) philanthropic, but also political and pragmatic. Administrators hoped thereby to remedy Sudan's under-population, seen as a legacy of famine and displacement caused by the preceding century of unrest, and aggravated by ignorance. They were eager to secure a native workforce for prospective cotton plantations like the Gezira Scheme, created to feed the Lancashire mills. And they sought to build a committed resident bulwark to Egyptian nationalist interests on the upper Nile, thus to furnish a living border between Egypt and Sudan.

Yet the problem was more perceptual than real: northern Sudan lacked not an ample population but a proletariat. Employable workers were scarce. Most families held some farmland and their menfolk could be induced to work for wages only intermittently and at high cost.[15] Though the British had fought to Khartoum on a promise of ending the slave trade, once in power they became convinced by the dearth of transactable labor that the economy depended on servitude, and adopted a permissive, indeed complicit stance toward domestic slavery so as, they said, to ensure the region's supply of food (Daly 1986:440; 1991:4).[16] More likely they feared an uprising of the Muslim population should the practice be suppressed. The Anti-Slavery Society, alerted to the hypocrisy by disgruntled junior officials, began a protest that culminated in the embarrassing exposure in Parliament of large-scale slave trading in 1928. Knowing this situation could not be sustained, Sudan officials had earlier begun to cultivate a cheap, abundant, and landless workforce by encouraging the settlement of West African pilgrims passing through Sudan *en route* to Mecca (Daly 1986; O'Brien 1986).

More subtle, biopolitical, transformations were left to British health and educational staff. As two decades of Pax Britannica had effected little growth in the northern population, officials became convinced that infibulation held the key. They blamed the practice for sustained low birthrates and high infant mortality, though, ironically, their own figures for the latter rivalled Britain's at the time. When the Director of the Sudan Medical Service disagreed, suggesting that malaria and venereal diseases were largely to blame, his opinion fell on disbelieving ears. Efficiently reproductive women were crucial to the colonial venture in Sudan, but their bodily reform required diplomacy, tact, and a flexible approach.[17] This the formidable Wolff sisters – whom officials dubbed 'the Wolves' – would arguably provide.

In a speech about the school's inaugural year, Mabel Wolff described her first case in the company of a trained local midwife thus:

On arriving at the house I found crowds of people gathered to approve or disapprove of me or my methods; against their customs I succeeded in inducing the patient to lie down on an angareeb but at the approach of the critical moment the women onlookers and even the menfolk became excited, there was a loud jabber of protests against the patient being delivered lying down. But in the meantime I was able to present to them a fine baby and all their anger was turned to deafening trills of joy.

The usual method of delivering the patient in this country is to suspend a rope from the ceiling, dig a hole in the ground over which is spread a special round mat plaited with a hole in the centre; the daya [midwife] squats on the mat with bared legs which she spreads out across the hole and has in readiness by her side a razor [to cut through the genital scar] with all but the tip of the blade wrapped round with, in most cases, a very dirty piece of rag. The patient stands over the hole and clings onto the rope and when she gets too tired or exhausted she is supported by various relations – none too gently as the poor things have often told me how they ached for days after.[18]

Though not mentioned here, someone did fling a *towb* over her head at said critical moment, which rendered her "quite helpless" for several seconds (Kendall 1952:44).

Note Wolff's use of the term "patient" to describe the laboring woman. By the time the sisters had begun to practice, the cultural construction of birth in the West had shifted: it was seen less as women's everyday feat and more as a pathological event requiring biomedical management. In some parts of Canada, for example, female midwifery had been outlawed since the mid-nineteenth century, under strong and continuous pressure from doctors seeking "to forge themselves into a unified profession" (Ontario Government 1987a:207). In settler communities women helped one another through delivery, and families relied on their own resources in coping with disease. Childbirth was an obvious route by which a physician could insert himself in a family's life cycle and begin to build a relationship by demonstrating his skills. Neighborhood midwives who did not practice for their living offered steep competition, and this doctors sought to remove by legal action (*ibid.*:207–8).

When threatened, however, not all of the midwives backed down. One Mrs. Bell, for example, dispatched a spirited reply:

When what you call midwifery was forced on me, I did it. No one was as glad as I was when your boys with the bag came along, but somehow they have proved not very satisfactory . . . Let me tell you, I will go to prison and stay there until I die before I pay a fine and acknowledge that I have done wrong . . . I have always advised them to get a doctor: I will never do so again . . . When a child comes, I will do my best and save it. I have saved 70. The mothers are all alive. Two boys are dead, but lived until nearly four years of age. Can your boys with the bag say that? . . . I am ready for trial any time, and if you have the power to imprison, I am ready.[19]

Even in Britain, where female midwifery was not suppressed as completely as in Canada and parts of the United States, midwives' autonomy was sharply curtailed when passage of the Midwives Act in 1902 required them to be licensed and subject to (overwhelmingly male) doctors' supervision; henceforth they were pressured to receive formal medical training as well (Tew 1990). Training in matters of hygiene was clearly welcome. Yet gradually, in both Britain and North America, births assisted by midwives were explicitly and successfully discouraged by newly consolidated medical establishments, in favor of hospital deliveries "managed," as today, by physicians. Biomedical practitioners, certain in their knowledge and ability and backed by the power of the state, spread the wings of an ascending hegemony and convinced lay women and men of the superiority of their methods; midwives, however skilled and knowledgeable, were discredited, portrayed as dirty and ignorant crones. Their status plummeted despite the fact that in the early decades of this century midwife-assisted home births were still statistically safer than doctor-assisted institutional and home deliveries, both.[20]

The disparity was due largely to philosophy. Most midwives practiced "masterful restraint," with the patience to let nature take its course. Physicians, on the other hand, were schooled to believe that human ingenuity could improve on the natural process; they were quicker to intervene with technology, some of it dubious, and such procedures, plus the fixed prone position required in anticipation of their use, introduced a whole new set of risks to giving birth (Rothman 1982; Martin 1987; Ontario Government 1987a; Tew 1990).

Barbara Rothman suggests that both Cartesian dualism (resulting in the notion of the human body-as-machine) and androcentric ideology (in which the [young] male body is the normative body-as-machine) are responsible for pathologizing women's bodies and physical processes in Western societies. Female reproductive events are seen as complications of that normative body, and as such appear to constitute systemic stresses requiring "treatment," "supervision" and "care" (1982:36–7). Moreover, early doctors were trained to deal mainly with abnormal deliveries; their view that birth without intervention is an aberrant process was a bias of experience that became generalized as they gained professional control (see Tew 1990:40).

Such processes, however, were part of a general bourgeois civilizing enterprise shaped by the culture and politics of empire in which the barbaric margins provided a foil for European self-definitions (Comaroff and Comaroff 1992; Stoler 1995). In Britain midwives practicing traditional methods of restraint and aid by manipulation if required were gradually superseded by medically trained midwives authorized to oversee only routine births and intervene rarely, if at all. Later still, they became obstetric assistants to physicians working in hospitals. But for both practical and ideological reasons, this pattern was not exported to the colonies whole; if local women's sensibilities required revision, their distinctness from Europeans was never presumed to be dissolved. Hence in the low-technology context of early twentieth-century Sudan, the Wolffs devised an ingenious synthesis of biomedical and lay approaches that bent to local custom even as it strove to undermine it.

Yet in the sisters' notable pragmatism and their perpetual struggle with officials to ensure that trainees were respected and adequately paid, one detects a note of resistance to the decline of midwifery at home as well as adaptation to conditions abroad; the sisters' relationship with the Sudanese was ambivalent, at once distanced and allied. A letter Mabel wrote to her sister while on inspection tour in 1931 makes the point:

> [R]eally it makes my blood boil to think that our [native] staff women should not be granted second class warrants [to ride the train], when they are doing such fine work, yet those blessed school teachers who really are not worth any more than our women are granted second class warrants . . . [B]esides, I feel strongly it is demeaning to our work and gives people a wrong impression of the social status of midwives in this country. I had quite an argument with [Mr.] Wallace on the subject . . . [who] said that midwives in all countries were rather looked down upon. It is a fact in most countries but it is not so in this, where they are respectable women and quite frequently related to the Mek, Omdah, or Sheikh, in fact the best in the land . . . I feel it almost as a personal affront to the good we are trying to aim at in raising the general standard of work. Of course the whole crux of the question is that we ourselves officially should be on an equal footing to the [Miss] Evans's, for after all isn't our work as important as female education, and as successful in every way within our control as theirs? "Fight, Fight, Fight!" that is my motto . . . [O]ne gets nowhere without PUSH.[21]

This hardly meant that Sudanese midwives, educated or not, would be permitted to retain their autonomy. Following the pattern in Britain, all existing practitioners were licensed and required to keep a register of attended deliveries. As many as could be accommodated received several months of medical training as well. Only women of sound moral character and non-slave status were selected,[22] and those who had not yet practiced had to obtain approval from indigenous male authorities in their districts. Yet insofar as these criteria were met, the tradition whereby the role passes from mother to daughter was retained. And the sisters did not attempt to interfere with the rituals of pregnancy and birth so long as these did not jeopardize their work. Indeed, they were keen ethnographers, keeping detailed notes and photographs that provide an invaluable record of women's lives during the colonial era.[23]

The visual emphasis of obstetric biomedicine – epitomized today by the ultrasound "photograph" of the unborn (see Duden 1993) – was necessarily compromised in the case of early midwifery training in

Sudan. Existing midwives had learned to deliver by feel, and many of them, being older and prone to cataracts, were blind. The tradition of working beneath a towb made seeing difficult in any case. This, of course, was intended to meet conventions of modesty. But it was also consonant with the sensory disposition of Sudanese women, a disposition oriented not primarily by visual reference, but also by touch, taste, smell, the sense of space and one's bearings within it (see Boddy 1989; cf. Duden 1993). When the Wolffs began their school, literate local women were rare; to keep their registers they required the help of educated men. Pupils were taught by rote and practical memory. They learned to identify medications by color, opacity, taste, texture, density, and scent; container shape and color were wisely deemed unreliable. They were taught how to wield scissors using "pieces of motor tyre . . . for practising slitting and suturing the vulval obstructions resulting from ritual circumcision" (Holland 1946:9). They practiced delivery with "full antiseptic precautions and prolonged washing"[24] on a "realistic" – if uninfibulated and Caucasian – model with movable parts and resident fetus, and learned infant bathing by handling Caucasian baby dolls. According to Wolff's report for 1926:

The midwives thus trained become in a minor way missionaries in the homes of people, in the cause of cleanliness and simple hygiene, and it is to their growing number and increasing influence that we must look not only to establish a standard of simple hygiene in the home, but also to combat the almost universal custom of complete circumcision which is so barbarous in its execution, and which is fraught with so much danger both to mother and child. It may be years before this custom is effectually checked, but in the meanwhile the first seeds of a silent revolution to cleanliness and hygiene are being sown in the homes of the people. (In Bayoumi 1979:150)

Clearly, the bodies and minds of pupil midwives were being shaped to new canons of normalcy and propriety. Ironically, the process may have been all the more effective in that the dummies exemplifying "the norm" adventitiously affirmed a local prejudice: white skin is considered a mark of holiness and nobility, an attribute of the Prophet Muhammad and his kin.

At first recruits were few, but by 1924 all Khartoum Province midwives had been trained, and schooling was extended to rural zones. Periodic inspections by the Wolffs identified backsliders, who chanced delicensing and the loss of their modest stipends and supplies. In 1932 prenatal care was added to midwives' responsibilities. This the sisters introduced by way of a simile:

[We asked,] when they put a cooking pot (halla) with food on the fire, did they leave it until the food was burnt and spoilt or was it usual to occasionally inspect the contents of the pot? Now amongst the womenfolk, the words "Kashf el Halla" [pot check] have become a recognized meaning for "Ante-Natal Examination" and attendances are so far very encouraging.[25]

Wittingly or not, in likening gestation to cooking the Wolffs had tapped into local meanings while shifting them to accommodate a biomedical view. Hofriyati, for example, tacitly compare pregnancy to making the batter for bread: mixing (female) fluid and (male) seed in an impervious container, something only women are properly able to do (Boddy 1982; 1989). As depicted by the Wolffs, pregnancy is like making a stew: a physical process to be monitored, helped along, indeed disciplined, by continuous visual surveillance (see also Kendall 1952:48). And note that agency has been reassigned: now the midwife, not the pregnant woman herself, is the "cook" responsible for care of the "pot."

Thus did the midwife, on whom every reproductive couple is compelled by infibulation to rely, become an agent of "civilization" backed by the authority of the colonial state. With time a partially Westernized habitus of pregnancy and birth became commonplace, entailing a modified set of corporeal dispositions with potential implications for identity and subjectivity.[26] Upright birth posture was deemed unnatural, brutish; and the reduction in maternal and child mortality that came with aseptic procedures lent its truth to this view. Even skepticism about colonial definitions did not prevent rope-delivery's demise: older women told me that although labor was quicker and less painful "on the rope," the anesthetic administered prior to being cut was an advantage available only to the recumbent. Their compliance was reluctant but assured.

The civilizing of midwifery was intended not only to expand the potential workforce, but also to ameliorate the "degraded" condition of women and effect a rise in their status that would signal "progress" for Sudan as a whole.[27] Yet it also effectively reaffirmed what the *fugara*, village clerics, declaimed: that women are inherently weak and dependent beings, at the mercy of physical processes beyond their ken and control. If anything, adopting a locally tempered biomedical view of their bodies may have fostered in women a sense of powerlessness, even as it boosted midwives' agency and independence. And here lay a paradox for colonial and postcolonial mandates: for it is precisely their dependence and material vulnerability that leads women to ignore the harm that attends female circumcision. Because childbearing in the context of marriage is the socially approved route to social and economic security, and infibulation renders women marriageable, most women of my acquaintance are still loath to risk their daughters' futures and continue to insist the procedure be done.[28]

Yet the Wolffs were astute, if not prescient. They seemed aware that the culturally configured female body has political import in northern Sudan; there a family's moral worth is tied closely to the discipline exercised by its womenfolk through modest dress, chaste behavior, and infibulation. What applies to the family applies also to the group and ultimately to Arab Sudan as a whole (see Boddy 1989; 1991). Local midwives perform infibulations and, rather than forbid them to continue the practice once trained, the Wolffs taught a modified operation that was less destructive than the "full pharaonic" type. The procedure came to be known as "intermediate" (*wasit*) or, tellingly, "government" (*hakuma*) circumcision, in contrast to Egyptian (*misri*) or – as the Wolffs put it – "Pharaoh's circumcision" (*tahur farowniya*), which was vilified. The sisters' intent was to encourage midwives to spread "propaganda" against genital surgery of any kind, while introducing progressively milder operations until the custom died out or was replaced by the religiously permitted form (*sunna*) wherein only the prepuce of the clitoris is cut.[29] The resulting distinction between "government" and "Egyptian" operations reflected colonial politics at a time when the Anglo-Egyptian Condominium ruling Sudan was under threat (see Daly 1986); and in the process, circumcision's relevance as a marker of northern Sudanese identity was implicitly endorsed.

The colonization of women's bodies, indeed, of consciousness writ large, was a contradictory, subtle, and eminently practical process, in the course of which the state, through its medical missionaries, extended surveillance into formerly uncolonized domestic space (cf. Arnold 1993). However incomplete, the process would prove relatively immune to challenge so long as it worked with, rather than against, indigenous ideas. Two developments make this clear. First, given the midwife's pivotal role, the partial medicalization of birth naturally entailed a partial medicalization of female circumcision. As the Wolffs' lesson book instructs: "Should a midwife do circumcisions . . . she must perform the operation with all cleanliness just as she would a labor case, and attend the case daily for seven days, or more if necessary, in order to avoid infection of the wound."[30]

Though life-saving, such precautions cultivate a medical mystique: local anesthetics, dissolving stitches, antiseptic solutions, and antibiotics are routine features of the practice today. Some wealthy and educated Sudanese, mindful of the need for sterile conditions, currently enlist physicians to perform circumcisions in hospital. Although this is anathema to the World Health Organization who warn against confusing the practice with biomedical surgery, many doctors feel morally bound to comply lest greater injury be done to the child elsewhere (Hall and Ismail 1981:99; WHO 1986:35). This too has lent the practice authorization and prestige, fostering syncretisms that seem likely to ensure its endurance. Now in Hofriyat, for example, infibulation is sometimes performed as a medical cure for a toddler's intractable illness because it is thought to encourage maturation.

Second, and by contrast, circumcision became a nationalist cause. In 1946 the colonial government, after years of groundwork, reversed its tactic and made performing an infibulation a criminal offense. It was a grave miscalculation. Soon after, two noncompliant midwives were remanded to trial, sparking a public outcry that led to anticolonial riots.[31] Enforcement of the law was quietly dropped. But unbeknownst to the protesters, and often behind the backs of the colonizing agents themselves, the transformation of consciousness was proceeding apace.

January 1984: An angry wind and pale, cold sun. Salima and I shiver as we walk the elevated railway track laid down by the British at the turn of the century and still the only excavated road in the north. We are on our way to visit Sheffa, the senior midwife who lives in a village several miles away.

We find her at work in an outlying hamlet. Sheffa seems delighted to see us and suggests I accompany her on her rounds. An 18-year-old is now in labor with her first pregnancy. The birth is likely to be prolonged and Sheffa offers to arrange transport if we get late. But first we must check on the laboring woman, then return to the clinic for Sheffa's regular prenatal appointments.

Sheffa astonishes me; she is unlike any rural woman I have met. Her clothes – a jeans skirt and tight fitting T-shirt – are urban and, apart from the white *towb* worn over top, more Western than Sudanese. Over her shoulders she has slung a sheepskin coat in case the day stays cold; instead of a midwife's traditional red and gold box, she uses a battered leather briefcase to carry her equipment. Sartorial iconoclasm enhances her commanding presence: she is tall, handsome, and radiates health, moving with unbridled energy, not the torpid gait considered feminine in these parts. And though only in her mid-thirties, what Sheffa says clearly goes: few would dare to oppose her.

We make our way to her patient's natal home where, as is the custom, she has returned to give birth. There we are served coffee to warm us, though the chill has left the morning and a strengthening sun has begun to shimmer the air. In the dark, still-cool reception room, Sheffa and I are directed to metal chairs set before the laboring girl, Nemad, who reclines on an *angareeb*. We are met by a junior midwife, Foziya, who reports that Nemad's contractions are still well spaced. As we sip they discuss the examination they will do in a few moments time. Now and then Nemad moans and as she does she grabs my hand. Sheffa comforts her, "It's alright, the pains are good. Soon it will be finished."

Gently, Foziya manipulates Nemad's belly to check the baby's location. The first position, she reports, head pointing down, face to the back, buttocks on mother's right side. But the body is high – common for a first delivery. Foziya inspects Nemad's mouth and gums for signs of illness, her eyes for anemia, her hair and scalp for lice which, if present, must be dealt with promptly lest they infect the baby after birth. All is well.

Sheffa scrubs her hands. Nemad is told to hoist herself aboard some rolled up mattresses on top of another *angareeb*. These have been spread with a vinyl cloth – blue to counter the evil eye, and laced with images of Pepsi bottle caps. Sheffa cautiously measures Nemad's dilation. "I circumcised her," she says. "Not too tight." (Nemad's eyes widen and she cries out in pain.) "I'd like to use surgical gloves for this, but we can't always get them in Sudan." One and a half fingers' width. Still the latent phase of the first stage of labor; there are several more hours to go. If the baby's head remains high at five o'clock, she must go to hospital in Shendi. Nemad is encouraged to walk; we leave her to it and move on to the clinic.

There, a 14-year-old girl is waiting to be seen. "I delivered her," says Sheffa. "She was my first local baby." The girl, she explains, was married at eleven, before she'd begun to menstruate; she's now five months pregnant. Natural delivery will be impossible as her pelvis is not fully formed and the baby quite large. This, Sheffa continues, is the tragedy of a recent trend: increasingly, parents in straightened circumstances are marrying their prepubescent daughters to suitors twice their age or more, who have lucrative jobs in Arabia. The men obtain compliant, partly educated, but indisputably virgin wives unlikely to question their domestic role. Since consummation takes place soon after menarche, the girls may conceive before their bones have matured. If so, their bodies channel energy from their own growth toward that of their babies, leaving stunted pelves prone to "disproportion" – too small for the baby's head to pass. Sheffa predicts a sharp rise in the number of cesareans over the next few years.

Years later I read in a World Health Organization piece that precocious childbearing and grand multiparity are "cultural practices" more pernicious even than female circumcision (1986:31). The latter con-

demns women to lives of suffering but is seldom lethal; early and
frequent births regularly kill.

Sheffa's office at the clinic has its own women's entrance and courtyard.
It is clean and freshly white-washed, with cheerful curtains and plastic
replicas of local produce strung along one wall. On the desk are jars
containing fava beans, lentils, rice, and peas − foods pregnant women
are encouraged to eat.

Sheffa speaks to a woman whose blood, like Amal's, has tested "light"
or anemic. Pointing to the jars, she warns her to eat properly so that
when the fetus becomes more demanding she will not suffer dizziness
caused by insufficient blood. Several others are tested for signs of
eclampsia, the disease of pregnancy that only last week sent a Hofriyati
woman into convulsions and caused her to abort twins. Sheffa takes
their blood pressure and pronounces them fit; however, she cautions
them to eat foods containing protein and return next week. But she
knows that few can afford meat and eggs on a regular basis, and even
lentils and beans are becoming expensive and increasingly scarce. The
harvest was below expectations. With less food entering the country
than is required to address the deficit, pregnant women and their
offspring are facing malnutrition.

It is now 2 p.m. and Sheffa, Salima, and I depart for lunch. Sheffa
lives with her mother and sister who help care for Sheffa's nine-month-
old son. Her husband, a clinician, is posted to a village nearer
Khartoum; he visits when he can. They wed two years ago when Sheffa
was beyond the usual age for marriage in Sudan. Her work and
education came first, she explains. Unlike most Sudanese couples, their
marriage was not arranged by kin. She and her husband are friends who
met at the medical school in Khartoum. "We chose each other," she
says.

Sheffa changes into loose-fitting garb to nurse her son, and plays a
tape of *zar* songs from Khartoum. A man's voice summons European
spirits − one who guzzles jugs of bootleg champagne; another whose
requests for drink are impossible to fulfill in newly abolitionist Sudan.
Sheffa is a strong believer in the power of spirits. I had not expected
this, thinking her medical training would have inclined her to disbelief.
In a few cases, she says, *zar* is *marad nafsiya*, psychological illness, but in
others it is not so easy to explain. An innumerate woman who requests a
watch while in trance is suddenly able to tell time; another can speak
English or knows what foods − clean foods − a European wants and how
to eat them with knife and fork. As for circumcision, she says that
although she is aware of its dangers, she must still perform the surgery

or risk losing villagers' trust. "I prefer just to nick the clitoris," she says, "but I do . . . whatever the parents wish. *Lazim* – I must."

Sheffa's own baby was delivered by doctors in Shendi hospital. Her pregnancy was not problematic, nor was the birth; she just preferred to make an appointment and do it that way.

September, 1983: A bright late summer evening. Little traffic clogs the lake shore as Melanie and I drive to the hospital in downtown Toronto. We are excited but apprehensive – I, over whether I can fulfill my promise to bear witness. As an undergraduate I'd volunteered to be a "droplette" at a blood donor clinic but had fainted at the sight of my first customer.

At the hospital Melanie is quickly braceleted and whisked upstairs to the maternity floor. Moments later I find her lying gowned and strapped to a fetal monitor attended by a nurse in surgical uniform. This is not a good sign. Though Melanie is hardly romantic about experiencing vaginal birth ("Bring on the technology!" she had been heard to say), things are not turning out as we had imagined. The room is a soulless box filled with gadgets and dials that have apparently detected fetal distress. Melanie is nervous, on the verge of tears. Another nurse enters the room and prepares to shave her. The anesthetist arrives to start an epidural block; the doctor and his team are scrubbing. I leave to phone Melanie's husband overseas.

January, 1984: As Sheffa changes back into work clothes a woman bursts into the courtyard. Nemad's labor is hot, she says. We must come quickly. Now!

We find Nemad lying on her red fertility mat. Again Sheffa washes and examines her. Two and a half fingers. Not quite there. Nemad's mother helps her walk back and forth across the room to bring the baby's head into position. Within half an hour she has dilated to three fingers, the head is down, and her pains are truly "hot." This will take time, cautions Sheffa, it will be several hours yet.

We drink syrupy tea and converse. I am asked how women give birth in Canada, and tell them about being Melanie's coach. "But normally," I say, "the woman's husband attends and helps." My companions are aghast, but think it rather sweet. In Sudan a woman's husband cannot set foot in the birth chamber the entire forty days of her confinement. He may not even hold his child until it is five months old. But this does not apply to all men, only the baby's father. Nemad's brothers are here today, impatient to welcome the baby.

Ninety minutes later Sheffa measures Nemad's pelvis relative to the width of the baby's head. She will be ready to deliver in an hour or two. As dusk descends we depart in search of a car to return us to Hofriyat; Salima and I are intent on staying to the end, but with no flashlight and no moon until morning, walking is out of the question. We set off for the Italian textile factory, built six years ago but never opened.

Inside a fenced compound on the desert fringe, massive wooden crates and bare machines are stacked and smothered by sand. Drifts have formed around derelict turbines, and with them gather the dissipated hopes of local families. An Italian manager and his Eritrean assistant live here, guarding the ghostly warehouse and equipment. They have placed their Landrover at Sheffa's disposal, and kindly agree to drive us home later on.

Before returning to Nemad's we visit a woman whom the Landrover saved a few days ago. She had delivered prematurely a stillborn child. Now she is home, and Sheffa wants to ensure she is taking her antibiotics to prevent puerperal fever and counteract the inflammation caused by remedial infibulation. The *nufasa* (post-partum woman) reclines resplendent in her wedding gold and the charms that deflect misfortune, her hair freshly plaited, her hands and feet stained with henna. Friends tease her about being in confinement, pampered like a bride and freed from chores for forty days. One quips that forty days are not enough to recover from being opened and resewn.

By 5:15 we are back and Nemad is close to giving birth. Sheffa readies the "delivery room." Working at a table near the south-facing windows – for now our only source of light – she places scissors, cotton gauze, plastic tubing and a length of string in a large enamel bowl and pours boiling water over all. She fills a clean syringe with anesthetic, then directs that an *angareeb* be placed in the centre of the room. A lawn chair is put at the end of the bed; this is where Sheffa will sit. Immediately behind it to the left is the *angareeb* where I am to observe and hold aloft the kerosene lamp when required. Beside me is another chair, with arms, that will serve as the baby's crib. Mattresses are piled up at one end of the birth bed and behind them in its center is placed a rope-strung stool. Over the mattresses the Pepsi mackintosh is laid as before.

Nemad is led into the room accompanied by four middle-aged women. The door is shut. Her mother's sister lifts herself onto the stool atop the *angareeb*, then extends her legs to either side of the mattress roll. The other aunts help Nemad onto the sheet before her. Nemad will give birth in her kinswoman's arms, her back leaning against her aunt's chest, her torso and hips angled upright. Sheffa, unlike Miriam, has modified the supine posture to better resemble rope delivery with its gravitational advantage.

The room is hot; its mud-brick walls, having absorbed the heat of the day, now emit it with a vengeance. A hint of breeze wafts through the north windows; we are lucky the wind has dropped and there is no blowing sand. The room is shadowy, muted in the fading light and alive with the humming of flies.

Nemad's legs are spread and held back, an aunt on either side of the *angareeb* to perform this task. The one nearest me is wearing Bruce Lee "Kung Fu" plastic sandals. Nemad's skirt is stretched between her elevated knees to provide modesty and prevent her from seeing what Sheffa might do. On instruction Nemad lifts her arms and locks them backward round her aunt's neck. Her mother stands by her side, fanning her face.

When I return to the monitored cubicle, Melanie has disappeared. A nurse escorts me to an antechamber where I don booties, hospital gown, and cap, and place a surgical mask over my nose and mouth. "They're about to begin," I'm told. "Go through the blue doors to your left."

The operating theatre is large, brightly lit, and chill. Figures in aphid green are clustered round an object ahead; they turn toward me and by their surprised expressions I know I've come through the wrong door. Now I see Melanie's body, stretched out and divided in two by a massive screen; people, lights and equipment are focused on her lower half, nearest me. The surgeon has already made a bright red incision through her belly and is about to clamp it back. I take a deep breath and walk to the chair by Melanie's head.

Sheffa tells Nemad to breathe; she wants her to cry out with the pain, rather than observe the custom of silence lest she hold her breath and deprive the baby of oxygen. A lamp is lit and passed to me through the window. I hold it high over Sheffa's shoulder. She inserts the syringe into the vaginal opening and makes several small injections around the area to be cut, much like a dentist freezing one's gums. Nemad is bearing down; Sheffa feels inside her and punctures the amniotic sac; fluid gushes onto the vinyl sheet and into a basin below. I fan away the flies. Soon the top of the baby's head shows through the opening. Sheffa pours water over the area to clean away some blood. She washes Nemad with carbolic soap then inserts two fingers between the head and the perineum. She waits until the head is crowning well, then quickly cuts through the muscle to the left and down. There is a spurt of blood. Kung Fu auntie swoons and leaves the room; Nemad's mother takes her place. The flies are growing thick; hands rhythmically brush them away.

After several more contractions the baby still cannot pass; Sheffa cuts a further inch or so. Next push, she eases back the muscle, gently grasps the baby's head and glides him into the world.

Melanie is flat on her back with her right arm strapped to a blood pressure cuff. Her free hand, attached to an intravenous drip, grabs my arm as I sit down. "I want to know when they're going to cut," she says. "Relax," I tell her, "you're already wide open." Beyond the screen the doctor's eyes crinkle in a grin. Melanie sinks back and closes her eyes; tension ebbs from her hand.

Sheffa sucks mucous from the baby's mouth with a small plastic pipe. He gives a hearty cry. Nemad's kinswomen are elated and congratulate her on the birth of a son. Sheffa ties the cord close to the baby and cuts it, then wraps him in a clean cloth and places him in the chair next to me. He whimpers and tests his legs, then puts his hand to his mouth and sucks. He is small but extremely alert. Sheffa closes the windows and returns her attention to Nemad. The afterbirth is delivered without mishap; now she threads a needle with suture and prepares to sew up the wound. I bring the lamp closer and wave away more flies.

The doctor tells Melanie she'll feel a moment of pressure as the baby is massaged from her womb. The anesthetist checks her instrument panel and adjusts a dial or two. She has oxygen ready should Melanie faint. Melanie moans with the oddity of the sensation, and a few seconds later she has a baby girl. A team of nurses shuttle her to an incubation table. They weigh her, put drops in her eyes, wrap her in a flannel blanket, and give her to me to hold. I lift her up for Melanie to see. "Hello, Julia." I hear myself say. "Wait till you see your room."

I telephone Melanie's husband as she and Julia are wheeled upstairs to a private room. When I rejoin them Melanie is in pain and about to receive medicine for its relief. The baby is taken to the nursery for the night, to be bathed and thoroughly examined. Melanie is attached to an intravenous drip. I leave as a large bouquet of roses arrives.

Nemad is helped down and supported by her aunts as Sheffa and her mother rearrange the room. The *angareeb* is moved back against the wall and Nemad soon put to bed. Sheffa uses oil to clean the baby of vernix and blood, then swaddles him in clean soft cotton and gives him to his mother to feed. I am taken by the simplicity of it all, and hope that when Amal's time comes it will be like this.

Nemad's mother stays with her as the rest of the delivery team go out onto the verandah for a breath of air. Incense is lit and placed beneath an *angareeb*. Nemad's brothers arrive, overjoyed that the child is a boy; her husband's family are heard cheering a few doors away. As we sip the celebratory coffee, women ask how birth in my country differs from what I've just seen. I am tired and emotional, and want to avoid a lengthy discussion. I reply that it's similar, but that we do not circumcise. "Baraka," someone says, "blessing," and the others murmur assent.

How different is giving birth in rural Sudan from doing so in urban Toronto? On one level the answer is obvious; on another it is not. In both places biomedicine shapes the process, yet in one more thoroughly than in the other. In Sudan, where persons are unthinkable save as members of a social whole, and spirit possession is a conventional event, the body and its parts may be less reified, less readily viewed as objects in themselves (Boddy 1989; 1994). Perhaps. The extent to which the natural process is respected may be greater there as well. But if Sudan is less interventionist, this seems more for want of means than by design. Moreover, it is hardly anti-interventionist: infibulation, after all, is underwritten by the view that the female body (like the male) is naturally flawed and must be perfected by human hand. In a deeper vein, we have much in common, it seems.

It is by now a truism that human bodies are everywhere subjectively informed by cultural meanings, including those labeled "scientific" and deemed unencumbered by ideology (Martin 1987; Young 1983). In so far as such meanings are backed by the power of the state and alternatives suppressed, bodies are "colonized" (Mohanty 1991) and "normalized" (Foucault 1979) as well. Moreover, as Foucault (1979; 1982) has pointed out, power in the modern state is masked and diffuse: it invests bodies, confers benefits as it disciplines, makes us subjects in the dual sense of that word. The gradual replacement of gynocentric birthing practices by those informed by assumptions of a tacitly androcentric biomedicine has taken place with the participation of women themselves. It has been an impressive colonization of consciousness – of selfhood – that of Western subjects most of all (cf. Martin 1987; Rothman 1982; Tew 1990).

Aggressive biomedicine in the West unarguably saves the lives of mothers and babies who would otherwise die; but the cost to the majority can be dear. In the novel *Surfacing*, Margaret Atwood's protagonist rages famously at the indignities of modern birth:

[T]hey shave the hair off you and tie your hands down and they don't let you see, they don't want you to understand, they want you to believe it's their power, not yours. They stick needles into you so you won't hear anything, you might as well be a dead pig, your legs are up in a metal frame, they bend over you, technicians, mechanics, butchers, students clumsy or sniggering practising on your body, they take the baby out with a fork like a pickle out of a pickle jar. After that they fill your veins up with red plastic, I saw it running down through the tube. I won't let them do that to me ever again. (1972:80)

Yet these words, we may presume, are those of a healthy, well-fed Canadian woman, who is unlikely to have been nutritionally compromised as a child, and whose privileged material position enables her to eschew technological intervention that she legitimately sees as intrusive. For her, home birth attended by an empathetic midwife is a reasonable alternative. Where it is the norm the options are different, and few.

In Sudan, biomedicine's advance has been uneven and slow. Yet its promise is alluring, and few who live and give birth under the country's parlous conditions want to resist what offers so much hope. But Sheffa's emphatic decision to deliver in Shendi hospital must be set against Amal's modest refusal to seek out the expertise available there. And both Sheffa and Miriam have forged different syntheses of local and biomedical techniques in their respective midwifery practices. Like the women they attend, Sudanese midwives are not all alike. Moreover, to view them as remnants of a golden age of women's power, in which women controlled the process of birth and delivered safely in their own or their mothers' homes, is to ignore both history and social context, and the inordinate risks and responsibilities of midwifery work.[32]

I remain convinced that Amal's chances of survival would have been better – not certain – had Sheffa rather than Miriam attended her from the start. But could she have been saved had she been whisked off to Canada for the moment of birth? I cannot say. While the duality of body and mind at the heart of biomedical science has enabled countless advances in knowledge, it has also encouraged an implicit confidence in the omnipotence of technology. We seem convinced that the more elaborate the procedure, the surer the positive outcome. Yet the assumption that institutional birth results in lower rates of maternal death is not wholly borne out even here.[33]

It is true that throughout the twentieth century maternal mortality has fallen in the West as rates of hospital delivery and technical intervention have increased. Counter-intuitively, however, the drop in maternal mortality owes more to rising standards of nutrition, overall health, and sanitation, than to ever-expanding institutional interventions (Tew 1990).[34] The effect is cumulative over the generations: a woman's physical fitness to reproduce depends on her mother's nutritional health while pregnant, as well as on her own from the time of her birth.

In Sudan, standards of living are low, and female circumcision plainly adds to reproductive distress. But in a country where material want is great, where women remain economically dependent on men and are expected to produce large families – in part so as to diversify their means of survival – and where male offspring are preferred, malnutrition alone likely rivals, perhaps exceeds, circumcision in this role.[35] It is estimated that a third of Sudanese children between the ages of two and five suffer from stunted growth.[36] In one study in Khartoum, 44 percent of children under 5 were infested with parasites, attributable to poor living conditions (Karrar and Rahim 1995). From my experience in the rural north, children consume few vegetables or fruits and very little meat, even in plentiful years; as people abandon traditional breads made from protein-rich sorghum or wholewheat flours, and adopt more "modern" foods like refined white baguettes (called *towst*),[37] this situation is likely to worsen (cf. Sukkar *et al.* 1975). Moreover, malnutrition compromises immunity, and is therefore linked to the prevalence of illnesses like dysentery, malaria, and hepatitis which add to childbearing risks and for which infibulation may be performed as a childhood cure. It is also responsible for rickets, which causes bone malformation leading to pelvic disproportion during pregnancy and, failing cesarean delivery, death. As Amal's country sinks deeper into poverty with the rest of the developing world, the nutritional status of its womenfolk is increasingly threatened. The economically motivated early marriage of daughters is becoming more common as well, adding precocious pregnancy to the litany of hazards women face. Yet there as elsewhere, technological fixes are offered for problems that are political and economic at heart.[38] The costly medicalization of birth continues to be seen as remedial, not palliative, touted as the appropriate response to high rates of maternal and infant mortality. Paradoxically, given the present inequitable distribution of power and global wealth, that view may be correct. And this, I think, is the true irony and tragedy of Amal's untimely death.

ACKNOWLEDGMENTS

For assistance with this article I am grateful to Carol and Jordan Eldred; Amal, the midwives, and other women of Kabushiya and Gedo Districts, Sudan; Julie Anderson; Rachel Bezner Kerr; Krzysztof Grzymski; Jacqueline Solway; Ronald Wright; El Haj Bilal Omer of the Institute of African and Asian Studies, University of Khartoum; Clare

Cowling, Archivist of the Royal College of Obstetricians and Gynaecologists; S. M. Dixon of the Wellcome Trust for the History of Medicine; the staffs of the Public Record Office, London, and the National Record Office, Khartoum; and Jane Hogan of the Sudan Archive, Durham University, whose help has been invaluable. Research was facilitated by the Social Sciences and Humanities Research Council of Canada, the Connaught Fellowship Fund of the University of Toronto, and the Harry Frank Guggenheim Foundation. My deepest thanks to them all; any faults are mine alone.

NOTES

1 See Boddy 1989, Part 1 for a discussion of the symbolism of food in Hofriyat and northern Sudan generally. See also note 35.

2 This is also the case elsewhere in North Africa and the Middle East. See, for examples, Abu-Lughod 1986; Delaney 1991. There are a number of female doctors in Sudan; however, none apparently practiced at Shendi hospital in the mid-1980s.

3 Cf. Handler 1988; Macpherson 1962; Toqueville 1835.

4 Figures for the 1980s are given as this is the period being considered. As the 1987 Ontario Government *Report of the Task Force on the Implementation of Midwifery in Ontario* notes, however, maternal mortality figures tend to be distorted by mistakes, doctors' desires to cover up deaths owing to faulty techniques, and inconsistent definitions. This does not diminish the fact that the rates are exceedingly low when compared to those in the developing world.

5 Spencer (1992; 1994), without specifying his source, puts it at 104 in 1992 (p. 119) and eighty-three in 1994 (p. 123). Because he is relying on a range of secondary sources which in turn rely on official statistics, both figures are likely to be low because of underreporting at the community level. See Sudan Government (1982:7). I see no reason to trust figures indicating a considerable drop in infant mortality during the early 1990s, when by all accounts Sudan's economic position continued to decline. Hofriyati I met in Sudan in 1994 confirmed that their livelihoods had dwindled since 1984. Cynically, one might wonder whether the current government is inflating its success.

6 NRO (National Record Office, Khartoum) Civsec 1/57/3/121, pp. 62, 28. The rates for 1973, 1926 and 1929 are not strictly speaking comparable, because the former reflects the entire country, the latter only the upper Nile. The reliability of the colonial figures is unclear.

7 Figures are summarised in Tew 1990.

8 From World Health Organization, *Maternal Mortality: A Global Factbook*, compiled by C. Abou Zahr and E. Royston, 1991:232. Figures vary by area and study.

9 Sudan Government 1982 (pp. 61–3) for the year 1973. The same study reports that some 11 percent of ever-married Sudanese women have never

been pregnant, and the rate of childlessness in the first five years of marriage is also relatively high (p. 63).

10 WHO estimates that fewer than half of maternal deaths are reported as such (Abou Zahr and Royston 1991:3). The same study notes that rates of maternal death are invariably higher in rural areas than in urban.

11 Assuming an adjusted maternal mortality rate just over twice the conservative level of reporting (Sudan Government 1982), at 140 per 10,000, and an adjusted average pregnancy (as opposed to live-birth) rate of 8: $10,000 \div 140 \div 8 = 8.92$.

12 N = 135 resident ever-married women.

13 This is a modified version of what is known as pharaonic circumcision; in "full" pharaonic operations the labia majora are also removed and any remaining skin stretched over the wound and sewn together as above.

14 Women suffer frequent urinary infections, even if married and therefore "opened": medical statistics suggest that some 28 percent of northern Sudanese women are affected at any one time (Shandall 1967). Voiding is excruciatingly slow. Moreover, when distorted tissue obliterates the urethra, the vagina may act as a secondary bladder; if a woman is pregnant, the fetus can be poisoned by a backup of urine, and miscarriage result. Estimates link between 20 and 25 percent of sterility cases to infibulation, with chronic pelvic infection and the difficulties of sexual intercourse cited as proximate causes (Mustafa 1966:304). Painful menstruation is a common complaint, occasioned by tight infibulation or chronic infection. Menses can accumulate, particularly in girls before marriage, causing abdominal swelling that requires surgical intervention. In the apparent absence of a monthly flow, this condition may raise the suspicion of premarital pregnancy for which the consequences, in northern Muslim Sudan where filial virginity is vital to the maintenance of family honor, can be dire (Dareer 1982:36–7; Dorkenoo and Elworthy 1992:8; WHO 1986:32).

15 This is not to suggest, however, that the north was "precapitalist" prior to this: as a colony of Ottoman Egypt in the nineteenth century, it had been part of the globalizing economy for some time. See Hill 1970.

16 Yet they insisted they were no longer "slaves" (*abid*) but now "servants" (*khudam*).

17 NRO Civsec 1/57/2/121, pp. 12ff, Report of the Sudan Medical Service, O. F. M. Atkey, Director: "Female Circumcision in the Sudan." April 7, 1930; NRO Civsec 1/44/2/12. See also Daly 1986.

18 SAD (Sudan Archive, Durham University, England) 579/3/24–25, punctuation altered for readability.

19 Ontario Government 1983:208, citing Manitoba Archives, College of Physicians and Surgeons of Manitoba, Correspondence File, MG10 A15, letter from Mrs. K. Bell, Belmont, December 5, 1899, to Dr. Gray, Registrar.

20 For example, "In Newark [New Jersey] a midwifery program in 1914–1916 achieved maternal mortality rates as low as 1.7 per thousand, while in Boston, in many ways a comparable city but where midwives were banned, the rate was 6.5 per thousand. The infant mortality rate in Newark was 8.5 per thousand, contrasted with 36.4 in Boston" (Rothman 1982:41).

21 SAD 582/7/45, punctuation altered for readability; original emphasis.
22 Most manumitted slaves remained dependent on their former masters, and the stigmatized status was not readily forgotten.
23 The information in this paragraph has been distilled from numerous Wolff files in the Sudan Archive, Durham.
24 From "Midwifery Service in the Sudan," Report of Dr. Fairbairn, Royal College of Obstetricians and Gynaecologists, 1936. SAD 581/4/1.
25 SAD 581/1/46.
26 My model builds upon the insights and phrasing of Pierre Bourdieu (1977; 1990).
27 See Arnold 1993:56.
28 See also Gruenbaum 1982; 1991.
29 See, for example, SAD 581/5/13.
30 SAD 581/5/13.
31 See, among others, files in the Public Record Office (Kew, London), FO 371/63047.
32 See Jeffery and Jeffery (1993) with regard to the status of midwives in Uttar Pradesh, India.
33 On one hand lies the problem of iatrogenesis. In a widely respected study of the effects of medicalized birth conducted by public health authorities in Aberdeen County, Scotland, between 1917 and 1927, when home birth was still common, some disturbing facts came to light. The findings were summarized in the *Canadian Medical Association Journal* in 1929: "The death rate per 1000 maternity cases delivered by midwives was 2.8, by doctors 6.9 and in institutions 14.9. The last figure, which includes only cases untouched before admission, is surprisingly high" (Blackader 1929:656). Moreover, as Tew (1990) points out, home delivery has remained statistically less dangerous even for older and multiparous mothers defined as higher risk. Discussing data published in the British Government's *Reports on Confidential Enquiries into Maternal Deaths* for the years 1964–75, she notes:

the ratio of hospital to home births changed from 78:22 in 1964–6 to 97:3 in 1973–5 for the older mothers and from 67:33 in 1964–6 to 93:7 in 1973–5 for the mothers of high parity. If hospital care was especially beneficial for these higher-risk groups, it should have caused their mortality rate (all birth places) to fall when it was given to a greater proportion of maternities. In fact the rate rose from 0.48 to 0.73 for the older and from 0.33 to 0.40 for the high-parous mothers. This increase was in contrast to the decrease in the rate for all risk groups from 0.185 to 0.166. Most of this decrease was attributable to births booked for home where the rate fell by 40 percent compared with a fall of 9 percent for hospital. (Tew 1990:222)

Despite such trends, doctors in Britain and North America pressure women toward hospital delivery with almost complete success. This is owing not only to physicians' belief in the superiority of heroic medical technology, of course, but also to that of their patients. We have a widespread sense of entitlement to perfect health. Doctors therefore feel bound to intervene in anticipation of being sued for not having taken all possible measures should something go wrong.
34 Tew (1990 *passim*) notes, for example, that maternal mortality rates had

already begun to fall dramatically in the decades before antibiotics were introduced.

35 UNICEF estimates that the daily per capita calorie supply in Sudan between 1984 and 1986 was 88 percent of requirements (in Abou Zahr and Royston 1991:229).

36 Sudan statistics, Electronic Arts 3–D Atlas CD-Rom, version 1.1.

37 Refined white flour is often called *lux*, after the soap. White foods are auspicious in northern Sudan: they are considered clean and pure, and are thought to "bring blood" (Boddy 1982; 1989). Their consumption is a mark of prestige.

38 Cf. the anthropological critique of development in Ferguson (1990). See also Morsy (1995) for an argument concerning women's health in Egypt that follows similar lines.

REFERENCES

Abdalla, Raqiya H. D. 1982, *Sisters in Affliction: Circumcision and Infibulation in Africa*, London: Zed.

Abou Zahr, Carla 1993, "Maternity care for all," *Orgyn* 4:12–16.

Abou Zahr, Carla and Royston, Erica (eds.) 1991, *Maternal Mortality: A Global Factbook*, Geneva: World Health Organization.

Abu Lughod, Lila 1986, *Veiled Sentiments: Honor and Poetry in a Bedouin Society*, Berkeley: University of California Press.

Arnold, David 1993, *Colonizing the Body: State Medicine and Epidemic Disease in Nineteenth-Century India*, Berkeley: University of California Press.

Atwood, Margaret 1972, *Surfacing*, Toronto: McClelland and Stewart.

Bayoumi, Ahmed 1979, *The History of the Sudan Health Services*, Nairobi: Kenya Literature Bureau.

Blackader, A. D. 1929, "Thoughts on maternal mortality," *Canadian Medical Association Journal* 25:656.

Boddy, Janice 1982, "Womb as oasis: the symbolic context of pharaonic circumcision in rural Northern Sudan," *American Ethnologist* 9(4):682–98.

1989, *Wombs and Alien Spirits: Women, Men, and the Zar Cult in Northern Sudan*, Madison: University of Wisconsin Press.

1991, "Body politics: continuing the anticircumcision crusade," *Medical Anthropology Quarterly* 5(1):15–17.

1994, "Spirit possession revisited: beyond instrumentality," *Annual Reviews in Anthropology* 23:407–34.

Bourdieu, Pierre 1977, *Outline of a Theory of Practice*, Richard Nice, trans., Cambridge: Cambridge University Press.

1990, *The Logic of Practice*, Richard Nice, trans., Oxford: Polity Press.

Comaroff, John and Comaroff, Jean 1992, *Ethnography and the Historical Imagination*, Boulder, Colorado: Westview Press.

Daly, Martin 1986, *Empire on the Nile: The Anglo-Egyptian Sudan, 1899–1934*, Cambridge: Cambridge University Press.

1991, *Imperial Sudan: The Anglo-Egyptian Condominium, 1934–56*, Cambridge: Cambridge University Press.

Dareer, Asma El 1982, *Woman Why Do You Weep? Circumcision and Its Consequences*, London: Zed.

Delaney, Carol 1991, *The Seed and the Soil: Gender and Cosmology in a Turkish Village*, Berkeley: University of California Press.

Dorkenoo, Efua and Elworthy, Scilla 1992, *Female Genital Mutilation: Proposals for Change*, London: Minority Rights Group.

Duden, Barbara 1993, *Disembodying Women: Perspectives on Pregnancy and the Unborn*, Cambridge: Harvard University Press.

Ferguson, James 1990, *The Anti-Politics Machine: "Development," Depoliticization, and Bureaucratic Power in Lesotho*, Cambridge: Cambridge University Press.

Foucault, Michel 1979, *Discipline and Punish: The Birth of the Prison*, Alan Sheridan trans., New York: Vintage.

    1982, "The subject and power," in H. L. Dreyfus and P. Rabinow (eds.), *Michel Foucault: Beyond Structuralism and Hermeneutics*, New York: Harvester Wheatsheaf, pp. 208–26.

Gruenbaum, Ellen 1982, "The movement against clitoridectomy and infibulation in Sudan: public health policy and the women's movement," *Medical Anthropology Newsletter* 13(2):4–12.

    1991, "The Islamic movement, development, and health education: recent changes in the health of rural women in central Sudan," *Social Science and Medicine* 33(6):637–45.

Hall, Marjorie and Ismail, Bakhita Amin 1981, *Sisters Under the Sun: The Story of Sudanese Women*, London: Longman.

Handler, Richard 1988, *Nationalism and the Politics of Culture in Quebec*, Madison: University of Wisconsin Press.

Hayes, Rose Oldfield 1975, "Female genital mutilation, fertility control, women's roles, and the patrilineage in modern Sudan: a functional analysis," *American Ethnologist* 2:617–33.

Hill, Richard 1970, *On the Frontiers of Islam*, Oxford: Clarendon.

Holland, Eardley 1946, "President's report on his visit to the Sudan, December, 1945," Annual Report of the Royal College of Physicians and Gynaecologists.

Jeffrey, Roger and Jeffrey, Patricia M. 1993, "Traditional birth attendants in rural north India," in Shirley Lindenbaum and Margaret Lock (eds.), *Knowledge, Power, and Practice: The Anthropology of Medicine and Everyday Life*, Berkeley: University of California Press, pp. 7–31.

Karrar, Z. A. and Rahim, F. A. 1995, "Prevalence and risk factors of parasitic infections among under-five Sudanese children: a community-based study," *East African Medical Journal* 72(2):103–9.

Kendall, E. M. 1952, "A short history of the training of midwives in the Sudan," *Sudan Notes and Records* 33(1):42–53.

Macpherson, C. B. 1962, *The Political Theory of Possessive Individualism*, Oxford: Oxford University Press.

Martin, Emily 1987, *The Woman in the Body*, Boston: Beacon Press.

Mohamud, Omar A. 1991, "Female circumcision and child mortality in urban Somalia," *Genus* 67:203–23.

Mohanty, Chandra Talpade 1991, "Under Western eyes: feminist scholarship and colonial discourses," in Chandra Talpade Mohanty, Ann Russo and Lourdes Torres (eds.), *Third World Women and the Politics of Feminism*, Bloomington: Indiana University Press, pp. 51–80.

Morsy, Soheir A. 1995, "Deadly reproduction among Egyptian women: maternal mortality and the medicalization of population control," in Faye D. Ginsburg and Rayna Rapp (eds.), *Conceiving the New World Order: The Global Politics of Reproduction*, Berkeley: University of California Press, pp. 162–76.

Mustafa, A. Z. 1966, "Female circumcision and infibulation in the Sudan," *Journal of Obstetrics and Gynaecology of the British Commonwealth* 73:302–6.

O'Brien, Jay 1986, "Toward a reconstitution of ethnicity: capitalist expansion and cultural dynamics in Sudan," *American Anthropologist* 88(4):898–907.

Ontario Government 1987a, *Report of the Task Force on the Implementation of Midwifery in Ontario*, Toronto: Ministry of Health and Ministry of Colleges and Universities.

1987b, *Reproductive Care: Towards the 1990's. Second Report of the Advisory Committee on Reproductive Care*, Toronto: Ministry of Health.

Rothman, Barbara Katz 1982, *In Labor: Women and Power in the Birthplace*, New York: W. W. Norton.

Shandall, A. A. 1967, "Circumcision and infibulation of females," *Sudan Medical Journal* 5:178–212.

Shaw, Evelyn 1985, "Female circumcision," *American Journal of Nursing* 85:684–7.

Spencer, William 1992, *Global Studies: The Middle East* (4th edn), Guilford, Connecticut: Dushkin.

1994, *Global Studies: The Middle East* (5th edn), Guilford, Connecticut: Dushkin.

Stoler, Ann L. 1995, *Race and the Education of Desire*, Durham, North Carolina: Duke University Press.

Sudan Government 1982, *The Sudan Fertility Survey, 1979*, Vol. 1, *Principal Report*, Khartoum: Department of Statistics.

Sukkar, M. Y., Boutros, J. Z. and Yousif, Karima M. 1975, "The composition of some common Sudanese foods," *Sudan Medical Journal* 13(2):51–62.

Tew, Marjorie 1990, *Safer Childbirth? A Critical History of Maternity Care*, London: Chapman and Hall.

Tocqueville, Alexis de 1835, *Democracy in America*, Henry Reeve, trans., 2 vols., New York: Knopf.

Toubia, Nahid 1994, "Female circumcision as a public health issue," *New England Journal of Medicine* 331(11):712–16.

van der Kwaak, Anke 1992, "Female circumcision and gender identity: a questionable alliance?," *Social Science and Medicine* 35(6):777–87.

World Health Organization 1986, "A traditional practice that threatens health: female circumcision," *WHO Chronicle* 40(1):31–6.

Young, Allan 1983, "Rethinking ideology," *International Journal of Health Sciences* 13:203–19.

3 Resistance and embrace: Sudanese rural women and systems of power

Ellen Gruenbaum

Studying rural Sudanese Muslim women's interactions with the health care system affords a very different perspective on "biopower" than that to which our critiques of the US health care system might lead us. While people in the industrial countries have experienced the medicalization of many health, illness, and healing processes, leading at times to a sense of disempowerment and a desire for alternatives, economically disadvantaged and rural people often see the situation differently. It is often the obstacles to access to medical services that seem to constitute disempowerment.

This situation is exacerbated for rural people in poor countries. My research on rural Sudanese Muslim women's interactions with the health care system affords such an expanded perspective on "biopower" and the complexity of power relations it entails. Inadequate political resources to demand adequate services in rural communities, costs, and cultural obstacles to use of such services leave many rural Sudanese, especially women and girls, without adequate access to the benefits of modern medical services. In this context, folk remedies and spiritual practices offer rural women not only sources of treatment for health problems but also a way to resist their dependency on the biomedical system and overcome their relative powerlessness in relation to government services.

At the same time, community-based techniques of handling illness and employing cultural practices considered medically harmful have been challenged both by the government medical system and by the forces of the Islamist movement, constituting not only another sort of disempowerment for rural women, but also a direct challenge to established patterns of resisting and giving meaning to their powerlessness. Examples of such challenges discussed here include the biomedical opposition to female circumcision practices (*tahur*) and the Islamist criticism of women's traditional spirit possession practices (*zar*).

Rural Sudanese women experience contradictory roles in the local systems of power in which their lives are embedded, and as a result experience tension between the desire to resist forms of power which subordinate them and yet simultaneously accept systems of power that afford them some degree of power over others, even if it means accepting restrictions of their autonomy. It is easy to see this in common patterns of familial relationships. For example, the subordinated wife who is fortunate to become the mother of sons will eventually achieve respect, prosperity, and power over daughters-in-law and grandchildren: it is the hope of that outcome that calms the frustrations of many a young wife.

But new contradictions have emerged from the rapid social changes rural communities are facing, especially in the areas of economic relations, religious movements, and health, that are linked to gender relations. In exploring these, I find that some forms of power seem to offer such positive benefits that women are disinclined to resist involvement in them, even when they must accept a degree of subordination or loss of autonomy. From one perspective, they seem to collude in their own oppression in order to gain some benefit. Yet from a different perspective their choice may be seen as a way to resist some other aspect of powerlessness and subordination. The question arises: is such resistance simply cooptation? Has their resistance been bought off for the benefit of those who hold greater power?

In this chapter, I consider what constitutes resistance and cooptation for Muslim women in two rural communities in central Sudan where I have observed numerous situations involving health problems and women's reactions to them. These two communities, one in the Gezira irrigated area and one in the Rahad area east of the Blue Nile, are experiencing profound changes in local structures of power.

I first did fieldwork in these communities in the late 1970s and returned again for short periods of follow-up research in 1989 and 1992. While the Gezira community was stable in terms of location, the degree of temporary or linked out-migration (that is, with frequent return visits and permanent ties) was significant. The Rahad community is part of a larger planned resettlement village; my earlier research had focused on two original villages (a collaborative project with Jay O'Brien and Salah El-Din El-Shazali) from which the resettlement community drew part of its population. Although the location has shifted, I have focused on the same families over the time span of my research.

As the two communities have increasingly been drawn into the capitalist economic system and have begun to utilize newly available government services (a clinic, immunization campaigns, a school), they have found themselves bound by new rules, new forms of stratification, and changing ideologies of morality. Although the people's basic human goals – health, security, dignity, pleasant family life, and religious virtue – remain unchanged and offer them a feeling of continuous identity, the paths to these goals have been changed in such a way that it appears to be more difficult for individuals to achieve any one goal without jeopardizing other goals. Many of the women I interviewed also perceived these contradictions and were struggling to respond appropriately. This response is partly due to paradoxical power relations, where resistance to subordination in one power relation entails subordination or deference to another form of power.

The areas of paradoxical power relations most closely entwined with women's and children's health include gender relations, economic stratification, ethnic relations, and contemporary religious challenges to cultural sources of female resistance such as *zar* spirit possession, and other impacts of the Islamist movement. In the following section, I first discuss how these power relations complicate women's access to the biomedical resources they desire. I then consider the dynamics among the different forms of power relations to see how resistance to one type of subordination may lead women to accept a role in a different type of power relation in their efforts to achieve satisfying lives.

Power and the problem of access to biomedical services

As in other poor countries, Sudan's government-sponsored medical care system is highly unevenly distributed throughout the country. The two rural areas where I worked – in the economically important seventy-year-old Gezira and fifteen-year-old Rahad irrigated agriculture schemes – were fortunate to have received primary health care service facilities. In the case of the older irrigation scheme, health services were first provided during the British colonial period in order to ensure the health of the workforce for the colonial economic "backbone" industry (cotton production for export to Great Britain) and to mitigate the potential for labor agitation by tenant farmers. Schools and medical clinics thus formed a key element of social control of the regions where colonial economic interests lay (Gruenbaum 1982). Other regions, such as the Rahad prior to the opening of the scheme in 1978, had very few health facilities accessible to rural populations. However, with the construction of the Rahad scheme in the 1970s, large resettlement communities were planned within the irrigated areas, with schools, clinics, markets, and water supplies promised as an inducement to farmers from small villages in the area to move their families to the initially rather desolate sites on the scheme and take up the risky tenancies and unfamiliar technology of irrigation to produce an export crop.

In the Rahad village where I worked, the clinic was staffed by two men, a medical assistant and his less-well-trained assistant. The Gezira village boasts a health center, staffed by approximately fifteen personnel, intended to serve several villages, each of which has its own small clinic. Located only 4 kilometers from a market town with a rural hospital, the health center is underutilized and overstaffed.

The services of rural government clinics are supposed to be open to all, but throughout this century, access to government health services has been tied to political and economic power.[1] With the country's current serious economic difficulties, small fees have been imposed in response to conditions set by international lending agencies, to recapture some costs of services. Now, drugs and supplies often have to be purchased rather than being provided free. Underpaid, low-status health care workers seeking to make ends meet and garner respect have created some other barriers, as the following example illustrates.

As an example of how economic barriers affect rural women, consider the handling of a post-partum medical problem in the Rahad village I observed in 1992. I arrived at the small round mud-walled thatched house of a tenant farming family several hours after the delivery of the baby to find a throng of well-wishers, mostly women, gathered inside drinking spiced coffee and sharing in the animated conversation that usually surrounds celebratory occasions such as this. The mother and newborn were screened behind a makeshift curtain – for warmth, modesty, and as a mosquito net at night.

The midwife – who had only informal training but considerable experience – was still there because the placenta had not yet been expelled. She and the family had sent for the medical assistant (the "doctor" as people called him) from the small local clinic. Customarily, a woman remains inside her house for forty days after childbirth, so even if it had not been in the hours immediately after birth, she would need a house call to get biomedical services. Much to my surprise the medical assistant arrived in a vehicle. There were relatively few vehicles in the village; most were Toyota pick-ups owned by men who had been migrant laborers in oil-rich countries, brought back for use in trade and transport. Such vehicles served as important symbols of wealth and prestige, especially for their owners, but also for those who were able to use them on personal business. The entire village was an easy walk from the clinic, but I was told the medical assistant would only make house calls if one hired a vehicle to fetch him.

He performed his cursory examination behind the screen, gave the mother an injection, and left without accepting the coffee that was offered. By declining the hospitality and requiring transportation, he thereby distanced himself in a way the midwife did not. Based on this and other contacts with this man, it was clear that this was part of his effort to cultivate a professional image in the community. In addition, it served to demarcate clearly the physical examination of the woman as a non-social contact. But the incident also revealed his power to create additional costs for the family. In short, to receive the benefits of biomedicine one must buy into the system where experts have power and can command a price.

The customary community nurturance by other women and especially by the midwife could be analyzed as a form of resistance to the imposition of such professional power. But it is clear that access to the biomedical services is also desired. Repeatedly in my interviews with the women of the Rahad village, who had had no local biomedical services prior to 1978, they expressed relief that they now had a clinic for the treatment of problems they could not handle through home remedies or spiritual healing.

Several additional barriers to receiving health care are also significant for village women, based on linguistic, ethnic, and gender obstacles. Yet these obstacles do not affect people uniformly. For instance, gender sometimes creates a barrier for women's treatment since most dressers, nurses, or medical assistants assigned to rural clinics are male. Female health care workers are not uncommon in towns, especially as nurses, but there are few women as primary caregivers in government health facilities in villages. Because health care is provided mostly by males, some Sudanese village families are reluctant to have women go for treatment unless it is minor (like a vaccination) or an emergency. However, women in the Gezira village, with its longer period of experience with a clinic, were relatively at ease about the clinic professionals and went whenever they thought it necessary. Even there, however, gender was a barrier for families of the West African-originating Hausa ethnic group, a minority enclave in the village. The Gezira village Hausa used the clinic less readily, owing to a combination of poverty, less education, ethnic subordination, and some families' stricter seclusion of women. In addition, most of the Hausa women did not speak Arabic as confidently as the men, making health care interactions far more difficult.

Lacking such barriers, the Arab-Sudanese majority in the Gezira village not only freely utilized the local health center, but also self-referred to the rural hospital where they expected care to be more expert and tests and medications more available than in the village facility. A government-trained midwife was available in the village to serve the reproductive health needs of the women and to circumcise the Arab girls. In addition, people of both ethnicities continued to make use of Islamic treatments by religious leaders (*shaykh*, sing.).[2]

Although the Rahad villagers in the past had sometimes traveled to the provincial capital for very serious medical problems requiring hospitalization, until the opening of the scheme in 1978 there were no rural facilities in their area. They had had to rely on itinerant "shot doctors" and tooth extractionists who occasionally visited their villages and on certain local men and women who served as repositories of traditional folk medical knowledge, including herbal treatments, Islamic practices, and some magical practices associated with Islamic piety. The local specialists in bone-setting and snake-bite treatments were men, but the traditional birth attendants who also performed female circumcision operations were all women. It was most often male religious specialists who offered Islamic treatments. Thus, Rahad women's experiences with government biomedical/health services prior to the scheme tended to be minimal except for those who had traveled.

The differences in the ethnicities of the two Rahad villages studied in the 1970s are significant: the West African-originating Zabarma people of one followed traditions of female seclusion which minimized the amount of travel women did outside the village, whereas the Kenana (Sudanese) Arab population of the other village were of nomadic origin, did not practice strict seclusion of women, and traveled more readily, including for seasonal wage labor as cotton-pickers on distant development projects. As a result, it was the Kenana Arab women who more readily accepted the services of the new clinic that became available when these two ethnic groups moved into the same Rahad irrigation scheme village in 1978–9. Yet despite their longer tradition of female mobility, resettlement to a multi-ethnic village had a somewhat mitigating effect, perhaps related to the presence of so many more people of differing groups. During my 1989 and 1992 research trips I found there was a reluctance, even on the part of the Arabic-speaking women, to venture away from their Kenana neighborhood through the more public market place to the clinic, and I observed some women delay going for a few days when they or their children were sick. Younger married or unmarried women who venture alone into a public place where men are gathered, such as the market, risk developing a reputation for being strong-willed – rather unfeminine – or even immoral, whereas older women seem to be able to do so with no comment. Zabarma women were even more reluctant to cross such public spaces.

Linguistic barriers to biomedical access arise when rural women are not Arabic-speakers. When they first resettled into the irrigation scheme (1978), the Zabarma men were bilingual but women spoke no Arabic (with only two women who had married into the village from urban West African groups as exceptions). This lack of Arabic ability, combined with the Zabarma people's traditional stricter seclusion (including fencing compounds and having to seek husbands' permission before leaving the compound for neighborhood visits), resulted in less likelihood of attending the clinic. By 1989, however, most of the Zabarma women had learned Arabic, some extremely well, and were visiting their Arabic-speaking neighbors and using the clinic when they needed it. I was unable to collect statistical data on attendance by the two groups, but the Zabarma women claimed they did not hesitate to seek medical services. Yet clinic staff observed that the Zabarma men, rather than the women, would usually bring the sick children for treatment. The medical assistant considered this a problem, since it would be a woman who would carry out the care of the sick child, and he did not believe the father would necessarily adequately convey his instructions to the caregiver. He reported that he sometimes insisted that the father with a sick child go back and bring the child's mother or grandmother.

Given the minimal level of services offered at the Rahad village's clinic and the chronic shortage of supplies and drugs, self-referral to a regional small hospital, e.g., at the irrigation scheme headquarters in El Fau, is not uncommon, but the bus or other transportation and possible overnight stay required would seldom be undertaken by a young woman alone or with a child. Older women might travel in the company of other women, but a young wife would be less likely to do so without her husband.

To summarize, the numerous obstacles to getting the biomedical services that women desire are related to power imbalances in gender, ethnic, linguistic, and economic domains, as well as to the general inadequacy of services in a poor country such as Sudan. In the sections which follow, I elaborate on some of these obstacles and explore the forms of challenge and resistance that Sudanese women are using, both to gain access to biomedical resources and to overcome the negative consequences of the forms of subordination to which they are subject.

Gender stratification and economic change

There are many ways in which the development of irrigation schemes has influenced both men and women, some of which cry out for further research: dramatic increases in malaria and schistosomiasis (malaria control improvements which were achieved in the 1980s appear to have been undermined in recent years), the harmful effects of the aerial spraying of pesticides, inadequate maintenance of clean water supplies, lack of sanitary facilities needed because of the denser settlement patterns organized by the scheme, and adverse changes in diet, to name a few. Several results of economic change have fallen most heavily on women – as water carriers and as providers of family meals, especially.

One area of particular interest here is women's economic vulnerability. Among all the ethnic groups represented in these communities, males are the acknowledged household heads, and their economic power in the family is reinforced both by the local interpretations of Islamic duties and by government policies that assigned land control – the tenancy – to male heads of households.[3] Even prior to the irrigation projects Muslim women were dependent on their linkages to men to guarantee access to economic resources, but women's work roles were recognized as essential to family provisioning. When the new economic arrangements of irrigation projects were established, most women found themselves more dependent on the men of their families than they had been before.

In the past, for example, Kenana women and children had sometimes worked in agriculture for wages (for neighbors or as migrants), but once the new scheme tenancies were assigned to male household heads, the women were expected to work without pay for the family enterprise. As a result, a woman's agricultural work contributed to a greater pot of disposable income for the male household head's discretionary spending rather than her own. Before women's responses to this situation can be fully explained, however, the part played by the Islamic context must be understood.

Islamic rules of divorce and child custody also contribute to women's vulnerability, particularly in situations of economic dependency, and a woman's conformity to morality rules is regarded as significant in maintaining her husband's respect and affection. If a woman violates rules that lead others to question her morality or if her behavior is construed as contributing to a loss of her husband's affection, she can expect little social support if her husband exercises his Islamic prerogative of unilateral divorce and the right to patrilineal child custody (after early childhood). She is also at risk of his taking a second or third wife, which women of most (but not all) families consider undesirable. Although a divorced woman has the right to return to her father's or brother's home, a woman without her children feels very vulnerable economically, because loyal children are the basis of old-age security and the foundation of a woman's social status.

A woman's social and economic vulnerability, then, is a combination of effects of Islamic traditions with local economic structures. Because the Rahad development planners assigned tenancies to males as heads of households, the annual lump sum cash pay-outs of the cotton profits are considered the husband's. This opportunity, combined with the desire for more children to help with the work or to engage in some of the new possibilities of education and employment – along with what men and women alike consider a natural male desire for younger women – has resulted in an increasing rate of polygynous marriages. Husbands find themselves economically better able than in the past to undertake the expenses incurred. Women, however, are concerned that polygyny will undermine their own and their children's economic security, as well as creating domestic tension.

Women react to this trend in Rahad with overt acceptance – both Kenana Arab and Zabarma women assert that polygyny is a man's right under Islam. But the women of the group which had not had much polygyny before, the Kenana, actively resist this trend in several ways: mild gossip and mockery (in which some of the men participated), increased child-bearing (to reduce a husband's reason for needing another wife to get more children), and reducing women's participation in agricultural production. As an example of the first of these, an elderly man who had a few years earlier taken a second wife wanted to take a third. Women I spoke with, and even some of the men, laughed about it and considered him a fool. His first wife, the other women reported to me in her presence, couldn't see why he would complicate their marriage with a second wife in the first place, and although she was careful not to speak ill of him, she looked as if she considered him positively senile.

The second form of resistance to polygyny is increased childbearing. Although I lack comprehensive demographic statistics to confirm it, there was a widespread impression among people of both ethnic groups that childbearing had increased in recent years and that birth intervals had become shorter (Gruenbaum 1996). My reproductive history interviews supported local observations of high rates of childbearing[4] and decreasing birth intervals. These trends were matched by an apparent increase in child survival, owing to better nutrition from the improved food production possible because of the scheme and to significant improvements in vaccination rates for women and children.

The goal of increased childbearing is to keep the husband satisfied by being fertile and attractive, giving birth to many children while still maintaining one's beauty and vitality. In a sense, the many cosmetic efforts of Sudanese married women that contribute to sexual attractiveness (henna dye decorations of the skin, hair plaiting, removing body hair, and incensing oneself) and even the tight reinfibulations following childbirth form part of the "resistance" to polygyny and divorce.

A third type of resistance by the Kenana women is their reduced participation in agricultural production. Most Kenana women said their husbands would not pay them if they worked in the fields. In their previous experience, prior to the scheme, the women had collected wages when they worked as migrant laborers for farmers in other areas where they were employed to pick cotton. Now, the Kenana women did not see the point in increasing the cotton profits by contributing their labor to cotton-picking because they might not be paid and it would only contribute to the likelihood of polygynous marriage. In the previous situation, women had control of their own incomes. Now, the husbands had control of the largest share of family income, and although they spent some of it on improved housing and somewhat better furnishings, which the women appreciated, husbands did not usually choose to invest heavily in the sorts of home improvements that would have eased women's work and improved their lives tremendously. It was the rare husband who undertook extending water pipes into the family courtyard or constructing a latrine. Instead, many men raised their levels of personal consumption and tried to take second wives.

In the Zabarma ethnic group, women's responses to economic vulnerability were different. Having experienced higher rates of polygyny in the past, the Zabarma were far more accepting of polygyny. Many (but not all) of the Zabarma women found advantages to having co-wives in terms of sharing of labor and offering respite from child care – and husband care. Paradoxically, these families, which had followed stricter seclusion of women before the scheme, had by 1989 and 1992 begun to increase women's agricultural participation (especially for older women without small children) and to reduce the degree of seclusion. Numerous Zabarma women harvested and marketed from their homes a share of the peanut harvest in a sharecropping arrangement with their husbands, the official tenants. Money earned was used for household equipment, furniture, and children's school expenses,[5] luxury items which husbands might not have supplied, and savings.

Polygyny was more acceptable not only because of prior experience with it, but because of the greater Islamic religious piety expected in the Zabarma community. Husbands seemed to strive to follow to the letter the Islamic injunction to treat multiple wives equally – eating and sleeping with the wives in strict rotation and buying them equal amounts of goods in the market. One pair of co-wives to whom I was particularly close often wore identical dresses – a sign of their husband's fairness – and referred to themselves as "twins." The amicability of the compound seemed to continue smoothly even after they were joined by a third wife.

Taken as a whole, the constellation of changing relations of production – from the family-organized subsistence/peasant production of the past, to the bureaucratized and market-oriented development schemes, whether in the older Gezira or newer Rahad scheme – has contributed to an increase in the power of men over the women of their families, while at the same time reducing most families' autonomy in the economy. For the older scheme, this has been offset to some extent by a gradual increase in the education rates for girls, which has led to government employment for quite a few of the women of this village (usually as teachers or clerks). Also, women of the Arab-Sudanese ethnic group in Gezira have benefited from their position in a stratified system marked by ethnic differences. The economic dominance of the Arab-Sudanese of the village relies on the utilization of a subordinated wage labor force, especially the resident West African Hausa proletarian population, but also the seasonal wage-earners who migrate from distant areas (including pastoralists, farmers, and refugees from droughts and wars). For both schemes, there has also been stratification built on pre-scheme advantages (such as the ownership of large land holdings, which entitled some farmers to the control of multiple tenancies on the irrigation scheme, or large herds that provide an off-scheme economic enterprise), as well as on the commercial investments of large, successful families. Thus, it is seldom the case that women of the advantaged families, classes, or ethnic groups would challenge their common subordination to men in alliance with women of the oppressed or less advantaged groups.

Resistance to gender subordination

Rural women in the past had relatively few avenues of resistance to gender subordination, perhaps because there were relatively few ways in which men's greater social power would be turned against wives, because of the support of close kin. Muslim men often say that they greatly respect their sisters and mothers, and, as repositories of the family honor, they must treat them well and look after their virtue lest any misbehavior bring shame upon them all; indeed, the virtuous kinswoman is said to be treasured. Numerous injunctions against cruelty toward women exist in Islam and are mentioned in rural Sudan, alongside the acceptance of a man's right – as the partner considered to possess greater rationality – to punish his wife physically if she has done something wrong. The strong preference for endogamous marriage also means that most village women have numerous male and female kin nearby, which helps to ensure fair treatment by husbands.

Nevertheless, for some women, male power has wreaked havoc with their lives. Among the women I knew were many examples: the unilateral divorce that had removed a woman's children; the infertile woman who found herself divorced and not able to remarry; the unlucky woman whose husband did not treat her equally with the other wife or whose co-wife was jealous; the wife who was divorced in retaliation for her brother's divorce of her husband's sister; the educated woman whose husband would not let her work, but derived prestige from her idleness; the women whose chronic illnesses or reproductive failures prevented them from fulfilling expected female roles (see also Boddy 1989 and Gruenbaum 1982).

For such women, one of the common social outlets to resist subordination was participation in the *zar* spirit-possession rituals (see Boddy 1989) or *zar* "coffee party" support groups (Gruenbaum 1991; Kenyon 1991). Muslims who practice *zar* in Sudan consider themselves to suffer from a possession by one of many quite different types of spirits, some capricious and relatively harmless, some pious, some dangerous, but all of them relatively stubborn. If symptoms of illness including infertility, miscarriages, chronic pain, fatigue, or mental problems are diagnosed as owing to possession by spirits, the individuals are advised to appease those spirits through sacrifices, participation with other devotees in ritual dancing with spirit-associated drumming, or other activities the spirit demands of them. Keeping the spirit(s) happy is expected to prevent further problems with health (or social ills) and in fact to bring blessing.

Janice Boddy's detailed study of *zar* practices in a village in northern Sudan demonstrated that women participants effectively use possession and trance as a form of resistance and an opportunity for solidarity with other women (1988; 1989). By allowing an opportunity for transcendent experience or at least supernaturally inspired consolation and advice, *zar* offers adherents leverage to gain certain liberties (smoking, drinking) or material benefits (special foods for ceremonies, special clothing, perfumes, or even gold) from worried husbands and kinsmen. As such it is a form of resistance to patriarchal gender relations, especially the expectation for women to produce many children (especially male heirs) – hence the higher affliction rates among childless and sonless women – and resistance to the economic and behavioral limitations normally imposed on women. As a key component of what some would call "women's culture" (Hale 1987) the *zar* offered an alternative way for women to give meaning to their experiences. Whereas I have not infrequently heard men say women are unaware of issues beyond their kitchens and children, the panoply of spirit characters, actions, and music involved in *zar* seems to offer creativity and perspective on Sudanese history and relations with outsider groups that allow for an enlarged, even transcendent, consciousness for the involved women (see Boddy 1989).

The ability of Sudanese women to engage in this particular form of resistance to their subordination is increasingly being undermined, as the legitimacy of these practices for Muslims is an area of ideological contention. Muslims who practice *zar* claim it is consonant with Islam, but adherents of the Islamic activist movement have been increasingly vocal in denouncing it as a pre-Islamic custom that is not "authentic" to Muslim culture (Hale 1996). Yet even prior to the contemporary Islamist movement, Muslims in Sudan varied in their attitudes toward *zar* and other unorthodox practices. Spirit possession and certain other quasi-religious customs (veneration of saints, visiting shrines, seeking blessing from dust of holy men's graves, etc.) were not pursued by the ethnic groups of West African origin (the Zabarma and the far more numerous Hausa, for example), who consider such practices irreligious.

For the Hausa and Zabarma, Islamic piety served as a form of resistance to the ethnic subordination and discrimination they faced as immigrants, usually labeled as foreigners despite long residence or birth in Sudan, and as victims of racial/ethnic discrimination against "fellata," a generic and rather derogatory term used in Sudan for West Africans. Zabarma piety was apparent to others in the Rahad village. The Zabarma men, as members of the Tijaniyya sect, engaged in frequent communal prayer in a neighborhood place of worship, which included chanting at specified times. Zabarma women, as their Kenana neighbors and I observed, performed their regular prayers faithfully and considered it salutary to listen to the prayers and chanting of the men. Zabarma women derived pride from their greater religious observance as compared with the Arab-Sudanese, and commented to me on the paradox that the Kenana – who they acknowledged as being of higher status since they are said to be descended from the Prophet Muhammad – were not as religious.

Although Zabarma and Hausa religious observances could be said to serve as resistance to their ethnic group subordination (reinforced economically and politically in ways that are beyond the scope of this chapter), there is also a potential for religious piety to be used ideologically both as a tool of resistance and as a means of subordination in the relations between the sexes. For example, once when discussing with some Zabarma women the existence of prostitutes in a nearby town, they acknowledged that it was not unknown for men to go to prostitutes. But this particular group of women was certain their own husbands were not involved. To underscore her confidence that Islam was on her side here, one of the women said that if her husband ever went to a prostitute she would sternly rebuke him with his duty to spend his money on his family and to have respect for them. Alternatively, religion is what is invoked in the very marriage, divorce, and child custody rules which can disadvantage women if they are unlucky enough to have a less than fair husband.

Impact of the Islamic movement

Accelerating since the early 1980s, the Islamist movement in Sudan has gained considerable influence on the society, particularly in urban areas.[6] Biomedicine has been an important avenue for the spread of the movement, since a major strategy for gaining adherents to Islamist goals and converts of Islam has been to offer private medical clinics (particularly in the urban areas) where free or inexpensive high-quality medical services are available.

Since the mid-1980s some of the long-standing forms of female resistance to male domination represented by *zar* and other activities of the subculture of women and girls (such as dancing for each other, practicing wedding songs and dances, fortune-telling, time-consuming cosmetic activities like henna applications, celebrating female circumcisions) have begun to be challenged by the movement for Islamic piety. Here the effects on the two areas I studied were markedly different. Although both areas have felt definite effects, the older Gezira scheme area was far more influenced by Islamism owing to the relatively high literacy rate, proximity to urban influences, experience of numerous labor migrants from the village who had worked abroad in oil-rich countries more central to the Islamic heartland (especially Saudi Arabia), and the possession of many televisions that carry the propaganda of the Islamist central government.

Women's roles and behaviors have been a major focus of the movement. The Islamists have pressured women to dress more modestly (including longer sleeves and more extensive veiling), to be restricted from public occupations, and to be subjected to more segregation. Their arguments are often framed in terms of cultural authenticity – getting rid of both "Western" influences and non-Islamic

Sudanese traditions alike. For them, the "authentic" culture is to be found in proper Islamic practices of the Arabian heritage. As a result, Sudanese cultural practices have begun to be disparaged by leaders of the movement, with the result that ordinary Muslims, cognizant of their lack of learning and not wanting to oppose what is said to be "true Islam," have found themselves either accepting the Islamists' advice or rationalizing their own presumed failures and delaying implementation of proper practices. Explicit opponents of the movement, including many of the urban intellectuals, find their political views delegitimized when they are labeled as "Westernized" for their educations, lifestyles, and lack of support for the regime. Worse, many have suffered detention (extra-judicial or governmental), been fired from their jobs, or been forced into exile for being "too secular" (Gruenbaum 1992).

What has been the effect of this political environment on women and on health care in the rural areas? First it must be said that the movement includes much genuine, thoughtful reflection on Islam and morality that goes beyond the heavy-handed political Islamism of the National Islamic Front leadership. Rural women in the Gezira village, for example, are seriously discussing the respectability and modesty of wearing long sleeves – when they can afford to get new clothes – versus the discomfort of such garb in their very hot climate. And in 1992, there was a noticeable increase in discussions of religion as well as frequent praying, even by young women. Two Gezira women I interviewed discussed different imams' teachings on whether women should pray in the mosque or at home. Such discussions have an interesting potential impact on gender relations. As women show themselves to be independently motivated to dress modestly and follow religious observances out of their own commitment, these women expect that the men of their families should not supervise their activities as closely as they did in the past, which could strengthen the women's positions in their families.

One result of the Islamic movement has been increased questioning of pharaonic circumcision.[7] In the Gezira village, the medical assistant has lectured separately to men and women against infibulation (which is done in the pharaonic form of the practice), on both health and religious grounds. The midwife no longer advocates pharaonic circumcision and has tried to switch to the modified "sunna" type that Sudanese Islamists accept, consisting of clitoridectomy at worst and removal of the clitoral hood at best. Clients still ask her to do the infibulations, however. Thus the Islamist movement, although advocating more stringent limitations on women's autonomy, might be a force for modifying these harmful practices.

For many Sudanese, female circumcision (*tahur*, purification) has important symbolic significance related to moral purity. Preservation of the most severe form is extremely important to some, such as the Kenana of Rahad. Their neighbors the Zabarma (like the Hausa in Gezira) have never adopted pharaonic circumcision in great numbers, while the Kenana continued (as of 1992) to practice pharaonic without either religious or health education challenges (Gruenbaum 1996). For the Kenana, infibulation is the embodiment of their moral superiority over their neighbors of West African ethnic groups. While this is not the only reason it is done, this particular meaning is a major obstacle to future health education efforts, and it may well be that strong religious arguments against it are needed if its significance is to be reduced.

Even though the clothing styles, dancing, female circumcision, and cosmetic practices so far have not changed significantly in the Rahad village, the Islamist movement has begun to undermine effectively one of the forms of women's resistance to the exercise of male and kin group power, the *zar* spirit-possession practices. Two spirit-possessed women, one in her forties and the other an elderly grandmother, complained to me that their families (especially the husband of the first and the son-in-law of the other) have prevented them from participating in any *zar* gatherings (none are being held in the village at present, so it would require travel). They also have not been able to meet the demands of their spirits – the wearing of a red hat for one, and a specific type of perfume and a pair of men's shorts for the other. In the past these would have been obtained by the men in their families to protect them against harmful consequences from the spirits.

Conclusion

In conclusion, human bodies are the site of ideological control in various ways in rural Sudan, and the biomedical services system is only one of several systems of power which women embrace or resist. Gender stratification, ethnic superiority, religious piety and authority, and social class differences are all situations of oppression that stimulate activities of resistance. But if resistance to one form of oppression involves embrace of another, women may find themselves taking on behaviors or roles that harm their health and well-being, even as they resist being used in another system of power. Understanding the embeddedness of these processes in competing power relations and conflicting ideologies helps to explain otherwise contradictory behaviors. Some women will accept and advocate female genital mutilation as a statement of ethnic superiority or as the emblem of their position in an honorable family. Others will resist it, recognizing the role of male dominance in perpetuating the conditions that provide obstacles to abandoning it, seeking support from a religious movement that withdraws cultural authenticity from certain Sudanese cultural practices. Resisting male power through the cultural repertoire of the *zar* requires resistance to the claims of Islamic superiority by those involved in the Islamist movement. Males can use the Islamist movement somewhat more effectively than women to assert their interests, and have done so with respect to the *zar*. Yet other women have succeeded in discovering interpretations of Islamic rules which are consonant with their well-being, holding men to Islamic expectations of moral behavior (Gruenbaum 1991). Some women have embraced systems of power based on social class privilege or on racial or ethnic discrimination, even though this requires accepting gender subordination; each of these forms of power could allow gender discrimination's effects to be mitigated in individual lives, even though they at the same time add to the burdens of others.

Although no tidy diagram of these social relations results, a dynamic analysis such as this is necessary to begin to understand the current cultural debates underway in rural Sudan. What this case suggests is that claiming a place in a power relation, even a subordinated position, may have something to offer – materially or ideologically – in resisting another form of oppression.

ACKNOWLEDGMENTS

This paper was originally presented at the American Ethnological Society Annual Meeting in Santa Monica in 1994 in a panel organized by Carole Browner on "Women and Biopower." I am grateful to the participants and discussants in that session for their comments on my ideas, and I thank Margaret Lock and Pat Kaufert for their concrete and most helpful comments during revision.

NOTES

1 Colonial services were intended primarily for the Europeans, important local leaders, groups targeted for "pacification," and workers needed by the administration. Hospital services were divided into first-, second-, and third-class wards, with the best care reserved for those who could pay higher fees. As rural services were developed, especially in the period since the 1940s, it has been the politically and economically important areas which have been able to get them. See Gruenbaum 1982.

2 Islamic treatments are widespread and variable. Although too numerous to detail here, common Sudanese folk Islamic treatments include such things as

wearing amulets of Qur'anic verses, burning of *bakhrat* (folded papers that have had verses or magical symbols written on them by a *faki*, or holy man) to produce healing smoke, drinking water infused with special ink that has been washed from a tablet where Qur'anic verses were written, rubbing dust from the grave of a holy man on painful areas of the body, drinking such dust with water, and being blessed by sprayed spittle from the mouth of a *faki*. Such practices are regarded with varying degrees of acceptance or disdain by other Muslims.

3 When the Gezira scheme was opened in 1925, tenancies were initially allocated to farmers (mostly male) and their dependants on the basis of prior land ownership in the area. Since the number of tenancies per person was limited, wealthy land owners, who were entitled to have many tenancies assigned for their land, had tenancies assigned to their kin and clients (especially former slaves). As these were later handed down through inheritance, some became controlled by women, since the usual Islamic inheritance rules (which would have divided the land into small plots of which sons would receive twice the share of daughters) did not apply and the management did not allow tenancies to be divided smaller than half their original size. In the Rahad, though, the only women who received tenancies in the initial allocation in the late 1970s were widows with dependants, and Rahad tenancies were much smaller than Gezira tenancies had been. Subsequent inheritance has not yet been extensive, and almost all has been to males; less than 1 percent of tenancies are estimated to be controlled by females.

4 The live births to the women in my sample who had completed childbearing averaged 8.0 for the Zabarma (n = 8) and 9.2 (n = 10) for the Kenana.

5 Relatively few Zabarma children went to school, although most boys attended the campfire-lit evening classes with the *shaykh* to learn to read and recite the Qu'ran.

6 What is often called "Islamic fundamentalism" by Western writers should actually be understood as a series of social and political activities, linked into a movement, which utilize a particular set of interpretations of the teachings of Islam. Although often referred to as "conservative" or "traditional," the proponents argue for new customs (e.g., heavy veiling of women) which are certainly not traditional within most of the societies in which they are being advocated. Thus, it is more accurate to call this a movement for Islamic piety, based on particular religious interpretations, many of which are disputed by members of the Muslim community (see An-Na'im 1990). The terms "Islamism" and "Islamist" are used here to distinguish the movement's interpretation of Islam and Islamic lifeways.

Cultural debates among adherents of the movement, other Muslims, and non-Muslim Sudanese, therefore, often take the form of arguments about what is "authentic" Islam, what is authentic Sudanese culture, and what is desirable for society – secular democracy with freedom of religion or the government promotion of Islamism. Although the divergent views are beyond the scope of this chapter, it should be noted that the ideological use of Islam is extremely powerful among Sudanese Muslims. (See Hale 1996 for a thorough discussion of these issues.)

7 "Female circumcision" is widely regarded as a euphemism for what is now often referred to as "female genital mutilation" or FGM. These terms include a wide range of surgeries from a relatively minor prepuce removal, to clitoridectomy, to intermediate partial closures, and to full infibulation. Pharaonic circumcision is the most serious form of these traditional female genital surgeries and is still widely practiced in Sudan. Infibulation leaves a smooth vulva of scar tissue resulting from the removal of the clitoris, prepuce, and labia, and the suturing of the labia together to occlude both the urethra and the vagina except for a single small opening for the passage of menses and urine. Modified surgeries that preserve erectile tissue beneath joined labia, only partially occluding the urethra and vagina, are also done by some practitioners (see Gruenbaum 1991).

REFERENCES

An-Na'im, Abdullahi Ahmed 1990, *Toward an Islamic Reformation: Civil Liberties, Human Rights, and International Law*, Syracuse, New York: Syracuse University Press.

Boddy, Janice 1988, "Spirits and selves in northern Sudan: the cultural therapeutics of possession and trance," *American Ethnologist* 15(1):4–27.

1989, *Wombs and Alien Spirits: Women, Men, and the* Zar *Cult in Northern Sudan*, Madison: University of Wisconsin Press.

Gruenbaum, Ellen 1982, "Health services, health, and development in Sudan: the impact of the Gezira irrigated scheme," Ph.D. dissertation, University of Connecticut.

1991, "The Islamic movement, development, and health education: recent changes in the health of rural women in central Sudan," *Social Science and Medicine* 33(6):637–45.

1992, "The Islamist state and Sudanese women," *Middle East Report* 179:29–32.

1996, "The cultural debate over female circumcision: the Sudanese are arguing this one out for themselves," *Medical Anthropology Quarterly* 10(4):1–21.

Hale, Sondra 1987, "Women's culture/men's culture: gender, separation, and space in Africa and North America," *American Behavioral Scientist* 13(1):115–34.

1996, *Gender Politics in Sudan: Islamism, Socialism, and the State*, Boulder, Colorado: Westview Press.

Kenyon, Susan M. 1991, "The story of a tin box: zar in the Sudanese town of Sennar," in I. M. Lewis, Ahmed Al-Safi and Sayyid Hurreiz (eds.), *Women's Medicine: The* Zar-Bori *Cult in Africa and Beyond*, Edinburgh: Edinburgh University Press for the International African Institute, pp. 100–17.

4 Not only women: science as resistance in open door Egypt

Soheir A. Morsy

> [I]n the constitution of [the] Other of Europe, great care was taken to obliterate the textual ingredients with which such a subject could cathect, could occupy (invest?) its itinerary . . . (including) ideological and scientific production. (Spivak 1988:280)

Introduction

In US academic circles evoking Foucault's name frequently serves to validate arguments related to power/resistance. Among feminist scholars some find promise in the Foucauldian ethic of permanent resistance. Others, transcending the intimidating complexity of the French master's language, recognize Foucault's work as nothing less than sexist. Beyond the perfunctory salutation to the women's movement, he is judged as "talk[ing] extensively about gender, but largely neglect[ing] to focus on women" (Hoff 1996:393). Moreover, Foucault's writings "offer no hint that female bodies targeted by bio-power are capable of resistance" (Simons 1995:6, 105–10).[1]

Particularly harsh condemnation of Foucault's conception of power/resistance has come from intellectual Others. His "challenge" to both hegemonic and oppositional intellectuals has been characterized as deceptive since it ignores the critic's institutional responsibility. In a major critique of Foucault's Eurocentrism, Gyatri Spivak brings attention to the conspicuous neglect of "the epistemic violence of imperialism." In generalizing about this neglect, she includes historical reference to the Female Other to illustrate the complicity of Western intellectual production with Western international economic interests.[2] In this vein she shows how imperialism's image "as the establisher of the good society" is reproduced by "the espousal of the woman as **object** of protection from her own kind" (Spivak 1988:299).

Sharing objection to the decentering of global structural power asymmetry, and the promotion of an illusionary international feminist consensus, many women activists of the South voiced rejection of the

77

restricted women's issues/reproductive health agenda of the 1994 International Conference on Population and Development[3] (WGNRR 1994:5–6). The Declaration of the Cairo NGO Forum (1994) demanded more attention to issues of development.[4]

Drawing on examples of development projects within the framework of Egypt's Open Door Economic Policy, this chapter addresses the deployment of scientific knowledge as mechanism of resistance. Based on participant observation, as well as readings of Arabic and English-language works, I address health-threatening projects which were promoted as the epitome of "progress," and elaborated in development-centered national debates during the 1980s. While the examples of resistance addressed in this paper involve and affect women, the associated debates are not formulated in terms of gender politics. Neither are these debates expressions of what Feher and Heller (1994) refer to as the "biopolitics" associated with the transition from class-based politics to the politicization of the body. Elements of identity politics other than gender, notably nationalism and professionalism, underlie the political postures of men and women addressed here.[5]

The forms of power/resistance documented in this chapter relate to the assault on Egypt as a whole. In relation to Egypt's current "openness," the targeting of Egyptian women's bodies within the framework of the North's international population control campaign (Morsy 1993)[6] is but one element of this multipronged assault which affects male and female adults, and, not least, Egypt's children (Morsy and El-Bayoumi 1993).

Among other political motivations, this paper is an expression of my own resistance to the control exercised by scholars and policy makers of the North over the determination of priorities of intellectual pursuit and development programming for the targeted Other. Thus the analysis which follows is purposefully presented as alternative to the North's self-assigned centrality, and the related tendency of subordinating South-generated data/experiences to its paradigmatic/programmatic priorities.

In relation to anthropology's authoritative metropolitan discourse, and related censorship through omission, this paper represents resistance to the power asymmetry underlying what Roger Sanjek (1993) describes as "anthropology's hidden colonialism." Even the discipline's feminist epistemology has not escaped the related silencing of globally representative Other voices. In this regard, the chapter's ungendered thrust, in reflecting fidelity to its empirical context, represents a challenge to metropolitan maternalism. As such the account of resistance which follows responds to Helan Page's (1994) urging of anthropologists to "question how our notions of the universal and the particular are put to political work." To this end Page counsels that we render transparent the structural relations and mechanisms which reproduce not only gender inequity, but also other forms of injustice.

Power/resistance: taking account of structure and hegemony

In relation to social movements, the deconstruction of systemic analysis threatens even further fragmentation as structural impediments to emancipatory projects are eclipsed by Foucault's notion of amorphous power. Arguing in this vein, A. Belden Fields warns that "we ought not to turn away from the most dogmatic interpretations of the (structuralist) metaphor only to walk into another metaphoric trap that prioritizes language or discourse and constructs theory-proof roofs over local sites of contestation" (Fields 1988:154).

In relation to global structures, rejection of Foucault's conception of power and resistance (e.g., Ahmad 1992; Parajuli 1993; Said 1987) extends to the related discourse on epistemes of cultural classification of the Other. Informed by cultural and historical specificity, some scholars caution that the latter may end up producing a new form of cultural globalization akin to classical Orientalism (Abaza and Stauth 1988:344; cf. Good and Good 1992). Spurr (1993) even argues that postmodernist deconstruction is more suited to exposing the overwhelming power of Western metaphysics than to identifying the exercise of power (and resistance) inherent in concrete human activity, especially in non-Western settings.

Attention extended to Others' "concrete human activity" in the context of hegemonic social and cultural relations has brought into focus resistance to the political instrumentality of biomedical/scientific knowledge. Documented accounts of such resistance during the colonial era lend credence to the judgment that the basic propositions of postmodernist sensibility are "not even new" (Noble Tesh 1990:60).[7] The rejection of the reproductive health agenda of metropolitan feminists by female Others is another variation of the protracted resistance to western hegemony.

At Commilla, in preparation for the Cairo ICPD, and in the stadium of the Egyptian capital, the voices of women activists of the South were raised in objection to "their" agenda for "our" bodies. In contradiction to universalized feminist biopolitics (Silverstein 1995), Evelyn Hong of the Third World Network, speaking for "women coming from the South" defined the "burning issues" as those of structural adjustment and debt servicing. Joining others who inquired about the whereabouts of the "D" in ICPD, women of Arab NGOs unanimously agreed that development, rather than the controversy around abortion and reproductive rights, should have been the focus of the ICPD. Gyatri Spivak labeled abortion as "the master symbol of reproductive rights . . . describ[ing] it as an alibi to the North to keep the world order as it is" (WGNRR 1994:5–6).[8]

While reproductive health continues to be the primary focus of hegemonic international feminist discourse, state-sanctioned "development" programs which threaten public health, i.e., the health of women, children, and men, remain relatively neglected. These programs are rarely the objects of analytical scrutiny in the sociomedical literature on Egypt. Instead, preferential consideration is given to women's reproductive health, studies of health service utilization and individualized therapeutic narratives, and occasional self-congratulatory accounts of expatriate do-gooders bearing the torch of enlightenment.

Assault/resistance: beyond "women's health" as gate keeping

In decreeing Egypt's Open Door Economic Policies (ODEP) President Sadat insisted that "the executive authority must be spared the burden of having to deal with political discontents" (Sadat as quoted in Jabara 1986). "Discontented" Egyptian researchers, whether women or men, had to face a situation where the regime became, to use Mark Kennedy's terminology, hermetically sealed except to foreign influences. Indeed, the Egyptian regime has "maintain[ed] a monopoly with its foreign donors over development planning, and . . . control over what shall and what shall not be investigated" (Kennedy 1991:79).

Since the mid-1970s some Northern professionals, in collaboration with Egyptian "counterparts," have played a central role in promoting research orientations and development programs commensurate with the state's ODEP. Illustrative of this development is Delwin Roy's commentary on the role of Ford Foundation staff in "restructuring the political economy of Egypt" (Roy 1985).

The exercise of inordinate power by international development institutions has had a profound impact on Egypt, affecting every facet of social and political life. This extends to women's reproductive health and other apparently humanitarian medical concerns (Morsy 1995). Whether such health-focused programs are judged as noble endeavors in pursuit of human rights, or objectionable expressions of the White Man's/Woman's Burden, questions remain as to the nature of the structural power relations toward which such efforts are channeled. In this regard it is important not to lose sight of the role of international institutions in promoting the privatization of Egypt's economy, including health resources, to the benefit of the few and the detriment of the many, men and women alike.

Under conditions of dependent development and political repression, collaboration between specialists and the public remains far from the ideal of a partnership between community and scientists. In general, the access of Egyptian political dissidents (including scientists) to the public has been limited to the publication of articles in the official opposition press or holding meetings at the headquarters of opposition political parties or other voluntary associations. All these activities take place under the close surveillance of the security forces. In spite of such restrictions, and at no small risk,[9] Egyptian scientists/activists managed to make use of their specialized knowledge to address problems of public health.[10]

Nuclear technology and public health concerns

In the 1980s, when the nuclear industry in the West experienced both threats from the political opposition and soaring costs, progress-bound Egypt, like other Third World countries, was seen as a less perilous terrain. In addition to direct corporate wooing, Egyptian nuclear professionals/state managers were supplied with promotional material. In the form of films and booklets, this depicts happy, healthy European (nuclear) families picnicking by ponds of goldfish and fields of beautiful flowers, all in the shadow of nuclear power plants. In turn, official Egyptian publications proclaiming the "inevitability of the nuclear program" reproduce the distinctive markings of commercial literature under the guise of impartial scientific commentary. Development and progress-centered symbol manipulations, proven effective in a variety of contexts, ranging from the sale of imported high-tar cigarettes to the promotion of women-centered family planning, extended to preparations for Egypt's "entry to the nuclear age."

Discussions of the implications of the proposed nuclear power program took place under the sponsorship of opposition parties and also involved professional associations, including the Engineers Syndicate, the Egyptian Society for Political Economy, Statistics, and Legislation, and university faculty associations. These discussions addressed a variety of concerns ranging from risks pertaining to women's reproductive health to the logic of technological fixes for Egypt's underdevelopment.

In Alexandria an *ad hoc* group dominated by women stood in opposition to the selection of nearby Sidi Krir as a nuclear power plant site. These women were not alone; for example, the Alexandria Local Council had voiced unanimous opposition to the Sidi Krir project in 1979. The arguments women used in the public opposition to the project in no way resembled the rhetoric of feminist biopolitics familiar in the North. Informed by a variety of specialist-generated information, including the expertise of professors from Alexandria University's faculties of Engineering and Science, the activist women drew attention to the potential ecological disaster which would befall the northern coast as a result of radioactive contamination. Raising the culturally charged banner of "protecting the welfare of our children," both male and female members of the *ad hoc* committee brought public health concerns into prominence. In addition to citing higher leukemia and death rates among children residing near nuclear power plants or exposed to radiation following nuclear accidents in the US and the UK, they described risks of birth defects, genetic mutations, and miscarriages.

Scientists from the Nuclear Energy Authority made good use of their easy access to the state-regulated press to reject criticisms based on the danger to health, asserting the safety of nuclear power. An effective counterargument was undertaken by other scientists who were well versed in the scientific language of the promoters of nuclear power, including the biomedical terminology pertaining to health risk assessment. As these critics also enjoyed culturally valued scientist status, they were especially effective in demystifying the rhetoric of those who supported nuclear power.

Using briefings prepared by some of these scientists, opposition members of the People's Assembly were able to present science-informed arguments against the establishment of nuclear power plants, interspersing their scientific references with culturally correct statements, including Quranic verses. Their invocation of nationalist sentiment took such forms as reference to our ancient Egyptian ancestors who "worshiped the sun" (to justify solar energy as alternative). They also contrasted the profit motive of foreign consultants with the proven patriotism of anti-nuclear Egyptian scientists (see People's Assembly 1984 Official Register).

The Minister of Electricity and Energy and his entourage of state managers/nuclear scientists continued to claim "specialist" monopoly, and tried to discredit opponents of nuclear power. They described the latter's criticisms of nuclear power as "scientific deception" and "alarmist," not to mention "communist." Nevertheless, expressions of opposition to nuclear power were voiced well beyond the confines of the corridors of power and headquarters of professional associations.

During election campaigns, anti-nuclear activists shared their concerns with crowds of ordinary Egyptians gathered in the alleys of Alexandria and Cairo, and in some provincial towns and rural areas. They popularized counterarguments to the claims of safety and assertions of "acceptable" levels of radiation exposure being made by government scientists. Some women listened to these arguments from their windows in the popular quarters of urban Alexandria; others met in the home of a leading anti-nuclear advocate, and in the city's Sporting Club.

As the nuclear energy debate continued, government scientists could not get away with comparing the risks to health from power plant leakage of ionizing radiation to those of daily sun exposure, flying in airplanes, and watching TV. Their credibility was attacked by their opponents who also pointed out that government scientists used the most conservative estimates of risk, even after these were superseded by a more recent and higher assessment. This criticism contradicted official scientists' claim that they used only the valorized "most recent scientific data" from Western centers of "advanced science" in defending nuclear power.

Egypt's nuclear power program has remained stalled. While some may like to credit anti-nuclear activists for this development, others present a more realistic reasoning: international institutions consider Egypt a poor investment risk. Meanwhile Egyptians, whether female or male, have not escaped the potential threat of radioactivity from other sources, including the burial of imported radioactive waste, and the importation of radioactive foodstuffs.

Open door Egypt as dump site: nuclear waste and radioactive food

A new threat to public health from nuclear technology was unleashed when Egypt was added to the list of other politically disempowered communities of the South considered appropriate dumping grounds for nuclear waste. Described by Stebbins (1992) as "garbage imperialism," this policy with its underlying racist logic relates to a variety of "imports" found in Open Door Egypt, ranging from the infamous Dalkon shield to radioactive infant formula.

Shortly after the launching of friendly relations between the US government and the Sadat regime, inquiries came to an Egyptian research center from a US academic institution requesting assistance in assessing a site for an international radioactive waste storage facility in the Western Desert near the Egyptian–Libyan border. While the Egyptian scientists who knew of this request generally found such "scientific collaboration" unthinkable, President Sadat agreed to the burial of Austria's nuclear waste in Egypt's Western Desert. This project was never implemented because the people of Austria voted down their country's proposed nuclear program. However, the very "openness" of Egypt as a dump site remained a serious threat to public health.[11]

After the Chernobyl nuclear accident of 1986 radioactive food imports, including infant formula, arrived in Egypt. Organized by a variety of professional associations, a campaign of public education was launched. Similar to the organized opposition to nuclear power plants, use was made of scientific and medical expertise. Official denials of the importation of radioactive foods were challenged at election rallies during 1987. Even members of security forces engaged in surveillance at these meetings were interested in learning which brands of radioactive infant formula had entered the country.

In Alexandria, Egypt's major port, the Faculty of Science took a leading role in proving that imported radioactive foodstuffs had been dumped in Egyptian markets. Professors of the Faculty challenged the definition of "safe" levels of radiation used by the government's scientists. In Alexandria and Cairo, conferences devoted to the health hazards of radioactive food imports were attended by scholars from different disciplines of the medical, physical, and social sciences. At these meetings, participants pointed out that a number of countries find the International Atomic Energy Commission's "safe" level of 350 becquerels/kg[12] of milk unacceptable. Even more importantly, international safety standards do not take into account the specificity of the Egyptian diet, and its variation over the life cycle.[13] These critics argued that the rampant malnutrition among children would amplify the adverse health impact of radioactive food consumption.

Criticism of the importation of radioactive food also came from economists who pointed to the more fundamental problem of food dependence associated with the agrarian policies of the era of economic liberalization.[14] Other specialists brought attention to the fact that imported food, particularly US stored surplus powdered milk and flour, reaches Egypt infested with insect pests. These critics cited references in the scientific literature which suggest a correlation between human malignancy and flour contaminated with the quinone-secreting tenebrinoid beetle (El-Mofty, Khudoley *et al.* 1992).

Debates on the structural framework of food importation included reasoned challenges to the familiar blaming of mothers' "ignorance" of sound nutritional principles made by the regime's loyal experts. The

national Nutrition Measure (which identifies the available food resources, both locally produced and imported) shows that there is no
deficiency in the national supply of food. But critics of this measure
argue that it does not address the maldistribution of food as a function
of income differential. Issues of food cost as a percentage of income,
decline in agricultural yields, and, more fundamentally, the predicted
adverse impact of *infitah*[15] are also ignored in this measure.

The health risks of agrarian production and food consumption

Although generally considered less hazardous than radioactivity, pesticide contamination represents a serious and widespread threat to the
health of male and female agricultural producers, and, more generally, to
the health of consumers. Of the many hazardous pesticides imported in
Egypt, Galecron (chlordimefor: N'-Chloro-0-tolyl-N,N-dimethyl-for-
mamidine) stands out as one surrounded by a complex controversy
owing to the contradictory interpretations of the experimental data
related to its use. Another part of this controversy is the concerted effort
made by health officials to conceal its testing on peasants by Ciba-Geigy.

News of Ciba-Geigy's testing of Galecron on rural children and youth
came to Egypt through European environmental activists in 1982. This
prompted allegations of corporate bribery of Egyptian officials, an
assertion once given credence by a Minister of Health who courageously
disclosed experiencing attempts at bribery by multinational pharmaceutical firms.

A protracted scientific/political/ethical debate followed the revelation
of the Ciba Geigy experimental use of Galecron. As in the case of
nuclear power plants, the opposition consisted of members of professional associations, university professors, and human rights activists.
Members of the Alexandria Association of Human Rights Advocates
actually visited the rural area where humans had been sprayed.
Although some of the researchers with expert knowledge on the adverse
health effects of Galecron, and experience with its promotion in Egypt,
were not directly involved in the public debate, they generously shared
their knowledge with those involved in the public dialogue (El-Bayoumi
1982:13).

Galecron had been used in Egypt prior to 1976 but the Ministry of
Health stopped its use after receiving Ciba-Geigy's documentation of its
carcinogenicity, and that of its metabolites (N-formyl-4-chloro-0-tolui-
dine and 4-chloro-0-toluidine) in white mice. My discussion with
environmental/health activist Marion Moses, MD in 1991 suggests that

Ciba-Geigy's experimentation in Egypt was related to the company's effort to comply with US regulations regarding "data gaps" when it was trying to reregister the pesticide. In the US, federal authorities had limited the use of Galecron to cotton, and to spraying by a registered technician. The US also banned the distribution of the seeds of the treated cotton plants. Even with these restrictions, Galecron was banned totally in California, despite the fact that Ciba-Geigy had built a California factory for the production of Galecron at the cost of 22 million dollars. The medical evidence had convinced many that Galecron should be banned even if there were no alternative pesticides (Maddy 1978).[16]

The Permanent Committee for Recommendations Related to Pesticides refused Ciba-Geigy's requests for field experimentation with Galecron sprayed from aeroplanes. The decision of this Egyptian committee, reached during its meeting of April 10, 1982, was informed by the California case and by data from one of its members' collaborative research project (El-Mofty *et al.* 1982). The Committee's decision had come after relentless efforts on the part of Ciba-Geigy's technical representative to convince its members of his company's "scientific" reasoning. For example, in a May 14, 1978 meeting with members of the Committee, his arguments were prefaced by the familiar paternalistic praise of the Third World audience's capacity for scientific exchange, but betrayed the equally familiar double standard operative in the international pesticide and development industry (PAN 1992). Although his company had used mice as experimental animals in its attempt to comply with US pre-registration testing procedures, the expert from Ciba-Geigy argued against the usage of derivative data for Egyptian humans. In fact he went so far as to try to use the US Environmental Protection Agency's ruling on Galecron to convince members of the committee that it should be used in Egypt. But he left out the restrictions imposed by the EPA, and its own documentation of accidents in spite of such restrictions. Moreover, he ignored the particularities of the Egyptian context of pesticide use.

In response to Egyptian scientists' documentation of residues of Galecron in cotton seeds, a major source of cooking oil locally, Ciba-Geigy's technical expert recommended purification to rid the oil of such residues and their telltale smell. He did not discuss either the effectiveness of such treatment, or its cost. He also undermined the health implications of Ciba-Geigy's own disclosure of anemia, and internal bleeding resulting from same-day exposure to Galecron. Yet, these conditions are not negligible affronts to health, particularly among parasite-infested, malnourished Egyptian peasants. By contrast, extensive use was made of impressive manipulation of statistical models and their conclusion that only one out of every 100 million persons exposed to Galecron is at risk.

By the end of 1983, the spraying of Egyptians with Galecron as part of Ciba-Geigy's experimentation could no longer be concealed even by the mainstream press. On December 26 of the same year *October*, a weekly, well known as a voice of the ruling National Democratic Party, published an extended article, using the comments of Egyptian specialists on the health hazards of pesticides, with specific reference to Galecron. The article stated that Ciba-Giegy had admitted to adverse health effects among Egyptian children who had been sprayed with Galecron in 1976. The Egyptian media also reported the public apology offered to Egyptians by a company representative appearing on Swiss television.

In a delayed and short response to questions raised by the press, the Ministry of Health insisted that it has never permitted, nor will it ever permit, experimentation on any Egyptian citizen. Despite Ciba-Geigy's own admission of experimentation on human subjects, the Ministry insisted that tests of the impact of Galecron on human health had involved the spraying of cotton, not humans. Yet, in contradiction of this claim the Ministry also denied "any adverse [health] effects" on humans as a result of the experiment. Ciba-Geigy's own Egyptian representative acknowledged the carcinogenic effects of Galecron on mice, and admitted to data showing adverse health effects on Egyptian children who followed the spray planes in the fields. Nevertheless the Egyptian Ministry of Health insisted on a favorable evaluation. Its document on the subject asserts that new data on this pesticide has vindicated it of responsibility for adverse health effects in animals and humans (El-Bayoumi 1983). As for the live human beings whose health status contradicts official wisdom, their suffering has prompted nothing more than Ciba-Geigy's public apology, not monetary compensation, as was the case in California.

As peasant agricultural producers, male and female alike, continued to be exposed to hazardous pesticides, consumers of the country's modernized food supply also remained at risk. For example, large-scale commercial producers of poultry add birth control pills to their feed. Experiments carried out at one of the many chicken factories by researchers from Alexandria University's Faculty of Science and Tanta University's Faculty of Medicine examined the effects of two antibiotics, chloramphenicol and oxytetracycline, given to hens in drinking water. The report from this study showed "significantly enhanced tumor formation in liver, kidney, spleen and heart" (El-Mofty, Abdel-Galil *et al.* 1992:205). This research added new credence to popular concerns over the health effects of consuming poultry raised in accordance with "modern" techniques.

"Worldly" production techniques have also been linked to a wave of unexplained maladies during the summer of 1992. Widespread abdominal pains, vomiting, and diarrhea prompted concern over the adverse health effects of consumption of "contaminated" food. While the usual official commentary asserted the absence of any cause for alarm, the opposition press published contrary opinion expressed by a number of specialists (*Al-Wafd* June 4, 1992, p. 3). Some scientists pointed to the many pesticides used on the fruits to which the maladies were linked. Other scientists criticized the hormonal treatment of orchards as a means of enhancing the size of fruits to an extent generally unprecedented for locally grown crops.

During a live interview on state television a professor of zoology from Alexandria University linked the maladies to profit motives on the part of commercial producers. A few months after this interview Professor El-Mofty shared with me its details during my visit to his laboratory at Alexandria University's Faculty of Science in the summer of 1992. In support of his argument regarding the potential health hazards of hormonal treatment of fruit plants, he cited laboratory research which demonstrates the induction of neoplasms in experimental animals by feeding them plant growth hormones. Although no harm befell the professor, the TV program hostess was called in for questioning by her superiors. In self-defense she resorted to the authority of science, requesting reprints of the professor's publications to present in her own defense.

Experimentation on human subjects

In contrast to the Ministry of Health's insistence to the contrary, there have been many accusations of the use of Egyptians as "experimental mice." Contrary to official denials, the state-regulated national press and scientific publications document experimental trials carried out on Egyptians within the framework of officially sanctioned "international scientific cooperation," and under the banner of "progress" and the "open door."

To Egyptian opponents of such collaboration, the issue is neither the goodwill of individual foreign researchers, nor local researchers' right to pursue scientific inquiry. Rather, the concerns are the framework of power relations within which such cooperation proceeds, the attendant determination of research priorities, and, not least, the right to real informed consent of human subjects in experimental trials. Such concerns are validated by the experimental trials of long-term contraceptive technology, and the testing of the efficacy of a molluscicide under US sponsorship.

Throughout the 1980s Egypt's lenders and international population experts continued to insist on a program of population control. The same type of experimental research on contraception, well documented for Puerto Rico and other parts of the global South, took place in Egypt and was touted as a form of modern health promotion. As part of international trials, Egyptian women have been injected with Depo-Provera and implanted with the five-year contraceptive Norplant (Morsy 1993). These trials occurred at a time when neither contraceptive had been approved by the FDA in the US.

Far from uniformly supporting experimental trials of contraceptives, the reaction of Egyptian physicians ranged from enthusiastic participation to outright rejection. Far from the engendered debates of biopolitics, rejection was expressed in terms of nationalistic fervor. While some biomedical specialists expressed concern over possible health risks, others were unequivocally opposed to any utilization of *Egyptian* women as "experimental mice" for drugs which had not been approved for contraceptive use in their country of origin (Morsy 1993). Through an Egyptian scientist/human rights advocate, opposition to the provider-controlled long term contraceptive known as Norplant was brought to the attention of an International Human Rights Conference held in Tunis in 1993. The opposition hoped to get the matter on the agenda of the UN-sponsored International Human Rights Conference held in Vienna a year later.

Human experimentation within the framework of international scientific collaboration is also illustrated by a research project on a molluscicide in rural Egypt. Designed to test the efficacy of topical niclosamide 1 percent lotion in the prevention of *Schistosoma haematobium* infection among Egyptian peasants/"volunteers," this project is headed by a North American infectious disease specialist as principal investigator. Independent verification of urine samples analysis involves the Walter Reed Army Institute of Research (Podgore 1991:3). The three Egyptian physicians/associate investigators involved in the project are affiliates of the Egypt-based US Naval Medical Research Unit 3 (NAMRU-3), whose commanding officer is responsible for medical monitoring.[17]

In his unpublished review of the project's application, which Professor El-Mofty shared with me, the professor presents reasoned rejection of the research protocol as outlined in the application (El-Mofty n.d.).

Citing collaborative research between scientists from Alexandria University and Maryland's Frederick Cancer Research Center, the reviewer states that "according to this work, it was shown for the first time that niclosamide (in a concentration similar to that used to control schistosoma snails in drainage canals) in Egypt has a carcinogenic effect on experimental animals."[18] He goes on to point out that the investigator's application makes no reference to this relevant research. Moreover, Professor El-Mofty notes that although earlier testing of the 1 percent niclosamide was carried out by the principal investigator/ applicant among another group of Egyptian peasants in Beheira governorate, "No reports were presented (in the application) to insure that no hazardous effects happened to experimental farmers."

Contrary to the Ministry of Health's above-noted assertion that it would not subject Egyptian citizens to experimentation, the application makes explicit the involvement of the Ministry in the testing of the molluscicide. Specification of eligibility reads as follows: "These volunteers will be drawn from a population of farmers identified by a prior Ministry of Health screening program as having *Schistosoma haematobium* and were subsequently treated with praziquantel therapy" (Podgore 1991:2). Evidently, and not unlike the cases of Norplant and Galecron, the Egyptian Ministry of Health has been instrumental in subjecting Egyptian "volunteers" to experimentation. Far from initiating this project itself, the Ministry's role has been no more than facilitator. In reference to the Beheira experiment the application makes clear that project monitoring was not the prerogative of Egyptian health authorities. Instead, "the sites received an on-site review and inspection by Maj. Gere of USAMMDA on June 9–13, 1991 for compliance with (US) FDA regulations" (Podgore 1991:4). This is in turn consistent with the fact that:

[the molluscicide] study is sponsored by the Surgeon General, Department of the [US] Army and conducted under Investigational New Drug application number 33,272 in effect with the United States Food and Drug Administration. [The] study of the effectiveness of 1 percent niclosamide lotion against *S. haematobium* is undertaken to fulfill FDA recommendations to test the lotion against at least two species of schistosomes to provide the necessary data in order to approve it for general schistosomiasis prevention. (Podgore 1991:4)

To Egyptian opponents of this type of experimentation the assertion of humanitarian intent of this scientific undertaking is easily dismissed in light of similar expressed interest in the eradication of schistosomiasis on the part of British colonial authorities (Farley 1988). Even minimal familiarity with the social position of Egyptian peasants prompts skepticism of the intent to obtain "written informed consent . . . [from research] subjects" (Podgore 1991:2). A visit to the Beheira site of the earlier phase of the proposed research by two Egyptian scientists, including a human rights activist, raises questions regarding appropriate measures of protection of human subjects and the feasibility of the proposed research protocol. More generally, Egyptian scientists' involvement in opposing this type of "international scientific coopera-tion" underscores the role of scientific knowledge as a tool of political resistance.

Discussion

[A]t the moment that the native intellectual comes into touch again with his people, this artificial sentinel (towards dominant "universal" values) is turned into dust . . . [T]hose values which seemed to uplift the soul are (towards dominant "universal" values) revealed as worthless, simply because they have nothing to do with the concrete conflict in which the people is engaged. (Franz Fanon 1963:47)

In recent years locally grounded social power relations have gained significance as the object of anthropological commentary, particularly its feminist variants. Yet, it seems that anthropology's distinctive-other "methodology" contributes to the preservation of the discipline's tradition of "the political as taboo" in relation to state policies. Critical commentary on state policies pertaining to "openness" to "international scientific collaboration" threatens anthropologists' continued access to the "field."

Anthropological studies which address the question of resistance to the Western economy, with its constituent systems of production, power, and signification, tend to focus primarily on social practices and symbolic mediation (Escobar 1987). Seldom is there reference to scientific knowledge or nationalism serving as instruments of resistance. Note-worthy in this regard is Sharabi's commentary on the work of Clifford Geertz, the prominent advocate of anthropological "thick description":

The nationalist or radical revolutionaries exist only on the margin of his scholarly interest; hence his distance from the central concerns of modern Muslim society. From this distant and patronizing perspective, Muslims, compared to Westerners, appear backward, ineffective, and self-deluding . . . He quotes a Muslim 'alim who tells him that the Declaration of Human Rights and the secret of the atom are to be found in the Qur'an, which leads him to this essentialist conclusion: "Islam, in this way becomes a justification for modernity without itself actually becoming modern. It promotes what it itself, to speak metaphorically, can neither embrace nor understand." (Sharabi 1990:11)

As for the sociomedical literature on Egypt, reference to modern science is generally restricted to accounts of programs designed to "introduce" or "upgrade" biomedical health services, particularly those related to women and children. In official circles the targeting of Egypt for internationally financed and executed women's health projects has been promoted as an expression of honor bestowed on the country.[19]

In contrast to the interpretations of compradorial intellectuals regarding women-targeted international health development projects, some Egyptians view "international scientific cooperation" as a channel for directing Egypt's development course to the benefit of the North. As such, "cooperation" related to women's reproductive health is judged as reminiscent of the exercise of power by colonial "educators" who sought to denationalize local women, rendering them intermediaries in transmitting colonial culture to local society (Chaudhuri and Strobel 1990:291). At the same time, Egyptian scientists/activists have relied on modern scientific knowledge in their attempt to counter the adverse impact of "opening up" to "worldly," science-inspired development.

Even the work of tradition-bound Islamist health institutions contradicts Foucault's assertion that the "forces created by [Islamic] religious spiritualism have marked a new stage of resistance against modern rationalism and power based on science and technology" (Abaza and Stauth 1988:354). Like other Egyptians who promote modern health care, Islamists are not blind to the benefits of biomedicine and other scientific knowledge, nor to modern technology. Their concerns differ from those of postmodernists whose admonishment of modernity as "discourse" proceeds from the privileged terrain of modern comforts which alleviate suffering and protect life.

For Egypt, as elsewhere, modernity as a "worldly" phenomenon, whether it pertains to biomedicine or to other specialized sciences, is simultaneously the product of the past and the present. The past includes the experiences of colonialism; the present entails "special relations" with the US whose "position as a model to be emulated remains hegemonic" (Rofel 1992:95; see also Abdel Fadil 1989). Neither of these complexes of experiences forms the basis of Foucault's historically specific European modern episteme which remains distant from the "epistemic violence of imperialism."

For opposition intellectuals in Egypt, whether male or female, it is their historically generated political consciousness, not Foucault's elaborate challenge to modern science, that renders comprehensible the counterdiscourse illustrated in this chapter. Informative in this regard is the case of China. Here memories of past relations have "taken on the hue of subversion in the context of economic reform" (Rofel 1992:95). A similar situation has been noted for Egypt where political economists came to occupy a political position of being "off-stage" with the abandonment of the policies of state planning/nationalism in favor of those of the "Opening." While some opposition intellectuals have been "waiting in the wings," as Kennedy (1991) puts it, others have engaged in more active forms of resistance, relying on a variety of scholarly knowledge.

Among those who resist global mechanisms of control and exploitation, including those generated through science, their efforts represent a historically derived political consciousness constituted of a complex of nationalist, religious, anti-imperialist, liberal, and socialist elements, not the philosophy of postmodernism. To accept postmodernism as a challenge to Western ideals of reason, progress, and truth entails implicit agreement that these values are unique to those who hold the Enlightenment as a central element of their cultural heritage, divorced from other philosophical orientations in human history. More importantly, postmodernism as Eurocentric "intellectual game" of textuality leaves us distanced from the historical and social context of the violence and dehumanization perpetrated against those who continue to be targeted for "enlightenment" within the framework of the Western civilizational project.

NOTES

1 While Foucault's work may well be illustrative of the personal–political dialectic cherished by feminists, the centrality of the former in instructing his intellectual pursuits is inescapable. As Simons recently noted, "it was Foucault's deepest personal concerns, his care for himself, that informed his intellectual work" (Simons 1995:9).
2 In relation to these interests Spivak reminds us that the entire over-determined global enterprise has been in the interest of a dynamic situation "requiring that interests, motives (desires), and power (or knowledge) be ruthlessly dislocated." She reasons that for European intellectuals to now invoke that dislocation as a radical discovery ("that should make us diagnose the economic as a piece of dated analytic machinery") serves, even if inadvertently, the reproduction of this very dislocation, and associated hegemonic relations.
3 The ICPD was held in Cairo in September 1994.
4 Similar concerns surrounding global structural relations and state policies informed the deliberations of feminists from both North and South at the 1993 Commilla Symposium which preceded the ICPD. These concerns were also manifest in some feminists' commentaries during preparations for Beijing. From this vantage point Vandana Shiva renders the Chiapas uprising relevant to poor Mexican women's welfare and Anastasia Posadskaya attributes Russian women's recently acquired status of second-class citizens to the "democratization" of their country and policies of market "reform."

5 In Egypt different forms of resistance to foreign domination include bureaucratic "inefficiency," which is maligned by international aid managers/development "experts."

6 Whether for Egyptian or for other women of the South, such population targeting represents a sharp contrast to the development of a thriving fertility promotion industry in the global North, and related technology (read commodity) transfer internationally.

7 For example, as Fanon reminds us in his account of medicine as instrument of racialism and humiliation in Algeria, colonized Arabs/Africans recognized, and *resisted*, biomedicine as an instrument of political control. The "natives" were well aware that statistics on sanitary improvements do not represent progress. Instead, they saw these as "fresh proof of the extension of the occupier's hold on the country" (Fanon 1978:229). For other examples of the continued relevance of Fanon's work see Gordon 1995:85–104.

8 Focusing on another "alibi"/gate-keeping phenomenon of sociomedical discourse, "genital mutilation," CNN indulged in taking license with the body of the Egyptian Other, a practice which extends to human subject experimentation by Northern scientists in partnership with local collaborators.

9 For example, in September 1981 President Sadat ordered the "transfer" of sixty-four professors outside Egypt's universities. More recently, in relation to the Gulf War, the imprisonment of an activist physician brought appeals from the Boston-based group Physicians for Human Rights.

10 In addition to being ungendered, the conception of these health problems differed from the formulations of compartmentalized academic disciplines. The arguments deployed in national debates involved shared transdisciplinary knowledge, including biomedical learning.

11 As recently as June 1992, in testimony before the Industry Committee of the People's Assembly, officials of the Ministry of Health and the Agency for Environmental Affairs stated that the burial of toxic and radioactive waste continues. They added that, in bypassing national regulations, "the advanced countries reach their objective through various means, including direct contacts with [individual] governors." The head of the Agency for Environmental Affairs added that Egyptian companies "continue to cut deals with foreign companies to bury nuclear waste in Egypt" (*Al-Shaab*, June 22, 1992).

12 A becquerel designates one nuclear disintegration/second.

13 "Safe" levels for bread in Europe cannot be accepted as such for the average Egyptian in whose diet bread makes up a major proportion.

14 While Egypt's food imports climbed to unprecedented levels the country witnessed the destruction of thousands of eggs, and what is regarded as the equally sinful "dumping of milk in ponds," both intended to maintain a high level of profit under conditions of "excess" supply.

15 The era of *infitah* ushered the privileging of rich peasants and capitalist farmers with subsidized feed for cattle and tax exemptions for poultry production and orchard cultivation. Encouraged by official economic logic, which is also legitimized by academic specialists, commercial production of vegetables, aromatic plants, poultry, red meat, and fruits underwent a

dramatic transformation, to the detriment of traditional field crops. In relation to wheat, of which Egypt is a major importer, this logic takes the form of juxtaposing of income from a *faddan* of wheat to its six-fold multiple from the same area of land devoted to exportable strawberries.

16 Included in the list of "Dirty Dozen" pesticides compiled by the international coalition of NGOs known as the Pesticide Action Network, the registration of Galecron in the US was voluntarily withdrawn by Ciba-Geigy in 1989.

17 NAMRU units "study diseases likely to endanger American troops" (Gallagher 1990:200).

18 This research was presented over a decade ago at a conference on the Prevention of Occupational Cancer held in Helsinki under the cosponsorship of the ILO, WHO, and the International Agency for Research on Cancer (see El-Mofty *et al.* 1981).

19 For example, at the 1988 celebrated "Egypt 2000" conference, professor Ibrahim Oweiss, president of the Association of Egyptian Scholars Abroad (which was established under the patronage of President Sadat) boasted about "the . . . choice of Egypt, among twelve nations, for the implementation of the biggest scientific medical program for control of world population growth, through the use of long-acting modern medical methods."

REFERENCES

Abaza, Mona and Stauth, Georg 1988, "Occidental reason, orientalism, Islamic fundamentalism: a critique," *International Journal of Sociology* 3(4):343–64.

Abdel Fadil, Mahmoud 1989, "The values of progress, and the values of underdevelopment," *Al-Ahram Al-Iqtisadi* 1044:20 [in Arabic].

Ahmad, Aijaz 1992, *In Theory: Classes, Nations, Literatures*, London: Verso.

Cairo NGO Forum 1994, Collective Declaration on Development and Economic Issues.

Chaudhuri, Nupur and Strobel, Margaret 1990, "Western women and imperialism," *Women's Studies International Forum* 13(4):289–93.

El-Bayoumi, Ashraf 1982, "Collaborative research and the scientific method," *Al-Ahram Al-Iqtisadi* November 15 [In Arabic].

  1983, "A return to the pesticide tragedy," *Al-Ahram Al-Iqtisadi*, January 24 [In Arabic].

El-Mofty, M. M., Abdel-Galil, A. M., Bayoumi, S. L., El-Zoheiry, A. M. and El-Kady, A. I. 1992, "Effects of some antibiotics on organs of hens (white selected leghorn)," *Journal of the Egyptian German Society of Zoology* 8(a):205–15.

El-Mofty, M. M., Galal, M. R., El-Sebae, A. and Essawy, A. 1982, "Liver neoplasms in toads (*Bufo regularis*) enforced fed with chlordimeform," in C. Vago and G. Matz (eds.), *Proceedings of the First International Colloquium on Pathology of Reptiles and Amphibians*, Angers, pp. 173–6.

El-Mofty, M. M., Reuber, M. A., El-Sebae, A. and Sabry, I. 1981, "Induction of neoplastic lesions in toads (*Bufo regularis*) with bayluscid (Bayer 73)," *Proceedings of the International Symposium on the Prevention of Occupational Cancer*, Helsinki, pp. 427–36.

El-Mofty, M. M., Khudoley, V. V., Sakr, S. A. and Fathala, N. G. 1992, "Flour infested with *Tribolium casatnewum*, biscuits made of this flour, and 1,4–benzoquinone induced neoplastic lesions in Swiss albino mice," *Nutrition and Cancer* 17(1):97–104.

Escobar, Arturo 1987, "Power and visibility: the invention and management of development in the Third World," Ph.D. dissertation, University of California, Berkeley.

Fanon, Franz 1963, *The Wretched of the Earth*, New York: Grove Press.

1978, "Medicine and colonialism," in J. Ehrenreich (ed.), *The Cultural Crisis of Modern Medicine*, New York: Monthly Review Press, pp. 229–51.

Farley, John 1988, "Bilharzia: a problem of 'native health,' 1900–1950," in David Arnold (ed.), *Imperial Medicine and Indigenous Societies*, Manchester: Manchester University Press, pp. 189–207.

Feher, Ferenc and Heller, Agnes 1994, *Biopolitics*, Aldershot: Avebury.

Fields, A. Belden 1988, "In defence of political economy and systemic analysis," in C. Nelson and L. Grossberg (eds.), *Marxism and the Interpretation of Culture*, Chicago: University of Illinois Press, pp. 141–56.

Gallagher, Nancy Elizabeth 1990, *Egypt's Other Wars*, Syracuse: Syracuse University Press.

Good, Mary-Jo DelVecchio and Good, Byron J. 1992, "The comparative study of Greco-Islamic medicine: the integration of medical knowledge into local symbolic contexts," in C. Leslie (ed.), *Paths to Asian Medical Knowledge*, Berkeley: University of California Press, pp. 257–71.

Gordon, Lewis R. 1995, *Fanon and the Crisis of European Man: An Essay on Philosophy and the Human Sciences*, New York: Routledge.

Hoff, Joan 1996, "The pernicious effects of poststructuralism on women's history," in Diane Bell and Renate Klein (eds.), *Radically Speaking: Feminism Reclaimed*, Melbourne: Spinifex Press, pp. 393–412.

Jabara, Abdeen 1986, "A shameful law," *Newsletter of the Association of Arab-American University Graduates* 13(2):5.

Kennedy, Mark 1991, "Dilemmas in middle eastern social sciences: contours of the problem of the relevance of western paradigms as guide to research, policy and practice," in E. L. Sullivan and J. S. Ismael (eds.), *The Contemporary Study of the Arab World*, Alberta: University of Alberta Press, pp. 65–80.

Maddy, K. T. 1978, "Acute hemorrhagic cystitis: industrial exposure to the pesticide chlordimeform (galecron)," *Journal of the American Medical Association* 239.

Morsy, Soheir A. and El-Bayoumi, Jehan 1993, "Risk as an analytical construct: implications for children's health in Arab societies, *Childhood: A Global Journal of Child Research* 1(2):75–86.

1995, "Deadly reproduction among Egyptian women: maternal mortality and the medicalization of population control," in F. D. Ginsburg and R. Rapp (eds.), *Conceiving the New World Order: The Global Politics of Reproduction*, Berkeley: University of California Press, pp. 162–76.

Morsy, Soheir 1993, "Bodies of choice: Norplant experimental trials on Egyptian women," in B. Mintzes, A. Hardon and J. Hanhart (eds.), *Norplant: Under Her Skin*, Amsterdam: Eburon, pp. 89–114.

Noble Tesh, Sylvia 1990, *Hidden Arguments: Political Ideology and Disease Prevention*, New Brunswick, New Jersey: Rutgers University Press.

Page, Helan E. 1994, "Breaking the silence on violence in academe," *Anthropology Newsletter* 35(3):44.

PAN (Pesticide Action Network) 1992, " 'Pollute the poor,' argues World Bank economist," *Global Pesticide Campaigner* 2(2):14.

Parajuli, Pramod 1993, "Beyond India the 'Orient' or India the 'Underdeveloped': footpaths towards a non-dominating knowledge," paper presented at the SSRC Conference on Questions of Modernity: Postorientalist Discourse in the Middle East and South Asia. Cairo, ARE, May 28–30.

People's Assembly 1984, *Registry of the Twenty-Eighth Session of the Fourth Legislative Session*, Cairo (in Arabic).

Podgore, J. K. 1991, "Placebo-controlled double-blind study to determine the efficacy of topical niclosamide 1 percent lotion in the prevention of naturally occurring Schistosoma haematobium infection in Egyptian farmers engaged in irrigation," (unpublished proposal).

Rofel, Lisa 1992, "Rethinking modernity: space and factory discipline in China," *Cultural Anthropology* 7(1):93–114.

Roy, Delwin A. 1985, "Restructuring the political economy of Egypt: Ford Foundation economic policy in the 1970s," *Journal of South Asian and Middle Eastern Studies* 9(2):20–42.

Said, Edward 1987, "Foucault and the imagination of power," in D. C. Hoy (ed.), *Foucault: A Critical Reader*, Oxford: Basil Blackwell, pp. 149–56.

Sanjek, Roger 1993, "Anthropology's hidden colonialism: assistants and their ethnographers," *Anthropology Today* 9(2):13–18.

Sharabi, Hisham 1990, "The scholarly point of view: politics, perspective, paradigm," in H. Sharabi (ed.), *Theory, Politics and the Arab World*, Washington, D.C.: Georgetown University, Center for Contemporary Arab Studies, pp. 1–51.

Silverstein, Leni 1995, "Guest essay: feminist policies and anthropological perspectives at the International Conference on Population and Development (ICPD) Cairo, Egypt, September 5–13, 1994," *Anthropology Newsletter* 36(3):11.

Simons, Jon 1995, *Foucault and the Political*, New York: Routledge.

Spivak, Gyatri Chakravorty 1988, "Can the subaltern speak?," in C. Nelson and L. Grossberg (eds.), *Marxism and the Interpretation of Culture*, Chicago: University of Illinois Press, pp. 271–313.

Spurr, David 1993, *The Rhetoric of Empire: Colonial Discourse in Journalism, Travel Writing, and Imperial Administration*, Durham, North Carolina: Duke University Press.

Stebbins, Kenyon R. 1992, "Garbage imperialism: health implications of dumping hazardous wastes in Third World countries," *Medical Anthropology* 15:81–102.

WGNRR 1994, "Women's groups from the South demand to be heard," *Women's Global Network for Reproductive Rights Newsletter* 47:5–6.

5   Inscribing the body politic: women and AIDS in Africa

Brooke Grundfest Schoepf

Introduction

Research on gender relations in Africa has long been informed by "the understanding of knowledge as power and of the ability of those in power to create and define knowledge. This understanding was culturally shared in many hierarchically organized pre-colonial societies" (Schoepf 1992a:204). Medical knowledge was integral to power and control. With life-threatening disease and other afflictions ascribed to disorders of the body politic, medicalization extended over a wide field.

Nineteenth-century missionary Christianity spread western healing practices in sub-Saharan Africa; in the Belgian Congo, biomedicine became a central justifying trope of the colonial discourse (Schoepf 1976). Then as now, however, access to quality care was extremely limited. Biomedical epistemology, power and efficacy continue to be vigorously contested by other healing traditions (Janzen 1978; Feierman 1985; Schoepf 1976; 1991a; 1992c; Taylor 1992; Comaroff and Comaroff 1993). In Zaire, the state's ideology of "authenticity" legitimates the special powers popularly attributed to diviners and witch-finders, who frequently scapegoat women by blaming them as the cause of affliction (Schoepf 1976; 1986a).

In the presence of persistent medical pluralism, moralist discourse conveys alternative interpretations of health and disease. Discourse about bodies often encapsulates metaphors about the body politic (Douglas 1966). In the case of AIDS, the bodies are female. Public health action proceeds on a terrain of contested meanings where different knowledges struggle for control. In the process, both medicalization and demedicalization occur.

This chapter examines biomedical and popular discourses and practices in the context of the AIDS epidemic in sub-Saharan Africa, where 19.2 million people were estimated to be infected with the HIV virus by the end of 1995 (Mann and Tarantola 1996:11). Of these, 8.4

million had developed AIDS, including two million children.[1] Heterosexual intercourse is the principal mode of transmission, and more
women than men are infected. In many African cities between 5 and 40
percent of sexually active adults are already infected. Propelled by
poverty and power, the virus spreads rapidly to new populations
through trade, labor migration, and wars. Effective prevention involves
enabling many among the general population to alter sexual relations
that are widely considered to be normal, "natural," and highly valued.
Related to sex, reproduction, and death, AIDS in Africa is freighted
with extraordinary symbolic power. While fieldwork data presented here
come from Kinshasa, similarities with research in other countries
indicate their broader applicability (reviews in de Bruyn 1992; Schoepf
1993a).

Societal responses to the epidemic, including disease control policies,
are propelled by cultural politics forged in the history of relations
between Africa and the West. AIDS brings forth representations that
support and reproduce already constituted gender, color, class, and
national hierarchies (see Schoepf 1988; 1991a; 1991c; Schoepf,
Rukarangira et al. 1988a; 1988b).

I draw upon research begun in 1985 by the collaborative medical
anthropology team, CONNAISSIDA.[2] The acronym, composed of the
French words for knowledge and AIDS, signifies popular knowledge
and our own; both were heterodox and changing. A similarly dialogic
epistemology informed our research methodology. The goal was to
convey biological knowledge in culturally accessible forms so as to
enable people to assess and reduce their risk of AIDS (Schoepf,
Rukarangira and Matumona 1986; Schoepf 1986b).

Ethnographic methods generated textured, first-hand accounts,
probed for representations and meanings, situating AIDS within the
context of cultural frameworks of affliction and disease. A "political
economy and culture" approach examined intersections of social
structure and human agency at many levels. Research assistants were
trained in action-research, a practice methodology which uses group
dynamics and structured projective exercises to produce new data and
empower change.

Role plays and simulation games are a genre of "performative
ethnography" (see Fabian 1990). They enable people to transcend
normative conventions and reach for deeper layers of meaning.[3] Sharing
these experiences, workshop participants showed how gender relations,
poverty, and sexual meanings – particularly with respect to power,
personhood, and desire – contribute to knowledge of HIV transmission.
Community-based risk-reduction support stratagems were devised and

practiced (Schoepf, Walu, Rukarangira *et al.* 1991; Schoepf 1992a; 1992b; 1993b; 1995a). Empowerment workshops also can provide a context for people to analyze broader issues related to health, household economics, and social justice and to organize for change (Hope *et al.* 1984). CONNAISSIDA demonstrated the usefulness for HIV prevention of a methodology which departs from informants' own knowledge of daily life, and links participant-observation of microlevel interaction to analysis of the macrolevel context.

Life histories of women are another way to understand why HIV infection spreads (Schoepf 1992b). They shed light on the social production and cultural construction of HIV risk. They show how women in various social settings resist infection within the limits of the possible. They reveal ways that stigmatizing discourse and practices of "race," gender, and class structure the epidemic in national and international arenas, acting to disempower women and diminish the effectiveness of their resistance to oppressive forms of medicalization. The practice methodology further demonstrates the possibilities and limits of women's resistance to infection. This knowledge "from below" is crucial both to understanding the spread of infection and to its prevention.

Together the methods also indicate ways that popular knowledges fuel misconceptions that public health campaigns must address. Personal narratives aid in understanding: "the ambiguities of everyday life . . . the overarching constraints of social structure on human agency, and the complex relationship of individual psychology to a culture-bounded social order" (Marks 1989:39).

Scholars recognize that both narrator and interpreter shape accounts of lived experience through the double filters of their respective consciousness. Their agendas may be distinct and not always compatible (Mbilinyi 1989; Romero 1988; Mizra and Strobel 1989; Personal Narratives Group 1989), particularly when the interpreter is also a translator. In this case however, compatibility appears to be high. My political agenda was made explicit to key informants. I sought to contextualize the social epidemiology of AIDS in Zaire as a means of widening discussion of international AIDS control policy, then dominated by epidemiologists and other biomedically trained Euro-American white men. I hypothesized that life histories could demonstrate how broad issues of gender relations, poverty, and development strategies are involved in preventing the spread of HIV. Women who told their stories were aware of these aims, and did not hesitate to express their own views.[4] A summary of the social epidemiology of AIDS in Kinshasa helps to situate the narratives.

Social epidemiology of AIDS

Disease epidemics generally erupt in times of crisis and AIDS is no exception. Most of sub-Saharan Africa, and much of the Third World, is in the throes of economic decline. While Zaire is probably a worst-case scenario, for many African nations falling terms of trade for tropical exports, the contradictions of distorted neo-colonial economies, with rapid class-formation and burdensome debt service have created permanent, ever-deepening macrolevel crisis. Zaire's crisis began in 1974 with the fall of the price of copper, the major export, and was fueled by widespread, crippling corruption. Per capita incomes are ranked among the world's lowest, averaging an estimated $150 per year in 1987 (World Bank 1989), and declining since. Moreover, average figures mask wide disparities in wealth. As Structural Adjustment Policies (SAP) shifted the burden of payment to users, already deficient health services became prohibitively expensive and school attendance declined. Many families in Kinshasa ate only once a day in the mid-1980s and malnutrition was widespread.

In the 1990s, hyperinflation and political violence destroyed the major industrial and commercial infrastructure of Kinshasa and other cities. The numbers of unemployed grew and the absorptive capacity of the already crowded informal sector diminished, becoming increasingly less profitable for many small operators. Incomes of the vast majority were outpaced by the cost of basic necessities and services. Many who could just scrape by in 1987 had fallen into more extreme poverty by 1990. Ever more desperate economic conditions since that time have shredded the social fabric formerly held together by extended kin networks. Banditry and gendered violence increased, with the poorly paid military cited as the worst offenders. Not only the poor, but many formerly middle-class families were reduced to "zones of non-existence."[5] Religious revivalism pervades both established and independent churches. The effects of grinding poverty upon the poorest who have abandoned hope are unknown.

Throughout Africa, poor women and children have experienced most severely the effects of structural adjustment policies and the deepening crisis. Economic crisis, the structure of employment, and laws inherited from the colonial period shape the present sociocultural configuration. They contribute to male dominance, to the feminization of poverty and consequently to the spread of AIDS (Schoepf 1988; Schoepf and Walu 1991; Schoepf, Walu, Russell and Schoepf 1991; Walu 1991). Although Zaire's cities contain as many women as men, women constitute only 4 percent of formal sector workers. An estimated 40–60 percent of urban men are without waged employment. They, and the majority of women who are without special job qualifications or political connections, resort to informal sector occupations. These include petty trade, food preparation, market gardening, sewing, domestic work, smuggling, and prostitution, occupations that yield very low incomes for most of those who practice them. Produce trade and smuggling take place over long distances within Zaire and across its borders. Women who are politically protected can earn high profits; they can sometimes avoid the multiple-partner sexual relationships that regularly accompany such trade (Schoepf 1978; Rukarangira and Schoepf 1991; Schoepf and Walu 1991).

Informants who formerly relied upon steady contributions from male sex partners or from their extended families reported that these sources had dwindled since others, too, are hard-pressed to make ends meet. Sexual patron–client relations and multiple partner strategies that maximize women's returns became crucial to survival. The health consequences of untreated "classic" sexually transmitted diseases (STDs) became much more serious because their presence increases HIV risk.

The presence of AIDS among Zaireans was identified in 1983. Infection is concentrated primarily in the cities, but has spread along trade routes to the rural areas. Not surprisingly, poor young urban women are at highest risk. More than 80 percent of poor prostitutes – women whose major source of subsistence comes from the sale of sex to multiple casual partners – are reported to be infected in several African cities. In Kinshasa the rate among sex workers rose from 27 percent of those tested in 1985 to 35 percent in 1988 (Nzila *et al.* 1991).

Commercial sex workers, however, are not the only women at risk. Samples of women delivering in Kinshasa hospitals in 1986 found 6 to 8 percent HIV infected (N'Galy *et al.* 1988; 1989; Ryder *et al.* 1989). Nearly 40 percent of infants born to seropositive women were infected and the majority died before the age of two years. Most of the mothers were married. Mothers age 20 to 30 years were most likely to be seropositive. Rates among women in this age group with formal sector jobs were higher still: 16.7 percent of hospital workers and 11.1 percent of textile factory workers tested were infected in 1986. Most were single and were paid below-subsistence wages. In Kigali, Rwanda, 30 percent of mothers were seropositive at delivery in 1986; the majority reported that they had had a single lifetime sexual partner (Lindan *et al.* 1991).

In sum, not only sex workers but many women of childbearing age are at high risk, as are young girls, many of whom are infected at first coitus. Without economic independence and social autonomy, most women can neither refuse risky sex nor impose condom use upon their partners. At some levels gender relations are subject to negotiation, but women's efforts to improve their condition take place in circumstances not of their own making. Public health campaigns can help to improve these circumstances or can render women's struggles more difficult.

Discourse about women and AIDS

The first two women on record as probably having died of HIV infection contracted in Zaire were a Zairian from Equator Region, and a surgeon from Denmark who worked in the same region in the 1970s. The contrast in the descriptions of the two women's lives in the biomedical literature is striking. The texts and their silences speak to cultural constructions of AIDS.

The Zairian woman is reported to have lived for some years as a "free woman" (meaning a woman not under the control of a father, brother, or husband),[6] in Kinshasa, where she is assumed to have been a prostitute. She then returned to the village, where her blood was collected in 1976 in a study of Ebola hemorrhagic fever. The woman died several years later of an AIDS-like disease, as did a 15-year-old youth. Three other people in the sample also had HIV antibodies, for a prevalence rate of 0.8 percent (Nzila et al. 1988).

The Danish woman practiced for several years at a mission hospital in the great forest. Because surgical gloves were in short supply, she often operated ungloved. Swollen glands without apparent cause were followed by a series of unusual infections, a cough, fever, and constant fatigue. Too weak to work, and worried by her inconclusive diagnosis, she returned to Denmark, where repeated diagnostic tests failed to establish a cause or a name for the mysterious symptoms. Her condition was described by a physician-friend who observed her long illness (Bygbjerg 1983). The anonymous African woman, by contrast, was mentioned only in an epidemiological report.

Juxtaposing the two texts of these presumed cases from the "pre-AIDS era" allows us to compare their underlying premises. The Zairian woman is assumed to have acquired the HIV while in Kinshasa and transmitted infection to others as a result of sexual intercourse. The Danish surgeon (also a "free woman" in the technical meaning of the term) is assumed to have acquired the disease from a patient's blood – in a rural area of stable low seroprevalence. The report is silent about the possibility that she might have transmitted infection to others. Different constructions of characteristics implicitly attributed to the women on the basis of gender, class, and color emerge.

The resulting dichotomies are Cartesian in their simplicity: white woman/black woman; missionary/sinner; heroic work/dirty work; innocent victim/perpetrator; valued, named/unvalued, unnamed; good woman/bad woman. In short, they form the prototypical we/other couplet, redoubled by the saint/whore dichotomy of western sexual morality. The possibility that an African woman presumed to be a sex worker might have acquired the infection from a blood transfusion is not entertained.[7] The possibility that a white professional woman might have become infected through sexual intercourse – in Zaire, or in Europe – is not entertained either. Unprotected by gloves or condoms, the occupations of both women carry considerable risk when background prevalence rises. Nevertheless, either of them might have become infected in the manner assumed for the other.

In the US, biomedical discourse is replete with metacommunication about gender, "race," and class prevalent in the wider society. It enters into clinical decision-making, shapes the ways patients, physicians, and the public view themselves and others, and influences public health policy (Schoepf 1969; 1975; 1979). This is especially the case with STDs (Brandt 1988). Freighted with emotionally charged issues of sex, blood, and death, AIDS is only the newest of disease metaphors in Western society.[8] It has unleashed stigmatizing metadiscursive practices and social action in both local and international arenas and within African nations as well.

Western popular and biomedical accounts of AIDS contain numerous examples of racist discourse about African cultures; these in turn have provoked defensive responses from African leaders and peoples (references in Schoepf 1991a; 1991b; 1991c). With Africa designated as the source of AIDS, exotic customs have been held responsible for passage of the virus from monkeys to humans and the sexuality of Africans has been characterized as "promiscuous" and different from that of peoples elsewhere. This discourse rapidly traveled to Africa via international news media and diffused from elites to masses. Western racism contributed to denial of AIDS by African leaders and slowed efforts to halt the spread of infection, as both leaders and publics defended African personhood against the stigmatizing attacks.

AIDS also became a stigmatizing condition within Africa, where popular and biomedical sentiment cast prostitutes as the major "reservoir" of disease. Stigma and anxiety led to denial of risk and to distancing, not only from the afflicted but from their families. As women in Kinshasa were aware by 1987, the majority of women are put at risk by their spouses. Since AIDS affects the general population of sexually active adults and adolescents, narrowly focused prevention strategies are not likely to stop the spread of infection.[9] Instead, because they associate AIDS with the stigma of prostitution, they increase the denial of risk and impede realistic prevention measures.[10]

In 1987 people began to report changes in their sexual lifestyles. In Kinshasa, monthly condom sales by a social marketing project rose to 300,000 per month in June 1988; nation-wide condom sales rose to 16 million in 1991. Condoms were used mainly by educated young men in casual encounters with women defined as prostitutes (Rukarangira and Schoepf 1989). This success notwithstanding, vignettes presented in the next section illustrate persistent obstacles to change which an effective prevention program must address. Each woman is from a different ethnic group; each story illustrates a common risk situation in which class differences exist but are not always what might be expected owing to gender inequality. Many obstacles identified in Kinshasa are common elsewhere in Africa.

Women at risk

In 1987 **Nsanga** was 26 and very poor. She had a 5-year-old girl and a boy aged 8, starting primary school. A younger sister also lived with Nsanga in the single room, part of a corrugated-iron-roofed block surrounding an open courtyard. The yard contained a shared water tap, a roofless bathing stall and a latrine, but no electricity. Nsanga and her neighbors washed their clothes, children, dishes, and vegetables in the courtyard. In good weather they moved their charcoal stoves outdoors to cook.

In this neighborhood typical of the poor quarters of Kinshasa, waste runs into the open drain in the lane. Yards, markets, and streets are unpaved; latrine pits are uncovered. Dust containing fecal matter blows in the dry season; latrines overflow in torrential rains. Malaria, intestinal worms, and diarrheal diseases are common; child mortality is high.

Nsanga wasn't always the head of her household. Village-raised, she married a schoolteacher in 1980, and managed – somehow – on his skimpy salary, despite galloping inflation of nearly 100 percent each year. In 1983 the IMF instituted a series of "economic recovery" measures designed to reduce government expenditures so that Zaire, like other Third World nations whose leaders had borrowed heavily in the 1970s, could make payments on its international debt. Support for public services fell sharply; user fees climbed. More than 80,000 teachers and health workers were made redundant by this "*assainisse-ment*" in 1984.[11] Nsanga's husband was one of those who, lacking a powerful patron to intercede for him, swelled the ranks of the unemployed. After six fruitless months of waiting in offices, his morale fell. He began to drink, selling off the household appliances to pay for beer and then *lutuku,* a cheap home-distilled alcohol. Nsanga berated him for wasting money; their relationship deteriorated. Often drunk and despondent, he beat his wife and children.

Meanwhile, Nsanga tried many things to earn money. Like most poor women in Kinshasa, she had had only a few years of formal schooling, and, like her husband, she was without powerful friends or relatives. Unable to find waged employment, Nsanga cooked food for men working in her neighborhood, she sold uncooked rice in small quantities and dried fish when she could obtain supplies cheaply. These efforts brought in only pennies at a time. She grew vegetables in a vacant lot, but soldiers stole her crop. In 1986 her husband left and Nsanga did not know of his whereabouts. When the children ate up her food stocks, she went into debt for the rent. She asked her elder brother for a loan, but he refused, pleading poverty. Although he had a steady job on the docks, he had two wives and nine children.

Without new start-up capital, exchanging sex for subsistence seemed the obvious solution. The first year Nsanga became a concubine or *"deuxième bureau,"* "occupied" by a lover who paid her rent and provided regular support. She also had occasional "spare tires" to help out. Then she got pregnant. Her *occupant* left. His salary couldn't stretch that far, he told her. Nsanga had to take on more partners – a fairly typical downward slide. The neighborhood rate was 50 cents per brief encounter in 1987 and Nsanga said that when she was lucky she could find two or three partners per working day, for a total of $30 a month – at most. Most were men whom she knew who returned several times each month; as her friends, they did not label her a prostitute.

Nsanga's new baby was sickly and died before her second birthday, following prolonged fever, diarrhea, and skin rashes. Nsanga believed it was because semen from so many men spoiled her milk. She reported a few bouts of STD for which she took tetracycline pills from the drugstore. In 1988 she had abdominal pains for several months, but without money to consult a doctor, she again self-medicated. Nsanga says that the European nuns at the neighborhood dispensary do not treat STDs. Diagnosis at the nearby university clinic in 1987 cost the equivalent of thirty encounters. None of the women Nsanga knew could afford quality biomedical health care.

Asked about condoms, Nsanga said that she had heard of but never actually seen one. She knew that men use them to prevent disease when they have sex with prostitutes. Nsanga rejected this morally stigmatizing label: "if a lover were to propose a condom, I would be angry. It would mean that he doesn't trust me." Many men now avoid sex workers because the government and mass media have warned against "prostitutes" as a source of infection. But in her own eyes and those of her lovers, Nsanga was not a prostitute, not a "bad woman." On the contrary, as a mother fallen on hard times through no fault of her own, she was trying her best, "breaking stones" (*kobeta libanga*), to meet family obligations. In the presence of HIV, however, Nsanga's survival strategy was transformed into a death strategy.[12]

In 1989 Nsanga became very thin and believed that people were whispering about her. In fact, her neighbors were sure Nsanga had AIDS. But then, Nsanga reasoned: "People say this about everyone who loses weight, even when it is just from hunger and worry. All these people who are dying nowadays, are they really all dying from AIDS?" Her defensiveness was shared by numerous women in similar circumstances, women for whom denial is a stratagem for coping with situations they see no way to change.

Tango is a college graduate who worked for twenty years for a European-owned firm in a high-visibility, gender-typed position. Her job demanded considerable technical and public relations skills. Unmarried, with a slim figure and wearing stylish European clothes, Tango had a succession of lovers. These included fellow-students and older professional men, Africans and expatriates. In 1986 Tango became pregnant and decided to keep the child, rather than seek an illegal abortion from a doctor in her network. Although her ethnic tradition strongly discouraged premarital pregnancy and imposed heavy sanctions on unwed mothers, Tango's parents were delighted with her decision.[13] They reasoned that she was unlikely to marry and would not have many more opportunities to bear a child to name after them.

The infant was robust, healthy, and much loved. When he was a year old, Tango was hospitalized for pneumonia, one type of which is frequently associated with AIDS. The sickness dragged on and she lost weight; tongues began to wag. Tango became frightened. Then she reassured herself: "My child is not sick; therefore I am not infected." After six months her health improved. Further reassured, she resisted HIV testing. Protracted sickness and the deaths of a former lover and numerous acquaintances nevertheless made her prudent. Although she did not believe widespread rumours to the effect that condoms are injurious to women's health, she had read that condoms do not provide 100 percent protection.[14] Tango preferred to forego sex altogether: "I have my child to think of," she said.

Tango remained unmarried by choice. She refused to place herself in the subordinate status and disadvantageous situations that marriage imposes on women. Before she learned of AIDS, Tango believed she had the best possible sort of life available to a woman without wealthy parents. She had a moderate-paying job which she enjoyed, health insurance, vacation travel, a low-rent apartment in the center of town, many friends and relations in the city, and the moral support of her parents living in a distant city. Tango also enjoyed having lovers, with dinner dates, dancing, and gifts. She suffered none of the heartbreak that comes from deep emotional involvement with one (she believed, inevitably) unfaithful man; no jealousy of rivals, nor the galling burden of having to support and care for children while their father divides his resources among several women.

Tango said that she missed both sexual satisfaction and the luxuries which her lovers provided. Trade might have brought additional income, but her private-sector job was too demanding. Unlike many people in government employment, Tango could not take time off to conduct business on the side. "Besides, everyone is selling something these days and nobody has money to buy." Tango voiced a common complaint. Whether she remained unflaggingly celibate is unknown, but because Tango was single and could manage on her salary, the choice was hers to make. If she decided to take a lover she could insist on regular condom use.

In 1985 Tango and her friends dismissed AIDS as an "Imaginary Syndrome Invented to Discourage Lovers."[15] Which lovers were being discouraged? Africans, of course. By whom? Europeans of course. Why? Because they believe that Africans have too much sex. Really, they are jealous! This denial served as a cultural defense against stigma. Then there were too many cases reported by physician-friends working at the three major hospitals in Kinshasa. Early in 1987 people in their relatively privileged circle acknowledged AIDS as real, fatal, and sexually transmitted. Some began to use condoms in casual encounters and with friends.

Tango and women like her are unusual. Owing to their relative economic and psychological independence, they can dispose of their sexuality and negotiate condom use. Since learning about AIDS, they have reduced significantly their level of risk. Not all employed single women are so fortunate. Most earn very low wages and often sexual clientship is a condition of employment or promotion. For Tango and several of her friends and colleagues, however, knowledge of AIDS came too late. Tango died in 1991 of "a long and painful illness," the euphemism used to speak of AIDS. Friends described Tango as "a saint," owing to her uncomplaining resignation in the throes of great pain and knowledge of impending death. A sister now cares for her son.

Vumba was a nurse who, aged 25 in 1987, earned $35 per month. She grew up in Kinshasa and is single, without children. She lived with her widowed mother and two younger sisters, still in school. The rent for two rooms in a courtyard very much like the one where Nsanga lives was $11. This courtyard had electricity, however, and Vumba split the bill with her neighbors. She paid $5 per month to run two dim lights, a two-coil hotplate, a radio, a fan, and an old refrigerator. (Nsanga had lost all these middle-class conveniences.) Vumba's mother sold beer in the yard, "but with everybody selling, there is very little profit." She looked around for something else to sell that would make more money. Meanwhile, Vumba was the family's mainstay.

She had a lover, a clerical worker who earned less than she. Although they had been together for nearly five years, he was in no hurry to get married. Vumba reasoned that he probably saw no advantage to marrying, since she would still have to use her pay to support her mother and sisters. She said she had talked to him about using condoms but he had refused: "'Because they aren't natural.' He said that condoms would interfere with his pleasure. He has never tried one, but friends who have complained they get less feeling. They say 'it's like eating a banana with the skin on,' or 'taking a shower in a raincoat.'[16] They want to go skin-to-skin." Her lover already had children with another woman and had no objection to Vumba taking contraceptive pills. In her experience this was unusual, and was an indication that he was "not serious about us, because children are the seal of a marriage."

In 1986 hospital workers were screened for HIV. Vumba was among those found seropositive. When she learned of her test results, Vumba was devastated, but when we visited in March, 1989, there were no signs of disease. Had she told her lover? "No, of course not. If he knew, he would probably disappear. I proposed to use condoms, but since he refused, the consequences are his lookout! (*Son affaire!*) Where do you think I got it, anyway?"

Vumba's defensiveness seemed related to her situation of relative powerlessness. Since many infected persons were shunned by friends and even by some family members, Vumba's behavior was self-protective. Like many people, she believed that sexual pleasure is essential to health and well-being. Moreover, Vumba believed that worry about AIDS would bring on the disease.

Actually Vumba *had* had other partners (she said she didn't remember how many). She began having sex in nursing school at age 17. Because she did not experience satisfaction in those encounters, she put them out of her mind. Vumba liked to dress well. In 1987 a 6 yard length of locally made wax print fabric and tailoring for an ensemble (blouse and two *pagnes*) cost two months' salary. By 1988, people had another name for AIDS (SIDA) that encapsulated their understanding of its social epidemiology: *Salaire Insuffisant Depuis des Années.* Moreover, Vumba said that sexual harassment at work was common. "The doctors . . . can cause endless complications for a nurse who refuses their advances." She heard that several doctors were infected, too. Quite a few were no longer at the hospital and two were said to have died of AIDS.

Vumba was afraid of the pain and the wasting. She was sad that she had not borne children, for "without offspring, one can never become an ancestor." Thus Vumba feared that she would die "an insignificant person" whose name would be forgotten, because she had no children to name their children after her. Because childbearing is so central to the female role and sense of self, many HIV-infected women become pregnant despite counselling. Not only do their husbands and families demand children; many women's self-esteem requires that they become mothers.

Vumba had other worries, too: "what will become of my younger sisters?" With many wealthy men looking for younger and younger partners whom they believe less likely to be infected, the temptations for girls from poor families are very strong. The deepening crisis leaves less money to pay school fees, buy clothes, and bribe poorly paid teachers to give them passing grades. Did her sisters know about condoms? Vumba wasn't sure. She hadn't told them, because she didn't want them to think she was encouraging them to have sex. Perhaps they learned about condom protection from Franco's song?[17] Vumba sighed:

Even if they know about *les Prudences* [this social marketing brand name became a popular euphemism for condoms], what's the use? Men won't use the things and the girls can't make them. Anyway, a young girl would be ashamed to ask her friend to use a condom. He would think she was a prostitute! It's the same as with birth control pills.

Men's disparagement of condoms and women's need for both economic support and social respectability increases sexual risk. Vumba's narrative underscores the need for activities which can effectively increase women's financial independence and their sense of self-worth, and lead to social empowerment over the long term.

Avoidance, denial, and notions of propriety combine with gender inequality to increase young women's vulnerability. Although at least half the adolescents in Kinshasa are sexually active by age 17 (Bertrand, Bakutuvwidi *et al.* 1991), many adults do not consider their sexuality legitimate. Their voices are silenced and parents avoid the subject. For many adolescent women, desire does not enter in; they are socialized for submission and frequently coerced into sex (Schoepf 1978; Verhaegen 1990; Walu 1992). Anatomical and physiological immaturity of the adolescent reproductive tract renders sex with older men, abusive or not, who may be HIV-infected, extremely risky. Together, these factors, rather than hormones raging out of control, explain why HIV spreads rapidly among poor adolescent women.

Mbeya was a stylish, carefully groomed woman in her late forties. She wore heavy gold jewelry, ensembles of imported Dutch wax print fabric, expensive handbags and matching shoes. She often drove a vintage Mercedes herself; a chauffeur ran errands and drove her youngest child to school. Three elder children studied at universities abroad.

Mbeya's husband was for many years an important figure in the ruling party's inner circle. For such men, the company of stylish young women is a perquisite of the job, part of the socializing integral to politics. Mistresses are often involved in the intelligence-gathering networks which no man in high politics can do without. The government's ideology of "authenticity," promulgated partly in order to undermine the influence of the Catholic Church, made both formal and informal polygyny respectable. As in the slaving period prior to this century, access to numerous women is a symbol of power and wealth. Mbeya said that she accepted her situation as a co-wife: "I was not too jealous because my husband always respected me as the first wife . . . and kept his other women away from the house. He never brought home any dirty diseases, either. There was plenty of money and I never felt done out of my rights. I have been very lucky, unlike many of my friends whose husbands are unfaithful." Mbeya spoke of her friend Anita, who couldn't abide her wealthy husband's public display of his outside wives and lovers: "Anita harangued him about this so much that finally he left. She divorced him, but he got back at her for insulting him publicly like that. He forbade their children to visit their mother when they came home from school in Europe . . . Everyone wonders why *that* man hasn't succumbed to AIDS!"

The fact that some notorious *coureurs* have remained healthy, and that some people get sick while their spouses do not, causes confusion. The lengthy period between disease and visible symptoms is not well understood. AIDS' apparent arbitrariness reinforces beliefs that implicate fate, luck, ancestral spirits, and sorcery in disease causation and contributes to denial of sexual risk. Nevertheless, Anita's former husband died in 1992 "of a long and painful illness." People expressed pity for his newest young wife whom they assumed to be infected.

In 1987 a wealthy physician-businessman living on Mbeya's street and two of his wives were reported to have died from AIDS. Neighbors blamed the first wife because she traded on her own account, traveling to Nigeria to purchase household appliances on commission for friends and acquaintances. Mbeya reflected: "It could just as well have been the husband who gave *her* AIDS! Who knows what younger wives do when their husband is away? And did he only sleep with his wives? After all, a doctor has many opportunities! Men are always quick to blame women, especially when women earn their own money!" AIDS has entered the complex terrain of gender struggles and competing moral discourses. Mbeya and her friends wondered where AIDS came from. They rejected the notion that the virus jumped to humans from monkey's blood purportedly used in love magic. They wondered if, as they had heard, the virus came to Africa from America (see Schoepf 1995b).

Several "traditional" healers claim that AIDS is an old disease which has become epidemic because women no longer observe the old sexual customs, such as fidelity and ritual bathing following intercourse. However, in Mbeya's ethnic group, as in many others, high-status women formerly controlled their own sexuality. "Tradition" has been reinvented many times over in aid of controlling women. A similar moral discourse emerged as some evangelical clergymen claimed AIDS to be a divine punishment which would strike down fornicators, leaving the innocent safe. Rejecting moralistic constructions in favor of a biomedical explanation, Mbeya said, and her friends agreed: "Innocent, monogamous wives can't keep husbands safe, so husbands pass infection on to them. And frequently a woman can't remain with just one partner throughout her lifetime. Men are most often the ones who repudiate their spouses, or die and leave them widowed and destitute."

In May 1987 Mbeya's husband brought home the first official notice about AIDS and left it on her bedside table. Mbeya laughed as she told us: "He just left it there, without saying anything." Although concerned, she was afraid to broach the subject of condom protection. "He would think I was accusing him." I spoke with her husband and several other officials at a funeral in August of that year. Despite the fact that they had received information from AIDS researchers well in advance of the general public, denial was their principal response.

Even elite women's knowledge is not always accompanied by the power to act. Toward the end of 1988, Mbeya became aware that her husband was sick and not getting any better. She began to suspect that it might be AIDS, and told him that she wanted to use condoms. Her husband refused. So she said that they should stop sexual relations. Her husband's family was outraged and he refused this, too. They threatened to throw her out and to take her youngest daughter. Mbeya acquiesced. Following her husband's death in 1990, her in-laws accused her of infecting him. Like many who give limited credence to biological knowledge, they believe that STDs result from "medicines" used by husbands to punish wives' infidelity. Mbeya protested that she married as a young virgin straight from a convent school and that, all through the years, she was a faithful wife. Mbeya believed that her affines' accusations were motivated by their self-interest. "The property is too valuable! The house will be sold and the money shared among my husband's brothers."

Mbeya was forced to leave the luxurious villa. Her husband's family took legal possession of the house, furnishings, cars, businesses, and rental properties upon his death. Formerly, her husband's younger brother might have allowed her to live in the house with his family, even if he did not become her actual husband. Turned out of her home with nothing but her clothes, bereaved and fearing herself to be infected, Mbeya went to her brother's where she became a dependant in his household.

Mbeya's story illustrates the ephemeral nature of women's class position when based upon a husband's ownership of resources. Formerly the manager of an extended family household with twenty-two people to feed, clothe, and care for, Mbeya said that she had no energy or time to start a business for herself. As a widow, she envied women who trade and earn money. "I never dreamt I would need to do that myself!"

When I saw her in 1989, Mbeya had not gotten very far with her planning. Emotionally, she was still reeling from her husband's death and in no shape to face the future. Although many in her circle believed that Mbeya was HIV infected, she might not have been. Why hadn't Mbeya gone to be tested? Although her husband was treated with expensive drugs which doctors said prolonged his life, Mbeya knew of nobody who had recovered from AIDS. She did not believe that the indigenous medicine about which the local press waxed enthusiastic actually offered a cure: "Even the doctor who is trying it does not claim success." Intellectually, she knew that AIDS is fatal, and that if infected she would die eventually. However, Mbeya preferred not to think about that. "If I am seropositive, then worrying would bring on the disease," she said. Many people invoke this idea to explain why they avoid learning their serostatus. Mbeya died in 1992. Had her husband agreed to use condoms, or had she the resources to leave him, she might still be alive.

Gisèle was a European woman with a professional degree, whose husband was seconded to Zaire as a member of a technical assistance mission in 1975. She lived a fairly luxurious life which, although it did not match that enjoyed by Mbeya while her husband was alive, was of a higher standard than she would have attained in her own country. Some years ago, Gisèle suspended her professional career to devote her energies to child-rearing. With her fourth child turning 4, she was thinking about returning to Europe and resuming her career. Fear of AIDS also was a motivating factor.

Gisèle was aware that her husband took advantage of the opportunities for sexual adventures conferred by his position. One liaison actually seemed serious enough to threaten her marriage, when her husband rented an apartment for a *"deuxième bureau."* However, that affair ended when the woman had a baby with another partner. Gisèle believed that she had reason to fear HIV infection. Although she was tested and found negative, her husband refused the test. When last seen in 1989, Gisèle had not yet decided what to do.

The Catholic Archdiocese of Kinshasa advised condom protection in 1987 for those who could not follow Church proscriptions (Schoepf, Rukarangira *et al.* 1988a).[18] However, the Pope subsequently forbade their use. Gisèle's strong faith precluded her violating a papal directive. She thought of presenting her husband with two alternatives: testing-and-fidelity (assuming an HIV negative result) or abstinence, to be enforced by her departure for Europe with the children. In the latter event, Gisèle hoped she could get a job, but recognized that the economic slump in her own country rendered this problematic for a woman in her forties. If she were to obtain employment, it would doubtless be at a lower level than her former position. She hoped that her husband would help with support payments for their children. Then again, she reasoned, perhaps that would not be necessary. Like many African women in Kinshasa, Gisèle prayed that risk of AIDS might convince her husband of the advantages of mutually faithful monogamy. In 1991, when riots by the military in Kinshasa and other cities caused European embassies to repatriate their citizens, Gisèle and her family departed.

Malu was 30 in 1987, a member of the Protestant Mothers' Club that sought AIDS training from CONNAISSIDA. Pregnant at 19, she had married Michel, a carpenter. Their fourth child was born in 1986, and Malu was still breast-feeding.[19] During the period of post-partum sexual abstinence prescribed by her culture, Michel sought other sex partners. Malu said:

Before I knew about AIDS I considered myself lucky because Michel did not take a second wife. He didn't get involved. But now I am afraid. Maybe he got infected by one of those women? I wanted him to use condoms at home with me. Then we could have sex without spoiling my milk, but he wouldn't hear of it. He jumped at me, shouting, "What? Don't you trust me?"

In the workshop we practiced talking about family planning as a way to get men to listen to the idea of condoms, so I tried that. I said, "My husband, we have four lovely children now. We need money to feed them and keep them healthy. We need money to send them to school. We could wait until times are better to have more children. Perhaps we should use condoms?" Remembering the last time I had raised the subject, I was a little afraid. But the workshop gave me the confidence to cajole him gently, and gradually he came around. Maybe he was thinking that if he is infected his children will need their mother?[20] Anyway, he went out and got the *Prudences* and we learned to use them. He let me put them on, the way [two sex workers] showed us in the workshop.

This stratagem assumes the husband's "suspicion awareness" of HIV risk. Rather than provoking confrontation, it shelters AIDS behind talk about family planning to create a situation in which the husband does not lose face. In addition to Malu's own enhanced confidence and skills, her husband may have become more amenable as a result of discussion with other men whose wives participated in the workshops at their church. A third of the church Mothers' Club participants were successful with this stratagem. Another third decided that their risks were minimal, while husbands of the remaining third would brook no discussion. Some women in the workshops gained confidence to address prevention issues with their adolescent children; one took home condoms for them. Although sex education was formerly undertaken by other kin, and considered taboo between parents and offspring, these mothers decided that their responsibility for children's health included protection from AIDS.

This and other women's groups found ways to use their new knowledge at home and in the community, extending the culturally accepted female role without overt confrontation of gender subordination. In light of state-supported male domestic power and most women's inability to acquire other means of support, confrontation can endanger them both physically and materially.

Structure and agency

The narratives lend texture to epidemiological data. They confirm the fact that the HIV virus spreads not because of exotic cultural practices, but because of many situations of everyday life. They also confirm the observation that many women at risk are not engaged in commercial sex work, and that most situations of sexual risk are not under women's control. Many women in Kinshasa were aware that prevention involves much more than simply telling people how to avoid risk. The experts, however, were not listening to women. In the context of pervasive social inequality, women's knowledge did not bring them power.

From the outset, the international AIDS control effort was dominated by the authority and resource-mobilizing capacity of biomedicine. Advised by the World Health Organization's new Global Programme on AIDS, African AIDS prevention campaigns focused on prostitutes and "promiscuity," and relied upon health information to change sexual behavior. The messages employed what, in the minds of many, were implicitly gendered key words: they warned (men) to "avoid prostitutes" and (women) to "remain faithful to a single partner." Condom promotion was targeted to what were conceived as "high risk groups." The driving hypothesis – that the epidemic could be controlled by reducing sexual transmission among "core transmitters" (sex workers and their clients, particularly migrant workers and truckers) likely to transmit HIV to more than one other person – was taken from earlier (failed) STD campaigns. Although married women who contract infection from their husbands may infect a child or two, they are not considered significant in sustaining the epidemic.[21]

Technically, this strategy was correct – or would have been had high-status men also been targeted – at the outset of the epidemic. But public health campaigns did not begin until the epidemic was well established in central and east Africa. Since population-based surveys found 5 percent of sexually active people in Kinshasa and 18 percent in Kigali to be HIV-infected in 1986, the appropriate technical message was quite simple. Everyone who had had sex with more than one partner in the past five years needed to use condoms to protect current partners (Fineberg 1988). This idea was uncongenial to many powerful men. The official campaign remained silent about personal risk assessment and the need for many to use condoms at home. It failed to address either the meanings in which AIDS is embedded or the political economy driving the pandemic. While its claim to an authoritative account was rejected on many fronts, stigmatizing moral discourse implicit in the official public health campaign was elaborated by many church leaders, lay moralists, and "traditional" healers (Schoepf 1988; 1992c; 1993b). In the face of competing discourses, the (bio)-medicalization of public health had unintended, although hardly unforeseen, consequences.

From the outset social scientists understood that information would not be sufficient to change complexly motivated behaviors leading to AIDS risk (Schoepf 1986b; Schoepf, Rukarangira and Matumona 1986). Indeed, studies made throughout the world find that mass media campaigns have increased knowledge of AIDS but seldom lead to widespread risk reduction. Nor do they change the situations that place people at risk.

Reid (1992) charges the biomedical community with a failure of epistemic responsibility because knowledge of women's risk was not investigated. Upon reflection, however, the physicians' failure to listen to independent-minded social scientists appears to have been over-determined, propelled by racism and sexism, by failures of political will at several levels, and by the self-interest of some researchers and bureaucrats, as well as by the arrogance of power (Schoepf 1991a; 1993a; 1995b).[22] With the help of the international donor community which channeled funds solely through health ministries, AIDS prevention was medicalized to the exclusion of other knowledges. Sexuality was constructed as a biologically driven individual behavior, divorced from culturally significant meanings, from social relations, from affect, and from power. People, objectified as "vectors" and "targets," were treated as empty vessels to be filled with "the facts" of health information.[23] Science was constructed solely as that which could be quantified through survey questionnaires. Ethnographic knowledge, deemed "merely anecdotal," revealed unwelcome complexities which, because they were not addressed, hampered prevention.

Preliminary findings led CONNAISSIDA to suggest that non-medical community-based animators be trained to use participatory methods to initiate talk about sexual health, AIDS prevention, gender, and culture change in a wide variety of settings. We proposed to involve members of revolving credit associations, clan gatherings, sports clubs, trade unions, youth groups, and market women's and business associations. We suggested workplaces, public conveyances, busy inter-sections, markets, and courtyards as possible sites for interactive problem-solving. The Zaire Government, through the Ministry of Higher Education and Scientific Research, approved the action-research for a period of five years, and in 1987 the Rockefeller Foundation granted three years' funding.[24]

The relationship between power and performance has been theorized for societies like Zaire in which brutal colonial domination was followed by quasi-totalitarian regimes. In these societies "the expression of opinion, social criticism and the free play of the imagination are severely restricted" (Fabian 1990:17–18). As used here, "performance" desig-nates both the ways people enact and become conscious of, or "realize," their culture, and the ways that anthropologists produce knowledge of cultures. Performance ethnography can be liberating for both anthro-pologists and informants who share in its production and thereby reap the fruits. So it was for us – for a time. Reflection about AIDS prevention as a matter of family and community survival enabled many people to come to terms with sexual risk, and to find creative ways to change their culture.

The Health Ministry suspended the project in April 1988. It appeared that some researchers envied the international attention attracted by this non-medical project; various officials sought to gain control of our funds. Privately I was told that, faced with the growing strength of pro-democracy forces, the regime had become increasingly concerned with security. CONNAISSIDA's community-based work could not survive in the political environment of Zaire.[25]

Ten years later, participatory, empowering prevention methods remain pertinent globally (Schneider and Stoller 1995), and the importance of non-medical avenues for prevention is internationally recognized. The feminist international health community has brought gender issues and women's empowerment to the fore. Some projects have adopted variants of the training-for-transformation approach to HIV/AIDS prevention in Africa.[26] Most recently, WHO's AIDS Communications Unit has issued a gender-oriented packet of experiential workshop guidelines (de Bruyn *et al.* 1995). Whether the non-governmental organizations to which these materials are addressed are able to use the approach creatively in a non-judgmental, sex-positive manner remains to be seen.[27] The AIDS crisis, with its myriad family tragedies and wide socioeconomic impact, may provide an impetus for culture change.

Conclusion

The spread of AIDS is determined by power/knowledge relations in the global and national political economy, culture, and society, as well as by the actions of individuals and groups. Given the wider context of gender relations and the enduring commitment of many men to the domination of wives, employees, and other women who fall within their power, the ability of women to avoid risky sex is a function of their ability to support themselves. Africa's ever-deepening economic crisis has fallen most heavily upon poor women, making economic opportunity scarcer, reducing the already low returns from petty trade, raising the cost of services, and reducing social support networks. Abating the HIV/AIDS epidemic requires fundamental changes in international development policies, national political economies, and state–society relations, as well as changes in domestic relations and social interaction.

This does not mean that nothing can be done in the absence of gender equality and social justice. Although poor women generally must dig deep to find their power, where popular initiatives are allowed to develop, collectives may discover options that allow women to overcome many obstacles, and group support can override women's socialization for subordination. The most likely arenas are in the traditional spheres of female activity, such as caretaking. Collectives which seek to empower wider social change require political space.

The narratives, and especially the workshops with their problem-oriented performances, suggest possibilities for developing local countercurrents of resistance to dominant ideologies and structures. Neither gender roles nor sexual relationships are static. While alternative discourses and practices at the local level do not alter power relationships pervading the wider society, they enable people to assess critically the sources of their oppression and to forge alliances based on newly perceived common interests.

The critical political space for change is not available in Zaire today. Although popular despair is deeper than ever, Zaire's pro-democracy movement has not yet won power. With support from international capital, the Mobutu dictatorship, the most long-lived in postcolonial Africa, and arguably the most corrupt, continues its many forms of political repression. New discourses of "tradition" in which women are scapegoated have emerged. Rape is used for men's personal satisfaction and as a political tool. In settings where human rights are violated routinely, collective action for health or for more egalitarian gender relations is unlikely to flourish.

The international public health effort initially avoided fundamental issues of the global economy and inequality which fuel the pandemic. It relied upon "messages" from biomedical authorities to reduce sexual transmission. Since communication systems are social systems, reception of information and the power to act on information received are differentially distributed. Official discourses generally mirror, reinforce, and reproduce structures of control. Recognized as such, they may generate counterhegemonic discourses of resistance.

When eventually they were heard, public health messages aimed primarily at low-status "target groups" increased their stigmatization. Fear of stigma contributed to denial of risk by many. Without widespread implementation of gender-sensitive community-based prevention strategies, the incidence of new HIV infections will continue to follow differences in power and knowledge.

Culturally informed empowering education which builds upon both biomedical knowledge and popular social knowledge is one necessary but not sufficient requisite of AIDS prevention or of any health and development strategy. The effects of deepening crisis, declining incomes, and rampant inflation are too pervasive to be resolved at the level of local communities; they continue to limit the possibilities of even highly motivated individuals to alter their behavior. Life history materials illustrate ways in which the condition of women, culturally constructed gender relations, and concepts of personhood are related to these processes.

Gender relations are emblematic of the process of capital accumulation which drains resources away from the villages, and upward from the urban poor to national ruling classes and outward to world markets. Analysis of texts and discourse about AIDS in the international arena provides a window on the contextual framing of historical and contemporary relations between Africa and the West. Sexual aspects of cultural politics continue to contribute ideological justification for inequality. Both the noise and the silences they create influence the spread of HIV. With its multilayered meanings, AIDS has inscribed the body politic on the bodies of women, creating, in the process, new forms of both medicalization and resistance.

NOTES

1 The Harvard AIDS Coalition estimates are higher than those of WHO, which placed the number of people infected or sick with AIDS at 14 million in November 1996 (Piot, cited by Altman 1996), up by 2 million from the end of 1994 (WHO/GPA 1995).

2 I wish to express my gratitude to colleagues of the core team composed of Professor Payanzo Ntsomo, sociologist, Dr. Rukarangira wa Nkera, public health specialist, Ms. Walu Engundu, anthropologist, and Claude Schoepf, development economist. None is responsible for the work presented here.

3 These characteristics set the method apart from "focus groups" favored by public health researchers as a technique for generating qualitative data.

4 A set of life histories of women collected in Lubumbashi and Kinshasa in 1977–9 found similarly compatible aims.

5 The phrase was coined by Professor Ilunga Kabongo in a 1982 address to the African Studies Association (Ilunga 1984). From the mid-1970s, with massive corruption, impoverishment, and repression of political opposition, the discourse of morality was captured by charismatic prayer groups oriented to resolving personal problems.

6 The term has been adopted in biomedical accounts from Belgian colonial law and discourse. It described a woman not living under the control of a male relative, who can therefore dispose of her own sexuality. The assumption that all free women are prostitutes is considered stigmatizing and is contested by many women (Schoepf 1978, 1981).

7 Transfusions are fairly common among poor African women with access to biomedical services. Chronic nutritional anemias are aggravated by malaria, pregnancy, intestinal parasites, and blood loss from menstruation, childbirth, and botched abortions.

8 Subsequent to this writing, the most recent outbreak of Ebola hamorrhagic fever temporarily superceded AIDS as the disease of "primitivity" in "the heart of darkness."

9 A World Bank team estimated that new infection in Kinshasa could be reduced by 75 percent by "eliminating prostitution" (Bulato and Bos 1988). They did not indicate how "prostitutes" are to be defined and identified. Nor are they concerned with other multiple-partner relationships.

10 The same is true of women in Mali (Bardem and Gobatto 1995), while Taverne (1995) finds a similar situation in the Sahel with respect to migrant workers who return from Ivory Coast.

11 The term *assainissement* is ironic; it means "cleaning up," and, by extension, making healthy. Bringing health to the budget, this housecleaning has brought malnutrition and ill health to hundreds of thousands, including low-paid government employees, their families, and those whom they formerly served. Many no longer have access to even minimal health care or education.

12 Leaders of a churchwomen's club pointed to abandonment, divorce, and widowhood as circumstances forcing women without other resources into commercial sex work.

13 Some cultures encouraged young women to bear one or two children for their fathers' patrilineage prior to marriage.

14 See earlier work (Schoepf 1991b; 1993a; 1993b) for examples of condom rumors encountered from the Sahel to South Africa.

15 *Syndrome Imaginaire pour Décourager les Amoureux*, SIDA is the French acronym for AIDS. Dismissal was a cultural defense against Western attribution of the disease to Africa, Africans, and "African (hyper-)sexuality."

16 The expression in Uganda was "eating a sweet [candy] with the wrapper on."

17 The late "Franco" (Luambo Makiadi), a renowned popular musician, issued a record of advice on AIDS prevention in May 1987. Set to music, his *SIDA* provided detailed information on transmission and prevention in accessible form. It was played in bars and taxi-buses throughout the city in advance of the government campaign (Schoepf, Rukarangira *et al.* 1988a).

18 The advice was prepared by Dr. Rukarangira, Co-director of CONNAIS-SIDA. Walu and I subsequently discovered that many educated men who served as "animators" of the base communities blocked the condom message on the grounds that "it would encourage immorality."

19 For trade-offs with respect to condom use and desired pregnancies, see Schoepf 1992b.

20 In 1991 I drew a humorous cartoon using her experience to suggest how to broach dialogue in couples for my "Draft AIDS Strategy Report" for UNICEF in Tanzania. The secretary took home a copy of the cartoon and used it with her husband. The next day we posted additional copies on bulletin boards around the building. Checking back two days later, each copy bore multiple pushpin holes. Women evidently had found the light touch a useful way to begin.

21 These mistakes are being repeated in the burgeoning epidemics of South

Africa and the Sahel, where biomedical public health professionals continue to dominate the allocation of resources.

22 Queried about this in 1994 in a lecture to the Harvard School of Public Health on "Women, AIDS, and Human Rights," Dr. Jonnathan Mann, architect of the WHO Global Programme on AIDS, attributed the failure to sexism alone.

23 Steven Polgar (1962) discussed this problem early in the history of medical anthropology.

24 Small grants also were provided by the Wenner Gren Foundation for Anthropological Research, OXFAM/UK, and the Maternal-Child Health Foundation. These allowed us to meet expenses and to double the salaries paid to Zairian collaborators from various research institutes and universities in Kinshasa and Lubumbashi. Claude Schoepf and I contributed our labor.

25 The core team carried on with the tacit approval of our own Ministry (Higher Education and Scientific Research) and the National Security Council. But there was no question of bringing the project to scale, as UNICEF had proposed.

26 *AIDS Health Promotion Exchange.* Issues 1 and 2 of 1994 contain pertinent articles.

27 Many are church-related or led by middle-class Christians whose moralizing approach may be counterproductive in prevention of sexual transmission.

REFERENCES

Altman, L. K. 1996, "UN Reports 3 Million New H.I.V. Cases Worldwide for '96," *New York Times*, 28 November, p. 10.

Bardem, I. and Gobatto, I. 1995, *Maux d'amour, vie des femmes: sexualité et prévention du SIDA en milieu urbain africain*, Paris: L'Harmattan.

Bertrand, J., Bakutuvwidi, M. *et al.* 1991, "AIDS related knowledge, sexual behavior and condom use among men and women in Kinshasa, Zaire," *American Journal of Public Health* 81:53–8.

Brandt, A. M. 1988, "The syphilis epidemic in relation to AIDS," *Science* 239:592–6.

Bulato, A. and Bos, A. 1988, "Cost-benefit analysis of AIDS interventions in Kinshasa, Zaire," unpublished paper. Washington, D.C.: The World Bank.

Bygbjerg, I. C. 1983, "AIDS in a Danish surgeon Zaire 1976," Letter. *The Lancet*, I:925.

Comaroff, J. and Comaroff, J. (eds.) 1993, *Modernity and Its Malcontents: Ritual and Power in Post-Colonial Africa*, Chicago: University of Chicago Press.

de Bruyn, M. 1992, "Women and AIDS in developing countries," *Social Science and Medicine* 34(3):249–62.

de Bruyn, M., Jackson, M., Wigermars, M., Knight, V. C. and Berkvens, R. 1995, *Facing the Challenges of HIV/AIDS/STDs: A Gender-Based Response*, Geneva: World Health Organization.

Douglas, M. 1966, *Purity and Danger: An Analysis of the Concepts of Pollution and Taboo*, London: Routledge and Kegan Paul.

Fabian, J. 1990, *Power and Performance: Ethnographic Explorations through*

Proverbial Wisdom and Theatre in Shaba, Zaire, Madison: University of Wisconsin Press.

Feierman, S. 1985, "Struggles for control: the social roots of health and healing in modern Africa," *African Studies Review* 28(2–3):73–147.

Fineberg, H. 1988, "Education to prevent AIDS: prospects and obstacles," *Science* 239:275–80.

Hope, A., Timmel, S. and Hodzi, P. 1984, *Training for Transformation: A Handbook for Community Development Workers*, Gweru, Zimbabwe: Mambo Press.

Ilunga, K. 1984, "Déroutante Afrique ou la syncope d'un discours," *Canadian Journal of African Studies* 18(1):13–22.

Janzen, J. 1978, *The Quest for Therapy in Zaire*, Los Angeles: University of California Press.

Lindan, C., Allen, S., Carael, M. *et al.* 1991, "Knowledge, attitudes and perceived risk of aids among urban Rwandese women," *AIDS* 5:993–1002.

Mann, J. M. and Tarantola, D. M. (eds.) 1996, *AIDS in the World II: Global Dimensions, Social Roots and Responses*, New York: Oxford University Press.

Marks, S. 1989, "The context of personal narrative: reflections on 'not either an experimental doll' – the separate worlds of three South African women," in Personal Narratives Group, pp. 39–58.

Mbilinyi, M. 1989, " 'I'd have been a man': politics and the labor process in producing personal narratives," in Personal Narratives Group, pp. 204–27.

Mizra, S. and Strobel, M. (eds.) 1989, *Three Swahili Women: Life Histories from Mombasa, Kenya*, Bloomington: Indiana University Press.

N'Galy, B., Ryder, R. W. and Bila, K. 1988, "Human immunodeficiency virus infection among employees in an African hospital," *New England Journal of Medicine* 319(17):1123–7.

N'Galy, B., Ryder, R. W. and Quinn, T. C. 1989, "Human immunodeficiency virus infection among employees in an African hospital (letter)," *New England Journal of Medicine* 320(24):1625.

Nzila, N., De Cock, K., Forthall, D. *et al.* 1988, "The prevalence of infection with human immunodeficiency virus over a 10-year period in rural Zaire," *New England Journal of Medicine* 318(5):276–9.

Nzila, N., Laga, M. *et al.* 1991, "HIV and other sexually transmitted diseases among female prostitutes in Kinshasa," *AIDS* 5:715–21.

Personal Narratives Group (ed.) 1989, *Interpreting Women's Lives: Feminist Theory and Personal Narrative*, Bloomington: Indiana University Press.

Polgar, S. 1962, "Health and human behavior: areas of common interest to the social and medical sciences," *Current Anthropology* 3(2):159–205.

Reid, E. 1992, "Gender, knowledge and responsibility," in J. Mann, D. Tarantola and T. Netter (eds.), *AIDS in the World*, Cambridge: Harvard University Press, pp. 657–66.

Romero, P. W. (ed.) 1988, "Introduction," in *Life Histories of African Women*, London: Ashfield Press, pp. 1–6.

Rukarangira, wN. and Schoepf, B. G. 1989, "Social marketing of condoms in Zaire," *AIDS Health Promotion Exchange* (3):2–4.

1991, "Unrecorded trade in Shaba and across Zaire's southern borders," in J. MacGaffey *et al.* (eds.), *The Real Economy in Zaire*, London: James Currey, pp.72–96.

Ryder, R. W., Wato, N., Hassig, S. *et al.* 1989, "Perinatal transmission of the HIV-I to infants of seropositive women in Zaire," *New England Journal of Medicine* 320(25):1637–42.

Schneider, B. and Stoller, N. (eds.) 1995, *Women Resisting AIDS: Feminist Strategies of Empowerment*, Philadelphia: Temple University Press.

Schoepf, B. G. 1969, "Doctor–patient communication and the medical social system," Ph.D. dissertation, Columbia University.

1975, "Human relations versus social relations in medical care," in S. R. Ingman and A. E. Thomas (eds.), *Topias and Utopias in Health: Policy Studies*, The Hague: Mouton, pp. 99–120.

1976, "Recherches en anthropologie médicale: théories et perspectives méthodologiques," *Bulletin d'Anthropologie Médicale* (Lubumbashi) 1(1):20–48.

1978, "Women in the informal economy of Lubumbashi," paper presented at 10th World Congress, International Union of Anthropological and Ethnological Sciences, Delhi, India.

1979, "Breaking through the looking glass: the view from below," in G. Huizer and B. Mannheim (eds.), *The Politics of Anthropology*, The Hague: Mouton, pp. 325–42.

1981, "Women and class formation in Zaire," paper presented at Annual Meeting of the US African Studies Association, October, Bloomington, Indiana.

1986a, "Primary health care in Zaire," *Review of African Political Economy* 36:54–8.

1986b, "CONNAISSIDA: AIDS control research and interventions in Zaire," proposal submitted to Rockefeller Foundation.

1988, "Women, AIDS and economic crisis in Zaire," *Canadian Journal of African Studies* 22(3):625–44.

1991a, "Ethical, methodological and political issues of AIDS research in Central Africa," *Social Science and Medicine* 33(7):749–93.

1991b, "Représentations du SIDA et pratiques populaires à Kinshasa," *Anthropologie et Sociétés* 15(2–3):149–66.

1991c, "Political economy, sex and cultural logics: a view from Zaire," *African Urban Quarterly* 6(1–2):94–106.

1992a, "Gender relations and development: political economy and culture," in A. Seidman and F. Anang (eds.), *21st Century Africa: Towards a New Vision of Self-Sustainable Development*, Trenton, New Jersey: Africa World Press, pp. 203–41.

1992b, "Women at risk: case studies from Zaire," in G. Herdt and S. Lindenbaum (eds.), *The Time of AIDS: Social Analysis, Theory and Method*, Newbury Park, California: Sage, pp. 259–86.

1992c, "AIDS, sex and condoms: African healers and the reinvention of tradition in Zaire," *Medical Anthropology* 13:1–18.

1993a, "Gender, development and AIDS: a political economy and culture approach," in R. Gallin, A. Ferguson and J. Harper (eds.), *The Women and*

International Development Annual, Vol. 3, Boulder, Colorado: Westview Press, pp. 55–85.

1993b, "AIDS action-research with women in Kinshasa," *Social Science and Medicine* 37(11):1401–13.

1995a, "Action-research and empowerment in Africa," in Schneider and Stoller, pp. 246–69.

1995b, "Culture, sex research and AIDS prevention in Africa," in H. ten Brummelhuis and G. Herdt (eds.), *Culture and Sexual Risk: Anthropological Perspectives on the Epidemic*, Philadelphia: Gordon and Breach, pp. 29–51.

Schoepf, B. G., Rukarangira, wN. and Matumona, M. M. 1986, "Etude des réactions à une nouvelle maladie transmissible SIDA et des possibilités de démarrage d'un programme d'éducation populaire," Research Proposal to Government of Zaire, WHO, and USAID.

Schoepf, B. G., Rukarangira, wN., Schoepf, C., Walu, E. and Payanzo, N. 1988a, "AIDS and society in central Africa: a view from Zaire," in N. Miller and R. Rockwell (eds.), *AIDS in Africa: Social and Policy Impact*, Lewiston, New York: E. Mellen, pp. 211–35.

1988b, "AIDS, women and society in central Africa," in R. Kulstad (ed.), *AIDS 1988: AAAS Symposium Papers*, Washington, D.C.: American Association for the Advancement of Science, pp. 175–81.

Schoepf, B. G. and Walu, E. 1991, "Women's trade and contribution to household budgets in Kinshasa," in J. MacGaffey *et al.* (eds.), *The Real Economy in Zaire*, London: James Currey, and Philadelphia: University of Pennsylvania Press.

Schoepf, B. G., Walu, E., Rukarangira, wN., Payanzo, N. and Schoepf, C. 1988, "Community-based risk reduction support in Zaire," paper presented at 1st IECS, Ixtapa, Mexico.

1991, "Gender, power and risk of AIDS in central Africa," in M. Turshen (ed.), *Women and Health in Africa*, Trenton, New Jersey: Africa World Press, pp. 187–203.

Schoepf, B. G., Walu, E., Russell, D. and Schoepf, C. 1991, "Women and structural adjustment in Zaire," in C. Gladwin (ed.), *Structural Adjustment and African Women Farmers*, Gainesville: University of Florida Press, pp. 151–68.

Tanzania Gender Networking Programme 1994, *Symposium Report on Structural Adjustment and Gender Empowerment or Disempowerment*, Dar-es-Salaam.

Taverne, B. 1995, "Stratégie de communication et groupe-cible: SIDA et migrants au Burkina Faso," *Sociétés d'Afrique et du SIDA* (GRID: Université de Bordeaux) 10:2.

Taylor, C. 1992, *Milk, Honey and Money: Changing Concepts of Healing in Rwanda*, Washington, D.C.: Smithsonian Institute.

Verhaegen, B. (ed.) 1990, *Femmes zairoises de Kisangani: combats pour la survie*, Paris: L'Harmattan.

Walu, E. 1991, "Women's survival strategies in Kinshasa," Master's thesis, Institute for Social Studies, The Hague.

1992, "Women's response to AIDS in Kinshasa, Zaire," paper prepared for the Conference on Culture, Sexual Behavior and AIDS, Amsterdam.

World Bank 1989, *Sub-Saharan Africa: From Crisis to Sustainable Growth*, Washington, DC: The World Bank.

World Health Organization/Global Program on AIDS (WHO/GPA) 1995, "Cumulative infections approach 20 million," *Global AIDS News* (Geneva) 1:5.

6   Barren ground: contesting identities of infertile women in Pemba, Tanzania

Karina Kielmann

> The overall fertility levels observed in Zanzibar have slightly decreased during the past ten years but are still among the highest in the world today . . . The Total Fertility Rates are . . . very high by international comparison, ranging between 6.9 in [Zanzibar] Town and 9.1 in Pemba.
>
> (Ministry of Health, Zanzibar 1988)

> Family planning efforts [in Zanzibar] have proven largely ineffective, a development officials blame on the country's religion – Islam . . . Government officials explain that Muslims consider family planning to run counter to God's commandments . . . Of the 16,665 women who registered for family planning services when the program began, about $\frac{1}{2}$ of them had dropped out by last December. Officials believe that the high attrition rate is due to an unfounded rumor that family planning makes women barren.
>
> (Chintowa 1991:3)

Introduction

Pemba is one of the two islands in the Indian Ocean that comprise Zanzibar, roughly 40 kilometres off the coast of mainland Tanzania.[1] Covering 868 square kilometres of hilly and fertile land, the island used to be known by the Arabs as El-Jazzirah, the Green Island. Infrastructure and tourism are far less developed than on the neighboring island of Unguja and Pemba has received comparatively little attention in the historical literature on the area.[2]

According to official statistics, however, Pemba appears as having one of the highest fertility rates in the world. In the language of global modernization theory, "high fertility" is a macrolevel indicator situating Pemba at the lower end of the "development" scale. In a more narrowly demographic discourse, it equates with poor performance, that is, a lag in the fertility transition. At the same time, high fertility connotes a microlevel attribute of individual women, the key targets of family planning programs in Zanzibar for roughly a decade.

Despite extensive family planning efforts on the island of Pemba, the so-called fertility rates remain high, a phenomenon that is often ascribed to the constraints of "culture" – Islamic law – or "beliefs" (as opposed to knowledge) concerning the negative effects of contraception on a woman's fertility. The extent to which "culture" and "beliefs," as presented in this view, are shared and constitute veritable obstacles to the adoption of contraceptive methods, is very much open to question. The more interesting question, however, stems from the recognition that women continue to bear and value many children in the face of national and international policies dictating that high fertility is a risk factor, not only for the woman and the child, but for the country's social and economic development. At the same time, there are women who are infertile, and who disappear altogether from the statistics and the discourse on fertility control.

What happens to women who remain childless in a so-called "high-fertility" area? What spaces do they occupy in local symbolic, moral, and social orders? How do they make sense of infertility and whom do they seek out for recognition and remedy of their condition? These were among the leading questions I explored in a study conducted in Pemba in 1994.[3] In addition to women who perceived themselves to be infertile, I interviewed a range of indigenous healers who had dealt with infertility cases as well as expatriate biomedical practitioners, most of whom deemed infertility to be unworthy of serious medical consideration.

The Irish midwife rolled her eyes in mock despair when I told her I was undertaking a study on infertility in Pemba, laughingly commenting that it was a "blessing in disguise." A year-old entry made in the Rotary Bank logbook of Flying Doctors at Wete Hospital noted: "many women come to the clinic complaining of infertility, but it is not something we should devote our efforts to given the high fertility rate." The Rotary Bank doctor present at the time of my stay in Pemba, a Swedish gynecologist, although sympathetic to the dilemma faced by individual childless women, did not necessarily see the treatment of infertility as a priority for the island. Attending his clinic at Wete Hospital, I sat patiently in a room at the side. On each of the two mornings of the week that clinic was held, the waiting room was packed with roughly 30–40 women sitting on wooden benches, waiting to see him for gynecological problems. Every so often, he would stop and let me know about women who complained of their inability to conceive. On two separate occasions, there were over ten "infertility clients." One of the cases that I interviewed was Amina, a slim, young woman with a lively sense of narration.

Amina is 19 years old and has a primary education. Married for three years, she lives with her husband in Kiuyu. Shortly after her marriage, she started to have very painful menstrual periods. In 1993, she missed her period for a few months, and went to the hospital after two days of heavy bleeding to "have herself cleaned out" (*amesafishwa*). She has not been able to conceive since and has consulted numerous practitioners for her abdominal pains, irregular and painful periods, and infertility. She believes that she is possessed by a spirit (*shetani*) who came one night in the form of her husband and "played sex" with her. She consulted an uncle who is a healer (*mganga*) in order to get rid of the spirit through a procedure of exorcism (*kupiga kilele*). She also consulted a midwife (*mkunga*), a doctor at Chake hospital, and another *mganga*. Her husband's family and the neighbors have put pressure on the husband to divorce or remarry, and she herself urges her husband to take on another wife, although he has said that she is young, and they can wait.

The discrepancy between a global discourse on population policy in sub-Saharan Africa which barely acknowledges infertility as a rumored problem and a local Pemban discourse that situates infertility as an indicator of disrupted social relations between men, women, and spirits, forms the subject of this chapter. This discrepancy rests partly on the axiomatic nature – global versus individual and medical versus social – of the envisaged problem. More fundamentally, however, it rests on the relative space occupied by women's knowledge and their narrative construction of events, including those which take place within the body.

In reaction to the tendency to portray women as passive victims of ascribed gender and reproductive regimes and institutionalized reproductive policies, there has been much recent work that addresses the question of women's agency within the constraints of discursive power. With a reconceptualization of power that is not only top-down, but continuous, subtle, and creating possibilities for knowledge in and through the production of discourses (Fisher and Davis 1993), the attention has shifted from the level of ideology and "culture" to practices – gestures, habits, and desires – that are grounded in the body. Women's everyday discourses and practices have been analyzed as bargaining and strategizing tactics (Bledsoe 1990; Bledsoe *et al.* 1994), and more radically as the sources of resistance and protest (Abu-Lughod 1990; Ong 1990; MacLeod 1991).

While discussions of women's agency, in particular resistance, are frequently linked to the medicalization of women's bodies,[4] I will argue in this chapter that it is the absence of a biomedical discourse on infertility in Pemba that has created the particularity of women's local knowledge on infertility. By acknowledging the possibility of medical roots of the problem, by conveying the distress of infertility through a distinct plethora of symptoms and etiological explanations which include biomedical referents, and finally, by increasingly resorting to doctors and clinics in seeking treatment for their condition, Pemban women's narrative accounts of infertility incorporate the very sites and discourses that contest their identities as infertile women. In doing so, the women testify not only to transformations taking place within Pemban society, that is "historical shifts in the configuration of power," but to a form of expression that is "neither outside of, nor independent from systems of power" (Abu-Lughod 1990:48).

In the first section, I consider the sites of biopower, that is, the regulatory mechanisms of a discourse on population in sub-Saharan Africa that denies a voice to infertile women. I explore how under-standings of "women," "fertility," and "culture," historically and politically situated in Western "developed" countries, have governed the rhetoric of population policies and guided both research and inter-ventions. At the same time, I critically review the work of interdisci-plinary anthropologists who have considered how these assumptions are challenged at the level of both the body politic and the social body. In doing so, I suggest that investing peoples' responses to the mechanisms of biopower with the motives of resistance is at least as problematic as rendering them compliant victims of "reproductive regimes."

The second section draws on ethnographic case material from Pemba. In studying how women and local practitioners manage infertility both conceptually and pragmatically in the face of a popula-tion policy that does not acknowledge infertility, I want to redress the problem of resistance. My intention is to show that infertility is a very tangible problem, grounded in manifestations of pain, jealousy, and possession and situated in both the individual and the social body. However, in contrast to authors who have decoded illness and posses-sion episodes as signs of protest (Boddy 1988; 1989; Ong 1988; Scheper-Hughes 1990), I suggest that it is not at this level of bodily suffering that one should seek resistance. Rather, meanings of resistance begin to emerge when Pemban women bring the sufferings of infertility to surface in the form of bodily knowledge: the elaboration of symptoms, the persistent search for recognition and divination of the problem, the narrative construction of past events, and the contestation of the ways in which the problem is interpreted by the larger community as well as by the practitioners consulted. Oscillating between the idioms of capricious spirits and unexplained symptoms, the articulation of this knowledge suggests a "syncretistic bricolage" (Comaroff 1985:6), a juxtaposition of organizational forms giving rise to new meanings and messages. Further, I suggest that local practitioners have a pivotal role in this production of subjugated knowledge. It is they who mediate, often with calculated ambiguity, between the social orders that monitor women's lives, including the discourse on family planning, and individual women's experiences of suffering and illness.

Regulating and resisting fertility regimes

While the anthropological study of fertility has traditionally centered on its symbolic associations, there has been recent impetus to consider its political and economic dimensions. In part, this results from the politicization of reproductive issues in the late twentieth century as well as the growth of political economy approaches in anthropology (Greenhalgh 1994). The study of the politics of reproduction has focused on "intersecting interests of states and other powerful institutions such as multinational and national corporations, international development agencies, Western medicine, and religious groups as they construct the contexts within which local reproductive relations are played out" (Ginsburg and Rapp 1992:312). These institutions, in so far as they are concerned with the regulation of individual, group, or population fertility and reproduction, represent mechanisms through which what Foucault calls "biopower" is exercised.

In particular, Foucault identified women's bodies as a key dimension in the history of a regulatory biopower inscribed in population policies and interventions (Sawicki 1991:68). Taking population policies in sub-Saharan Africa as an exemplary channel of regulatory biopower, this section examines the assumptions and rhetoric underlying a dominant paradigm of African women as "overproducers." This paradigm has guided programs as well as research towards the determinants of, and the means to reduce, high fertility, thus overshadowing the significance of infertility as a public health problem.

Paradigms of fertility and the politics of fertility control

Selected medical literature indicates that while female infertility in sub-Saharan Africa presents a serious problem,[5] much of what is known as secondary, or post-infectious infertility, is amenable to prevention (WHO 1987:966; Wasserheit 1989:145). Yet the causes, consequences, and management of infertility in sub-Saharan Africa are largely neglected areas of public health (Wasserheit 1989:146; Bergstrom

1992). In part, female infertility has been ignored because it remains hidden: women with sexually transmitted diseases (STD) and reproductive tract infections (RTI) that can lead to infertility are frequently asymptomatic and thus remain undiagnosed until the damage is irreparable. At the same time, however, the dearth of information and interventions pertaining to infertility in Africa testifies to a "global climate of concern over population growth and high fertility [that] is not conducive to the perception of infertility as a real problem" (Frank 1983:142).

Population policies in sub-Saharan Africa have been primarily concerned with fertility reduction (Sherbenin *et al.* 1994). This goal is grounded in a vision of excessive and ultimately self-destructive African sexuality and fertility that has directed research and interventions in a particular manner. On the one hand, medical representations of sexuality and sexual health continue to suffer either from an overtly Victorian or "ethnopornographic" viewpoint (Barton 1989), or, at best, have maintained a narrow Eurocentric perspective. For example, the notion of a distinctly African sexual system has been used to interpret lagging fertility decline as well as the spread of sexually transmitted diseases in sub-Saharan Africa (Caldwell *et al.* 1989).[6] In demographic literature, on the other hand, sexuality is oddly sanitized and replaced by more ominous metaphors of technology and production such as "reproduction" and "risk of exposure" (Watkins 1993:558–9). An emphasis on biological reproduction, analyzed through the concept of fertility and its proximate determinants, has deflected attention away from women's subjective experiences of sexuality and childbearing as well as from the social and symbolic frameworks within which these experiences are given meaning.

In the process of objectification, fertility becomes a disembodied attribute of individual women, and thus manageable through technical procedures. This is evident, for example, in the notion of "unmet need," a parameter used to measure the number of women who claim they do not want further children, but are not currently using contraceptives (Bongaarts 1991). The underlying assumption is that more and better contraceptive services will necessarily lead to a decline in fertility, a conclusion that has been challenged for its failure to consider the social, economic, and political context of women's sexuality and childbearing experiences (Nathanson and Hill 1994).

When fertility levels remain high despite effective distribution of contraceptives, much of the demographic literature resorts to an explanation of "culture." In the population explosion rhetoric of the 1960s, a dominant theme was the struggle between forces of modernization, represented by the organizations distributing modern contraceptives, and forces of resistance, characterized as macrolevel attributes – the "weight of custom and tradition" – or individual attributes such as "apathy and inertia" (Watkins 1993:556). In the late 1960s and early 1970s, the leading theory of demographic transition was called into question and there have since been attempts to operationalize "culture" as language, ethnicity, or geographical region in order to explain high and low "fertility regimes."[7] As Greenhalgh points out, the result has been a worryingly reductionist approach that treats culture as divorced from social, economic and political organization: "something that facilitates or obstructs contraceptive communication" (Greenhalgh 1994:15).

The overwhelming focus on excessive fertility has meant that women who cannot have children are only of interest in so far as they affect overall fertility levels. In the demographic literature, infertility or sterility appears as a "low-priority proximate determinant" of fertility (Bongaarts cited in Ebigbola and van de Walle 1987). Even those who acknowledge that infertility affects a considerable number of women in sub-Saharan Africa see it as a hindrance to the success of population policies, rather than a problem deserving attention in its own right:

Infertility will represent a major obstacle to Africa's fertility transition, because uncertainty in childbearing inhibits response to intrinsic and extrinsic pressures to reduce fertility goals. Infertility could remain *a strong source of resistance* even when other barriers to fertility regulation are coming down, since certain aspects of modernization . . . foster the diffusion of venereal disease. (Frank 1983:143; emphasis added)

The paradigm of excessive fertility has wide-reaching implications for the quality, accessibility, and utilization of women's health services. Family planning services have tended to be falsely separated from other services including STD control and maternal and child health (MCH) facilities. This has clearly influenced their acceptability, as is evident in the case of STD clinics that remain highly stigmatized, and therefore avoided. Since services for women's health are deficient or poorly integrated, women's RTI and STD continue to be hidden problems, or not even recognized as such because they are widely shared and seen as the natural consequences of being a woman (Dixon-Mueller and Wasserheit 1991).

At the same time, the technical solutions proposed in family planning programs are often poorly understood or divorced from the realities of women's lives. As Maina-Ahlberg describes for the Kenyan setting, modern family planning had limited impact because it was based on decontextualized knowledge. Focusing on the fertility of married women, it ignored other social groups relevant to fertility outcomes, as well as the power structures within which decisions concerning sexuality and fertility were made. In addition, the program overlooked "reproductive problems such as infertility and sexually transmitted diseases which are of major concern to women . . . plans were based on the conviction that prevailing high fertility is supported by cultural values and attitudes favoring high fertility" (1991:201).

In the late 1980s, increasing criticism toward the narrow focus of population programs led to the coining of the more comprehensive "reproductive health services." The premise of this shift in attention has been that every woman has a right to "regulate her fertility safely and effectively; to understand and enjoy her own sexuality; to remain free of disease, disability, or death associated with her sexuality and reproduction; and to bear and rear healthy children" (Dixon-Mueller 1993:269). The orientation toward reproductive rights, while ethically more correct, does not stray far from the narrowly mechanistic view of women as reproducers (Townshend and McElroy 1992). Despite the use of empowering euphemisms like "reproductive choice" and "reproductive decision-making" which imply that women have the power to control their fertility, the expectation is that they use this power to control world population growth (Watkins 1993:557). At the same time, the very notion of rights must be understood here as a "culturally specific product of a legal system premised on individual rights" as indicated for the American case justifying abortion as a woman's right to bodily autonomy (Ginsburg and Rapp 1992:317). The appropriateness of this strongly individualistic and objectified view of "reproduction" in a non-Western setting such as Zanzibar is questionable.

"World-system demography," a term coined by Riedmann (1993) to denote First World bureaucratic surveillance of Third World fertility, continues to have a pervasive influence on population and reproductive health policies targeting women. However, the portrayal of women as victims of culture-bound "reproductive regimes" that constitute obstacles to the acceptance of modern contraception has been challenged, in particular by researchers who arbitrate between the fields of demography and anthropology.[8] It is argued that women actively use resources at their disposal and devise strategies not only to challenge, but to alter oppressive systems (Greenhalgh 1994:31). In the following section, I examine the usefulness of recent social science writing on resistance in addressing women's responses to so-called reproductive regimes and reproductive policies.

Recasting the seeds of resistance

While the notion of "biopower" has been used to identify the ways in which government reproductive policies and technologies threaten women's control over their lives, it is also understood to provide the grounds for creating and maintaining forms of everyday resistance to this control. In contrast to large-scale, collectively organized, and visible resistance movements, forms of everyday resistance are manifest in "subjugated knowledges", that is, experiences and knowledges that have been "disqualified as inadequate . . . or insufficiently elaborated: naive knowledges, located down in the hierarchy beneath the required level of cognition or scientificity" (Foucault 1978 in Sawicki 1991:87). This suggests shifting attention from the sites of biopower, that is the institutions that develop and sustain discourses on the regulation of the social body, to the sites at which these discourses are internalized, transformed, or resisted by the women who are affected by them, namely their reproductive experiences.

In social science and feminist studies of women's micro-level resistance, the analytical starting point is the relationship between structured forms of constraint and women's agency. A central theoretical and methodological question is: how does one investigate the ways in which women's bodily knowledge and practices are limited through asymmetrical power structures, and at the same time treat women as knowledgeable actors in the constitution of social life? (Mahoney and Yngvesson 1992; Abu-Lughod 1990; Fisher and Davis 1993). For Moore, the question is posed more starkly: "How is it possible for people both to consent to and dissent from the dominant representations for gender when they are encoded in the material world all around them?" (Moore 1994:75).

In searching to explain this apparent contradiction, medical anthropologists have turned to the body and body praxis (Scheper-Hughes and Lock 1987; Scheper-Hughes 1990). In place of the inert biomedical body, there is a recognition of "anarchic" bodies that "refuse to conform to universal concepts of disease, distress, and medical efficacy" (Scheper-Hughes 1990:44). The reintroduction of subjective experience into the study of illness has allowed the body to become "mindful," and thus both the "immediate terrain where social truths are forged and social contradictions played out, as well as the locus of personal resistance, creativity, and struggle" (Scheper-Hughes 1990:49). The implication is a body that actively expresses what the conscious mind is unable to voice:

What can no longer be spoken is repeated in behaviour. It seems clear, then, that body knowledge can both refuse us and traduce us. It can insist on things that we would like to leave behind and it can continue to guide us when we have lost all sense of strategy and purpose. What emerges from this is that resistance does not need to be discursive, coherent or conscious. (Moore 1994:81–2)

My argument here is that endowing particular bodily practices such as gestures, habits, and symptoms with the meanings of resistance and subversive action is both troubling and problematic. The so-called "anarchic" body, divorced from the presentation of self and the subjective meanings that individuals invest in their actions and reactions, is far from anarchic when inscribed with raw and unconscious (however noble) intent. Beyond the notions of a disempowering medicalization and a defiant body, I suggest that we can only start to attribute meanings of resistance when women themselves envisage and express the possibility of options diverging from orthodox frameworks of meanings surrounding the body, body knowledge, and bodily practices.

Mahoney and Yngvesson have argued that conventional accounts of resistance fail to account for motivation, that is, what propels certain individuals, and not others, to resist domination and to make change. Their argument, relying heavily on concepts from cognitive psychology, may be limited in its applicability to non-Western settings. Nonetheless, it introduces a previously neglected and essential dimension of reflexivity. In the sites where struggles with power and dependence take place, including women's bodies, they suggest that "the invention of new forms is shown to be shaped by and dependent on old meanings, and the interplay of resistance and determination produces practices and understandings that are simultaneously of an existing order and a reimagining of it" (Mahoney and Yngvesson 1992:63).

In discussions of the response to global population policies, the theme of resistance is played out at political and social levels. The global discourse of high fertility is a highly sensitive political issue, and local government resistance to US-dominated population policies is read in the repeated failure of countries to meet fertility reduction goals, as in Egypt (Inhorn 1994) or in the puzzle of rising birthrates in Malaysia (Ong 1990). While these statistics are loosely interpreted as symptoms of resistance, the more interesting signs of public dissent are "vocal efforts by Islamic 'fundamentalist' reform groups in Egypt to increase rather than to decrease the absolute number of Muslims" (Inhorn 1994:503), or the evidence from Malaysia that "although teachers and other state servants might be practicing contraception in private, in public they loudly proclaimed the practice contrary to Islam" (Ong

1990:264). At the same time, government recognition of high levels of infertility, as for example in Central Africa, have resulted in the maintenance of strongly pro-natalist ideologies (Nkounkou 1989).

In addition to locating resistance at the level of the body politic, recent work in the field of demographic anthropology points to the social construction and contestation of demographic truths. Bledsoe, for example, argues that "individuals constantly tinker with family structures in ways that cumbersome biological acts of fertility cannot" (1990:97–8), drawing on examples of how people influence demographic outcomes by restructuring household compositions and influencing children's obligations through particular patterns of marriage, child spacing, and child fosterage. Greenhalgh (1994) points to examples from north India, where women secretly defy their husbands and in-laws to arrange for contraception and abortions, and from China, where women resist the state's one-child-per-family policy to negotiate a revised version of the policy more consistent with their needs.

Here again, the question arises to what extent women (and men) who work *within* the constraints of a system are pursuing strategies, let alone resisting the system. It seems that less ambiguous forms of resistance can be found in those situations where different systems of meanings surrounding the body confront each other, allowing for a reinterpretation of both past and present events. The possibility of a new order of things permits individuals consciously to reaffirm the "old" and familiar order as one that is integral to their identity (individual and social), or alternately to modify or reject the "old" order in a deliberate appeal for change. Thus for example, Abu-Lughod (1990) sees new forms of resistance in young Bedouin women who adopt the consumerist lifestyle of mainstream Egyptian society. Wearing Egyptian fashions and staging elaborate Egyptian-style wedding ceremonies, of which older Bedouins disapprove, they both emulate and reject dominant orders. A similar example is provided by Fuglesang (1994) who looks at the role of videos in the lives of Swahili women in Lamu, Kenya. Watching Hindi and Western films is an enormously popular form of recreation for women, she argues, because it contributes in part to "making the traditional universe a reality which is neither inevitable nor necessary" (Fuglesang 1994:180–1). They furnish the images and a language which women use to make sense of, but also to contest, their emotions and relationships with men.

Examples of resistance to state regulation of women's bodies can be drawn from the experience of field research, where the discrepancy between researcher's and subject's understandings of fertility are brought into sharp focus. Riedmann's critical analysis (1993) of

Caldwell's CAFN (Changing African Family – Nigeria) project illustrates how the subjects of fertility research used various techniques to evade, challenge, or undermine researchers' questions on the "problem" of too many children. In another fertility study, a researcher investigating cultural obstacles to contraceptive use in Zimbabwe was confronted with women who asked: "Why is it that the government wants to intervene when it means limiting our fertility, and abstains when we have infertility problems?" (Mhloyi 1987:139). Women also challenge researchers' narrow problematization of fertility by shifting attention to the political and socioeconomic backdrop. Thus, African-American women interviewed on the "problem" of teenage pregnancy in Baltimore angrily point to the high rate of homicide in the area[9] and women in eastern Germany recast the "problem" of declining birthrates as a premeditated, albeit drastic, reaction to the economic crisis since reunification.[10]

What is apparent in all of these examples is that women derive and articulate different, sometimes opposing, possibilities for meaning and conduct *on the margins* of dominant discourses regulating their bodies. It is this position that allows them to defend their knowledge of the body, to mediate between social orders and to invent new forms of knowledge. In the second half of this chapter, I turn to the case of infertile women in Pemba, Tanzania. Here, women resist the dominant rhetoric that they are by nature (or for that matter by culture) "overproducers" in two ways. First, they are aware of this rhetoric and subvert it through a variety of discursive techniques. Second, they move comfortably, in their search for treatment, between conflicting sites and bodies of knowledge (biomedical and local) on fertility and infertility.

Sheikhs, spirits, and symptoms: transformations of local knowledge on female infertility in Pemba

Arrived in Micheweni today to find the hospital completely abandoned and much commotion on the road through town. Met with Bi Nadia, the MCH-coordinator, who told us that Sheikh Shariff, the 8-year-old wonder child from Dar es Salaam, was there for the day. Just behind the hospital, a huge crowd of at least 500: women in brightly-coloured *khangas* [printed cloths] and babies on their back on one side; men and children on the other. The boy-sheikh's older brother was delivering a sermon on the miracle of Sheikh Shariff who apparently converted his entire family to Islam at the age of six. A long harangue, punctuated by occasional shouts of *"Kibeer!"* [mighty] and *"Allah ho akhbar!"* [God is great] by the crowd, some religious incantations, and finally Sheikh Shariff appeared seated on a raised stage. People were asked to present their questions to him, however not in written form as he cannot read. The boy-sheikh gave short and stammering answers, which were interpreted by his brother. Out of the handful of people who asked questions, two related their problems of childlessness. One man lamented his four wives' inability to give him a child; another woman said that she had been married for some time without conceiving. Both were brushed aside rather vehemently and told that these were not proper questions. When the woman asked the boy-sheikh to perform a *dua* [invocatory prayer] for her, he refused. S.'s [my field assistant] explanation is that people were expected to ask questions about *dinya* [religion] and not to dispute matters that were in God's control. Later, the crowd dispersed with much chatter and amazement. (author's fieldnotes, November 29, 1994)

Selected anthropological references point to an overarching concern with infertility in areas of so-called high fertility in Africa.[11] In the above story, the anxiety created by infertility is such that it is voiced in the public sphere. Despite a certain rhetorical ambivalence regarding whether the matter is one of human or divine intervention, it is women who are implicated in cases of infertility and who bear the consequences, including the responsibility for seeking treatment.

In coastal Tanzania (Swantz 1986), Ghana (Ebin 1982), and Kenya (Katz and Katz 1984), areas where barrenness occurs relatively commonly, women constitute the majority of clients of indigenous health services including healers, herbalists, and spirit mediums. In other societies, therapeutic fertility cults reflect the pervasive preoccupation with the cause and the prevention of infertility. Examples are the *kifudu*, a female fertility cult among the Giriama of Kenya (Udvardy 1990) and the *khita* fertility cult among the Yaka of Zaire (Devisch 1993) within which the relief of gynecological disorders, including infertility and anomalous births, is sought.

In general, anthropologists have tended to look at infertility through an exclusively symbolic lens, focusing on metaphors (Feldman-Savelsberg 1994) and ritual processes (Inhorn 1994; Neff 1994) surrounding childlessness. Infertility is seen as the dialectical counterpart of fertility which in turn is reified as a pervasive trope in much of sub-Saharan Africa. While this framework of interpretation has led to provocative speculations on how infertility threatens the social order and the body politic, it is limited in its understanding of what infertility represents for individual women. The underlying view of the body as imprint of society fails to consider how infertile women interpret bodily experience, sometimes reinforcing, at other times rejecting the symbolic order. At the same time, the emphasis on fertility and infertility as cultural symbols deflects attention away from the more tangible concerns that infertility embodies such as compromised health conditions and disturbed social relations.

In three months of fieldwork in Pemba,[12] I interviewed twenty-five women who perceived themselves to be infertile, many for over two years preceding the interview (n = 22). Often rumored about and rejected in their immediate social networks, they initially confided most frequently in their mothers and sisters. Over the years, they proceeded to seek recognition, explanation, and treatment of their condition from midwives (*wakunga*), healers (*waganga*) and sheikhs (*masheikh*), some eventually turning to local and expatriate biomedical practitioners. The extensive range of practitioners consulted suggests that a local discourse on infertility in Pemba is composed of diverse strands of knowledge. Before examining how women contribute to shaping and modifying this discourse, I situate local perceptions of infertility within the broader framework of social relations in Pemba.

Men, women and spirits: the social context of infertility[13]

Despite the recognition that both men and women contribute to producing children, infertility in Pemba is perceived to be an exclusively female problem. Men are considered infertile only if they are unable to maintain an erection and ejaculate, in which case they tend to remain unmarried. Women, on the other hand, marry young and are expected to bear a child within the first year of marriage.

If a woman is unable to conceive within a given period of time, she is deemed infertile (*tasa*). While there are numerous reasons why one and not another woman is infertile, it is generally agreed that the problem is a "disease of the stomach area" (*ugonjwa wa tumbo*). Ethnophysiological descriptions of infertility centre on particular reproductive organs (*uchango wa uzazi* or *viungo vya uzazi*):

> There is a swelling of the uterus [*mayoma*]. (MCH-aide, Ole)
>
> The woman has too much fat; an obesity of pregnancy [*kitambi cha mimba*]. (*Mkunga*, Micheweni)
>
> There are changes in the intestine concerned with reproduction. It has red fluid [*Kubadalika chango. Kuwa chango lina maji mikundu*]. (*Mganga*, Kiuyu)
>
> The abdomen is not clean. It cannot hold the foetus [*Tumbo chafu. Uchango wa uzazi haupokei watoto*]. (*Mkunga*, Kiuyu)
>
> The organs are lying upside down [*Viungo vya uzazi umekaa upande*]. (*Mkunga*, Ole)
>
> The abdominal area is ruined, it cannot hold anything. The blood is not good [*Tumbo huwa ni bovu, halikai kitu. Damu inakuwa si mzuri*]. (*Mkunga*, Micheweni)

Taunted as a *fuu tomo* or *fuu zubu*, a coconut shell with a hole, it is said that the infertile woman eats without producing any fruit. She is considered useless because she has not experienced labor pains and often treated with contempt by her husband's relatives, especially her mother-in-law and her sister-in-law. Her husband may be advised to undertake a temporary "medicinal" divorce (*kachwa dawa*), to remarry, or to take on another wife. Out of the twenty-five women interviewed, over two-thirds had been married more than once (n = 18) and eleven had been divorced by their husbands specifically because of the problem of infertility. Roughly half (n = 12) were in polygynous marriages.

The high rate of divorce and remarriage among infertile women is a stark indicator of social relations and expectations that are threatened by childless women. For Pemban women, successful marriages and childbearing remain highly important criteria for achieving social status, partly because the female education and employment opportunities are restricted. Despite the existence of free and compulsory education in Zanzibar since 1964, female illiteracy is high at 47.5 percent (MOH Zanzibar 1988) and the number of girls at higher levels of education extremely low. These numbers are explained in part by early marriages or premarital pregnancies forcing girls to drop out of school (Puja and Kassimoto 1994).

Marriages among the predominantly Muslim families of Pemba are traditionally arranged by the parents soon after the girl is considered mature,[14] although girls nowadays have more choice in their marriage partners. Bridewealth (*mahari*) is paid to the girl's family and, depending on the family income, can range from 10,000 to 100,000 Tanzanian shillings.[15] As most families know each other, careful attention is paid to the choice of the bride and the preferred marriage is between cross-cousins. Families conduct investigations (*mchunguzi*) in order to determine whether the girl is polite, respectful, and most importantly, modest in her behavior. Close attention is paid to the constellation of stars at the time of the wedding. Certain months, often those in which Muslim holidays such as *Aid el Fikr* and *Aid el Hadj* are celebrated, are considered more auspicious than others for marriage.

The relatively early age of marriage and the social pressure to marry the right man or woman at the right time leads to conflictual situations. Rumors circulate about families choosing marriage partners against the will of their daughters and girls resisting arranged marriages by suicide threats.[16] Infertility is often linked to a couple's blood not being related (*damu zao haziendani*)[17] and to the inappropriate timing of the marriage, at the wrong time of either the day or the month.

Children are expected within the first year of marriage and celebrated. For most of the women, the number of children desired depends on

God's will. A common saying is that "each child has its own *riziki,*" meaning that each child will be provided for by God. Accordingly, when a woman is unable to bear children, it is often said that God is not yet ready or willing (*Mungo hajamjalia*) for her to conceive.

In Pemba, the importance of children extends beyond the immediate family. Most married couples live with their children in a household. However, if there are many children or close spacing of births in a household, relatives and neighbors share the responsibility in taking care of and feeding children. According to Rose, these widespread relations of exchange in child-care cooperation, known as *kuleleana,* act as an important theme in the "management of placing and spacing of children within families . . . Children have a central place within the household and because they are its most mobile members, act as a link between kin in close geographical proximity or across large distances" (Rose 1994:28).

Although it is not customary law, the failure to conceive within a given period of time can lead to divorce. Divorce is relatively easy and acceptable, the most common grounds being adultery and failure of the husband to provide for the family. If a woman is mistreated by her husband, she can go back to her parents, who then try to negotiate with the husband and convince him to take her back. If it is the woman who demands the divorce, the family must return the money, and the girl may even lose clothes and other possessions she might have acquired during the marriage.

Jealousy (*wivo*) is a frequent theme in the discussion of conflicts between men and women, especially between spouses in polygynous marriages. Although the first wife is supposed to be the most powerful, she is often neglected, and it is said that her jealousy can lead to the casting of spells in order to attract the husband, who has to work out a timetable for sleeping with his wives (*zamu*). Often, jealousy and adultery lead to accusations of witchcraft. Love-drugs can be obtained from local healers (*waganga*) and, in more dramatic situations, wizards (*wachawi*) may be called upon to punish the offending husband or wife by casting "bad words" (*maneno mabaya*) and bewitching (*urogaji*).[18] Many cases of infertility recounted to me second-hand established the conceptual links between infertility, jealousy, and sorcery:

S. spoke of a woman who could not be treated by a doctor at the hospital and went to a *mganga* for her pains in the uterus. He claimed it was a case of jealousy of the second wife, who did not have any children. The second wife feared that all wealth would go to the first wife and her children. (author's fieldnotes, November 14, 1994).

One woman in the waiting room [clinic at Wete hospital] mentioned the case of a young girl who was married to an old man by force. She refused to sleep with him and divorced, later marrying another man. The first man failed to have children with his subsequent wives and believes that he is bewitched. (*amerogwa*) (author's fieldnotes, November 18, 1994)

One of the *wakunga* [midwives] from Ole told me the story of a woman who had come to her after repeated abortions. She was convinced that she had been bewitched by her neighbor who was infertile. (author's fieldnotes, November 22, 1994)

A further dimension of social relations on Pemba is constituted by the "personal bodily possession and the family possession of spirits" (Rose 1994:24). The island is said to be inhabited by spirits of the sea (*mashetani*) and of the land (*pepo*) that occupy a central position in local perceptions of illness and healing.[19] A spirit (*shetani*) may be inherited, or may possess someone, whereby the human body becomes its vehicle. It manifests itself directly by speaking through the body, more commonly, however, indirectly through physical and mental illness, misfortune, and barrenness (Giles 1987:240). While *mashetani* are recognized in Orthodox Islamic doctrine, there is disagreement among the *walimu* (Islamic teachers) as to whether they can cause death of a victim, a power generally attributed to God alone.

Spirit possession is first suspected by the emergence of symptoms of illness or abnormal behaviour including paralysis (*subiani*) and fits of shouting or crying fits (*kuchagawa*). The victims of possession are usually women; indeed spirit possession is generally regarded as the most common cause of sickness in women (Gray 1969:171).[20] While many conventional studies of spirit possession have understood the phenomenon to be an anomaly, an "individualistic strategy of redress by poor and marginalized people . . . especially women" (Scheper-Hughes 1990:55), Boddy (1988) points out the taken-for-grantedness of spirits in the everyday lives of Sudanese women and Giles (1987) maintains that the *shetani* cult is an integral part of Swahili culture.

In Pemba, local healers frequently attribute pregnancy complications and infertility to the presence of *mashetani*. Invariably, these spirits are male, and their entry into women's bodies is often explicitly described as sexual:[21]

Those who are having bleeding during pregnancy (*wamwagaji*); they usually say "something came during the night and touched my abdomen." For these cases, I read a *duwa* to make the *shetani* leave the body. (*Sheikh*, Ole)

Male spirits (*mashetani dume*) can get inside the abdomen and touch it so that there is no chance of conceiving. (*Mkunga*, Micheweni)

Mashetani can resemble the body of the husband. They try to play sex with the woman and destroy the pregnancy. (*Mkunga*, Wete)

The *shetani* stays at the site where the foetus is supposed to lie and drinks the semen produced by the husband. (*Mganga*, Kiuyu)

While women bear the onus of responsibility for infertility, most local explanations situate the problem within the larger context of social relations, thus allowing women to seek remedy in the public arena. There are signs, however, of the development of a modernist discourse that individualizes and moralizes the problem of infertility. Women in Wete, a higher number of whom are educated and employed than those in Ole, Kiuyu, or Micheweni, suggest that infertility is a consequence of unacceptable behaviors on the part of the woman. These included being sexually promiscuous (*asherati*), drinking alcohol, using contraception, and having a "criminal" abortion, summarized by one woman to be "un-Islamic" activities.

The absence of an overtly biomedical discourse on infertility in Pemba has indirectly encouraged women to turn repeatedly to local practitioners for advice and help. According to Rose (1994), patterns of resort are adopted depending on whether the illness is seen as a "local" matter (*mambo ya kiswahili* or *kienyeji*) or a "hospital" problem (*matatizo ya hospitali*). As one *mkunga* from Kiuyu commented, when infertility is considered a "local" problem, many practitioners are consulted to determine the source of the problem (*Tatizo ni kienyeji huwa kuna jambo mpaka wamalize wengi*). Out of the twenty-four women in the study who sought any form of treatment, half (n = 12) had consulted three or more practitioners. In the course of the study, however, it became clear that the boundaries between "local" and "hospital" problems are hazy. While only four out of the twenty-four women chose to consult a biomedical practitioner *first*, over half of the women (n = 13) did visit a clinic or hospital at some point in their search for treatment.

The next section draws on individual cases of women and practitioners to illustrate the eclectic ways in which infertility in Pemba is managed. Patterns of resort for infertility have less to do with cost, distance, or a distinct etiology than with the reputation of the practitioner as well as circumstances that allow women to acknowledge other options of explaining the problem.

The Swedish doctor and the sheikh: managing infertility in Pemba[22]

Estimated at a negligible 2 percent, infertility has received little attention in health planning priorities set for the island of Pemba (MOH, Zanzibar 1988).[23] It is overshadowed by high fertility rates, the consequences of which are seen to have a negative impact on the quality of women's lives, their status, and their development in Tanzania (DHS, Tanzania 1993; Mbilyini 1985) and Zanzibar (Chintowa 1991; Tumbo-Masabo and Liljestrom 1994). As a result, policy statements regarding women's health have focused on the control of fertility.

Family planning activities in Pemba started in 1985, with three clinics staffed by family planning motivators in Chake-Chake, Wete, and Micheweni. At present, all PHC-units[24] have a family planning component, and are run by MCH-aids who are trained in the applications of so-called "natural" and "modern" contraceptive methods. At the time of the study, local midwives, now officially recognized by the WHO as "traditional birth attendants" (TBA), were also being provided with family planning training seminars through the Ministry of Health.

While family planning methods are widely familiar and accessible as a result of these efforts, their acceptance remains very low.[25] Belying an ideology that has equated their health and welfare with control of their fertility, women emphatically declare that to have many children is not only important for the mother and father but for the nation as a whole (*ni muhimu kwa taifa*). They openly affirm that the number of children a woman bears depends on God, and that to interfere with fertility is against Islamic law.

Fertility regulation is publicly discussed with much ambivalence. "Natural" family planning such as the "mucus" and "calendar" methods are a source of amusement and mockery among women, who see them as incompatible with the unpredictable timing of both men's and women's sexual needs. On the other hand, commonly mentioned "modern methods" including the pill, the loop, and tubal ligation (*kufunga kabisa* = "to close completely") are unexplained, and there-fore threatening. Women claim that the pill is rarely used because it is not known "where it goes and how it works." Contraceptive use in general is associated with the risk of cancer, infertility, and excessive bleeding.

Privately, however, as many *wakunga* admit, an array of "traditional" means are employed to influence the course of a woman's fertility. The *mkunga* can provide medicinal herbs made from roots and plants and a *mganga* may be sought out to perform a particular Islamic healing ritual. There is a perceived hierarchy, however, in the control of means to reduce or to enhance fertility. One *mkunga* pointed out that the *masheikh* were the most knowledgeable about fertility-reducing drugs, but did not provide them to the people.

The public resistance toward an ideology of high fertility and fertility control is buttressed by local practitioners in subtle ways. For example,

MCH-aids who serve as the family planning distributors often transform the intended use of Western contraceptives.[26] They tend not to prescribe the pill as a birth control method to a woman until after the birth of the third or fourth child. It is more frequently given to women for the spacing of childbirths, and as a means of regulating irregular and thus infertile menstrual periods.

At the same time, many of the women who perceive themselves to be infertile persistently seek out the very sites that disclaim their status as patients. They travel by *dala-dala*, the local public taxis, from villages in the north of Pemba down to Wete Hospital to see the Swedish gynecologist or to the southern tip of the island to consult the Chinese doctors at Mkoani Hospital. Some take the ferry to Unguja, to seek advice from doctors at Masimoja Hospital while others continue their journey to Muhimbili Medical Centre in Dar es Salaam.

As indicated earlier, most of the twenty-five infertile women in the study were interviewed at a health facility. For the twelve women who had never consulted a biomedical practitioner for their infertility, the structured context of the interview setting and of the interviews reproduced, to some extent, a first "clinical" encounter, allowing me insight into the manner in which women articulate their suffering. In the face of practitioners who diagnose illness on the basis of bodily signs, women use the language of symptoms to gain recognition of their problem. For over a third of the women in the study (n = 9), symptoms of infertility were attributed to a general illness in the body (*mshipa*), or to a problem of the abdominal area (*matatizo ya tumboni*). Other women, who related the problem to causes external to the body nonetheless localized pains within the body. Specific areas of pain included the abdomen (n = 15), waist, and upper thighs (n = 6). Pains were also specified in time, usually before or during their menses (n = 9), but also during sexual intercourse (n = 2). Painful sensations were described in considerable detail, as "pains that start high and come down"; "pain that cuts like a knife" (*kama kisito*); "pain down below that feels like a lump" (*kama donge*); "pain that is sharp" (*kata*); "shivering (*kina vuma*) during sex because of pain"; "a heavy head [that buzzes] like a car" (*kama gari*); and "heat in the stomach" (*inasokota*).

Despite the many women who present this complex of symptoms, expatriate health workers remain skeptical about the amount of time and resources that should be devoted to infertility, given its official low numbers. Local biomedical practitioners, on the other hand, note the increasing visibility of the problem in their clinics with anxiety. They link the unexplained symptoms with past complications compromising women's health.

We have [infertility] in every clinic [PHC unit] . . . in Micheweni and Chake, even in Konde. As soon as the Swedish doctor comes, they come. Most don't say what is wrong directly. They try to hide the problem and show other symptoms . . . dysfunctional bleeding, pain during menses and stomach pains. The main reasons for infertility are PID [pelvic inflammatory disease], mainly because of home deliveries, and sometimes male infertility, although men are generally not followed. (Medical assistant, Wete Hospital)

Nearly 50 percent of the patients seen by the gynecologist are infertility cases. Many women have tried elsewhere, and decide to come to the clinic. They are not referred but come through word-of-mouth. Often, the causes for infertility are not known, as we have no facilities for diagnosis . . . The most common causes [of secondary infertility] are PID and abortions. PID is a very severe infection, the women usually come as emergency cases. Some need operations, for example, when there are fibroid tumors or ovarian cysts; some may need plastic surgery when there is a narrowing of the tube. (Surgeon, Wete Hospital)

We encounter the problem frequently, although women are reluctant to say that they have come to seek help for infertility. Most say they are sick and have abdominal pains. Upon further questioning, the problem is revealed . . . We used to have an Infertility Clinic every Thursday and see at least five women per day. (Family Planning Coordinator, Masimoja Hospital)

The reading of infertility as a sign of hidden health complications provides a critical dimension in understanding how knowledge on infertility is shaped in Pemba. According to medical assistants[27] at Wete Hospital, pelvic inflammatory disease (PID), repeated spontaneous abortions,[28] and post-abortion infections are the most common gyneco-logical complications seen in women that attend the hospital and the key causes of secondary infertility. In turn, the hospital practitioners link these complications to STD[29] and illegitimate or illicit pregnancies, issues reluctantly spoken about in public, and thus difficult to gauge in terms of their magnitude.

In the Kiswahili posters produced by the Ministry of Health, STD are referred to as *wagonjwa wa asherati*, literally "diseases of [sexual] promiscuity", and are thus understandably stigmatized.[30] As such, they tend to remain hidden and therefore untreated, despite the availability of drugs. Hospital staff pointed out the large quantities of STD drugs donated by the EEC that lie unused in the storeroom because STD patients prefer to procure the drugs privately.

Local biomedical practitioners also point to hidden induced abortions in the case of pre- and extramarital pregnancies. Although induced abortions are officially illegal, I was told that some assistant medical officers would attend to cases outside of the hospital. On the other hand:

Septic abortion often happens as a result of self-induced methods. One woman arrived at the hospital with her cervix tattered and pus draining. The pregnancy was from a relative and they had tried to use a stick to terminate it. (Surgeon, Wete Hospital)

As integrated members of the community from which their patients stem, these practitioners have a privileged vantage point on the social factors conditioning medical etiologies of infertility. They are also aware of other dimensions shaping local knowledge and women's patterns of resort for infertility:

Women are supposed to conceive as soon as possible, usually within one year of marriage. They always think they are the ones to be infertile and there is much resistance to bring the husband, even from the woman's side. By the time the woman comes to the hospital, she has already been to the witchdoctor. (Family Planning Coordinator, Masimoja Hospital)

Religion complicates many matters . . . the problem of [untreated STD] has its roots in polygyny, and the causes of transmission are often men. I try to advise the woman to bring along her husband, but it is not easy. It is easier to get the husband to bring along his wife . . . There was a lady who was divorced because she failed to bear a child. She had a child with her second husband, while the first husband failed to have a child with his second wife. Probably a case of male infertility, although these cases are rarely presented. (Surgeon, Wete Hospital)

Most [women] tend to go to local doctors first because of belief. They believe that they were bewitched or that the problem is due to *mashetani*. (Medical assistant, Wete Hospital)

The fragmented case stories allude to the flexibility of local practitioners in expanding the definition and scope of infertility. Their ambiguous position is even more evident in the role of MCH-aids, local women who are posted at the PHC units after two years of formal training in maternal and child health. When I asked the MCH-aid at Micheweni what she thought the causes of infertility in her area were, she inquired whether I wanted to know the medical or the local reasons. In general, MCH-aids are well versed in biomedical explanations and specified STD, PID, "infections in the uterus," "infection that is transmitted to the Fallopian tubes," an "inverted uterus," "repeated abortions," "hormonal problems" as causes of infertility. However, asked about the source of the problem, they pointed to the intervention of spirits (*mashetani*), bad timing of the marriage, jealousy in the case of more than one wife, and general uncleanliness of house and body. One MCH-aid, herself infertile for six years, believes that she had been bewitched by her husband's first wife. She first sought advice from a *mkunga* and has since decided to consult a gynecologist.

MCH-aids are not regarded as influential or independent practitioners. They do, however, serve as important mediators of information and key referral persons in women's patterns of resort for infertility.

Often, they are the first person from whom advice is sought after female relatives. For infertility cases, they can do little more than a ritual physical examination. Occasionally, in an ironic reversal of roles, they prescribe one or more cycles of a contraceptive pill, believed to normalize the woman's fertility cycle, thus helping her to identify her most fertile period.

Apart from these essentially symbolic gestures, MCH-aids refer women to reputed local healers if the cause of the problem is obscure. If the woman has already seen a number of local practitioners without success, they may refer her to the hospital, although, as one MCH-aid stated, "there is no special doctor for these cases," referring to the chronic shortage of gynecologists and medical facilities.

In contrast to biomedical practitioners, local healers play an established role in patterns of resort for infertility, partly owing to their long-standing reputation on the island. Some of Pemba's healers, in practice for over twenty years, are famed and feared as far as the mainland and neighboring countries.[31] Many of these practitioners are syncretic, bearing witness to centuries of immigration from the Arab and the Persian Middle East, the Asian subcontinent and the African mainland (Mazrui and Shariff 1994). They combine Islamic and African healing traditions and a pharmacopeia that they claim originates in India and China.

Among local healers, the *wakunga* are the most frequently consulted for diagnosis and treatment of women's problems relating to fertility and childbearing. The term *mkunga* means any woman who has experience in delivering babies although there is a distinction drawn between women with different levels of experience, knowledge, and skills. *Wakunga* not only deliver babies but advise on women's and children's sicknesses and administer a variety of herbal medicines (Rose 1994).

For nearly half of the women who sought any form of treatment (n = 11), a *mkunga* was the first practitioner consulted. In contrast to the oblique way that infertility is revealed to biomedical practitioners, women present the problem directly to local healers. In order to diagnose the exact location of the problem, the *wakunga* use a technique of palpating and massaging the abdomen (*kukanda tumbo*). They recognize abdominal pains (*zingizi*), severe pain during menstruation, and irregular periods (*siku zake si za kawaida*, "her bleeding is not as normal") to be common "symptoms" of infertility that will not disappear until the woman has conceived. Treatment, given to alleviate these symptoms, consists mainly of medicinal roots and plants (*dawa za mzizi* and *dawa za miti shamba*).[32]

Wakunga commonly perceive the causes of infertility to lie within the reproductive organs. They are among the few local practitioners to suggest that the problem may be with the husband, who has weak sperm (*mbegu hazi kubaliani*) or no sperm (*mume hana mbegu*). However, if they are unable to determine the bodily cause, they will refer the woman to a *mganga* or a *sheikh* for diagnosis. If the cause is known, but the problem is perceived to be too complicated, the woman may be referred to the hospital. There are indications that the *wakunga* are losing their exclusive hold over the domain of women's illnesses, especially since their integration into the formal health sector as TBA. Women increasingly turn to the hospital for complications of pregnancy and childbearing, and many *wakunga* claim that they refer women to the hospital when the problem is beyond their knowledge or skills. Bi Mwamize, a very old and respected *mkunga* from Micheweni, told us that her skills would die with her, as no one of the younger generation wanted to learn the trade of the *wakunga*.

Following the *wakunga*, the most common pattern of resort for infertility are the *waganga*. A third of the women in the study (n = 8) chose to consult a *mganga* initially. The *waganga* are differentiated through their training in a variety of skills, including spirit exorcism, divination, herbalism, and the preparation of medicines to encourage the successful outcome of illness, marriages, love, and business affairs. Those with divinatory skills refer to astrology (specifically known as *waganga ya falaki*), divining boards (*ramli* and *bao*), pots (*vitungu*), or spirits to help them diagnose and prescribe an appropriate course of action.

In cases of infertility, the *waganga* are most frequently sought out when the interference of *mashetani* is suspected. Strictly speaking, before the suspected *shetani* can be exorcized, its existence has to be confirmed through a diviner, who holds the Islamic office of *sheikh* or *mwalimu* (teacher). Following a confirmed divination, the woman may choose to consult a *mganga* or another *sheikh* in order to expel the spirit. The *mganga* acts as a spirit medium, compelling the spirit to leave the body by talking to it or through a longer procedure of exorcism involving ritual dance (*ngoma*) and the sacrifice of a small animal, usually a goat. The *sheikh* or *mwalimu*, on the other hand, compels the spirit to leave by wielding the spiritual power of Islam in the form of religious chants, prayers (*dua*), and the preparation of protective devices (*hirinzi* and *kombe*[33]).

In principle, the functions of *mwalimu*, *sheikh*, and *mganga* are distinct. Tension exists between the roles they occupy[34] and the ideological systems they represent; the *mganga* has roots in African healing traditions, the *mwalimu* and the *sheikh* are of Islamic origin. In Pemba, distinctions are further drawn between the *masheikh*. Some are merely elders *(mzee)*, while others are learned men *(mtu ghalim)* who are literate in Arabic and have undertaken Koranic studies abroad. In practice, however, the roles of these healers are less easy to separate. Their strongly syncretic nature is illustrated in the case of two sheikhs who deal with infertility.

Sheikh A., famous throughout the island, is a learned man who spent many years studying Arabic and religion in Yemen. He is most often consulted for complications during pregnancy, including bleeding during pregnancy *(wamwagaji)*, delayed delivery, "wrong" positioning of the foetus *(mtoto amelala vibaya*, "the child is lying badly") as well as for infertility. While he says that conception ultimately depends on God's will, complications during pregnancy and the failure to conceive can be due to diseases inside the abdomen *(ugonjwa wa tumbo)* and the interference of *mashetani*. For these problems, he appeals to God by reading a *duwa*, or preparing *hirinzi* for the woman to wear until she is able to carry a pregnancy to term. He also gives the woman a mixture of medicines (thirteen plants from India) mixed with octopus, which is believed to clean the fallopian tubes *(mivija ya fuko la uzazi)*. He distances himself from the *waganga*, whom he claims are liars and money-makers, and from the sorcerers *(wachawi)* who deal in evil forces.

Sheikh H. is an *imam* and a *mganga ya kitabu (mganga* of the "book," i.e., the Koran), and was taught Arabic by another sheikh from Ole. He treats most children's diseases and women's problems by giving them herbal medicines *(dawa za majani)* and *kombe*. He attributes infertility to wrong stars during the time of marriage, changes in the reproductive organs, and *mashetani*, who drink the blood and the sperm of the husband. He is able to divine whether the woman will be able to conceive by looking at her head *(falaki ya kichwa)*. If there is a chance, he prepares a *hirinzi* wrapped in a black sheet around a thin rope which is administered in a number of ways. It can be put around the woman's abdomen at night for seven to twenty-one days, around the neck of a hen who has never lain eggs, or around a tree which bears no fruit. When the hen lays eggs, or the tree bears fruit, the woman should become pregnant.

A common theme in the discussion of how various local practitioners manage infertility is their functioning at the interface of different systems of explanation. The biomedical practitioners are able to link medical etiologies of infertility to social conditions that compromise health. The MCH-aids and the *wakunga* mediate between biomedical and ethnomedical explanations, and the *masheikh* and the *waganga* reconcile religious and lay interpretations of infertility. Despite the implicit antagonism in these dual roles, these practitioners coexist with mutual acknowledgment, if not respect. They collaborate in unspoken ways in the formation of a body of knowledge on infertility that is coherent because it responds to shifts in the local configuration of power.

The adaptive character of many local practitioners encourages an articulation of women's fertility problems that clearly surpasses the officially documented 2 percent infertility. The narrow scope of clinically defined infertility is exploded, on the one hand, by the range of socially legitimate concerns of women seeking treatment for infertility. In Pemba, infertility "cases" include not only women unable to have children in the lifetime of a marriage, but also very young women who fail to conceive within a few months of their marriage, women who have children from a previous marriage and have remarried, women whose children have died, and in some cases women who have no sons. On the other hand, women envisage alternate frameworks of explanation for infertility, enabling other legitimate patterns of resort. In the following cases[35] of women who had been unable to conceive for many years, the range of possible meanings of infertility[36] allowed the women a certain bargaining power within the circle of family, neighbors and practitioners who made up their therapy management network.

Fatma, roughly 35 years old, has never been to school. She lives in Kiuyu with her third husband, with whom she has been married for two and a half years. She was divorced twice because she was unable to bear a child. She first consulted a *mkunga*, who told her that she had no visible problem with her reproductive organs, and referred her to a *mganga*. He told her that she was possessed by a *shetani*. Her husband's family urged her to undergo a special treatment to exorcize the *shetani*, but the spirit did not appear to ask for something. She herself does not believe that she is possessed but links her infertility to an ectopic pregnancy that she had roughly six years ago. She had severe abdominal pains followed by a period during which she missed her monthly bleeding and later heavy bleeding. She does not remember the operation as she was unconscious when taken to the hospital and believes that the doctor may have removed her uterus and cervix at the time. (Case 12; December 12, 1994)

Asha, 29 years old, has a Form 3 education.[37] She was divorced once because of her infertility and now lives with her second husband. Her husband has another wife with whom he has no children. Asha thinks that her inability to conceive may be linked to an infection that she had a few years ago, for which she had to go to Chake Hospital. The infection (*kisonoo* = gonorrhea) caused her severe abdominal pains and discharge and she was given penicillin injections. Some time later, following the advice of her first husband, she consulted a doctor at

Wete Hospital. He said that her infertility was due to a "mass in the uterus" (*donge*) and that she should have an operation to remove it. She refused because there was no guarantee that she would be able to conceive, and because of the pressure of her mother who insisted that the problem was a local one (*matatizo ya kiswahili*). She consulted a well-known *mganga*, who said that she was possessed by *mashetani*. A second *mganga* told her that her husband was possessed, as he had no children with his other wife. Both times, she was given *kombe* and some herbal medicines (*dawa ya miti shamba*). After spending almost 5000 TSH [US$ 10] on various *waganga*, she decided to follow the advice of a nurse from Wete Hospital who recommended that she get the pill (*dawa za majira*) from a PHC unit. She started to take these but stopped because of the side effects they produced. (Case 14; December 12, 1994)

Halima, 22 years old, has been married to her first husband for eight years. Her husband has another wife who has five children. She says that her infertility is due to a problem (*mshipa*) inside of her uterus. She first went to see a *mkunga*, who, after examining her, said that she had a ruined abdomen (*tumbo bovu*). She then consulted the Chinese doctor at Mkoani Hospital, who examined her and gave her drugs to stimulate ovulation. She "conceived" for one month, but then started to bleed. Her husband accompanied her to see a *mganga*, who said that she was possessed by land spirits (*pepo*). The mganga gave her a *kombe* to drink for seven days and staged a ceremony (*ngoma*) to expel the spirits, where she was told to dance until the *pepo* came out. After the *pepo* failed to appear, she went with her sister to see the MCH-aid. She was told to go to Wete Hospital, where she was examined by the Swedish doctor [at the time of this interview]. He told her it was a case of primary infertility and recommended that she have a tubal blow. (Case 25; December 21, 1994).

As local medical assistants, nurses, MCH-aids, *wakunga, waganga* and *masheikh* mediate between systems for explaining illness – internalizing and externalizing (Young 1983), local and imported, earthly and divine – the symbolic weight of infertility is transformed. The above women's awareness of multiple etiologies and the implication of other individuals within these etiologies allows them to negotiate their socially devalued status to some extent[38] through new alliances and the options to accept or reject a set of "diagnostic criteria." The simultaneous logic of greedy spirits and faulty organs objectifies the meaning of infertility, thus deflecting blame from individual women and encouraging them to persist in their search for treatment and therapy.

   As my focus in the study was on women who perceived themselves to be infertile at the time, it was difficult to evaluate the relative "success" rates of local healers in treating infertility. Local biomedical practitioners, however, readily express their frustrations with the limits of managing infertility effectively:

All we can do is to take gynecological histories, temperature, and mucal status [and] tell women how to determine their fertile period. We cannot deal with it adequately at the moment . . . we need to train medical assistants and doctors in infertility management. (Family Planning Coordinator, Masimoja Hospital)

Every woman wants to have more children. All I can do is give psychological treatment . . . there is a lack of trained doctors and facilities, even for doing a hysterosalpinography. (Medical assistant, Wete Hospital)

Suspended between a clinical understanding of infertility and a common empathy with women's longing for children, these practitioners are on the horns of the dilemma of resource allocation in reproductive health policies. They are acutely aware that as long as children remain a primary indicator for women's status and a vital link between kin and neighboring households, the threat of infertility is a paramount concern.

Conclusions: contesting identities and etiologies

The fact that she had not yet conceived at the age of twenty-six added to her frustration. She was said to suffer from *baridi yabisi*, a state characterised by depression, apathy and irritation. Naima longed for a baby, and for a while she thought she was pregnant. However, it turned out to be a false pregnancy, a spirit (*pepo*). (Fuglesang 1994:272)

A twenty-two-year-old girl was brought to the maternity ward at Muhimibili by close neighbors: an elderly lady and a young woman. When the obstetrician on duty enquired about her problems, the girl claimed to have delivered a baby three hours before, but she had neither seen the child nor heard it cry. The old lady added on that the girl had delivered a baby. They had brought her to hospital for medical help because she suffered from abdominal pains. The old lady presented a lump wrapped in sheets. When it was unfolded, a dead, old chicken with long, sharp claws and brown feathers was displayed . . . When the girl saw the chicken, she became distressed and broke down in tears. In utter disbelief, the obstetrician calmed her down first, then proceeded to take down her obstetric history . . . The patient in discussion appeared hysterical in personality. She firmly believed to be pregnant without the presence of a foetus . . . The presentation of a dead chicken as a baby appears to be secretive, obscure manipulations of the old lady, whose motive, in part, was to evoke mysterious powers of witchcraft. Although the chicken was illogical and incongruent to the situation, it served a cultural psychosocial function of lending credibility to the false belief . . . *severe personal stress could have accentuated the precipitation of a new identity simulating symptoms of pregnancy.* The phantom pregnancy could be seen as the affective equivalent of the wish for pregnancy. (Ndosi and Lema 1992:539–41; emphasis added)

The first documented case of a mysterious "phantom pregnancy" at Muhimbili Medical Centre in Dar es Salaam hints at "historical shifts in the configuration of power" (Abu-Lughod 1990:90) that affect the way women's concerns with fertility are articulated and managed. As women seek recognition and treatment of their problems, the signs, meanings, and consequences of impaired fertility are framed and reframed in the diagnostic criteria of the local practitioner. Reflecting women's subjugated knowledge about the body, the ghosts of unfulfilled pregnancies present a thorn in the eye of a largely foreign public health discourse that does not acknowledge their existence. In so far as infertility is recognized in this discourse, it is seen as a "source of resistance" to achieving the modernist goal of fertility transition (Frank 1983).

At a symbolic level, fertility in Pemba constitutes an important social theme in the management of individual and collective lives. It represents the continuity of a healthy body in multiple dimensions: the individual body of the woman, the social body of interpersonal relations, and the body politic of religious and state discourses on the population. Consequently, infertility stands for an ailing body, for disturbed social relations, and for threatened boundaries. At the same time, women in Pemba contest a global rhetoric on fertility control by emphasizing its destructiveness to all levels of the "healthy body": contraception is unacceptable because it causes bodily illness, because it disrupts sexual relations, and because it is against religious proscriptions.

At an individual level, the objectified causes and symptoms of infertility and the subtle mockery of the discourse on fertility control may be interpreted as signs of "ritualized resistance" (Comaroff 1985; Boddy 1989; Lock 1993). In contrast to Boddy, however, who sees spirit possession as mediating the "historical dialectic of acquiescence and resistance" (1989:347), I maintain that consciousness of the "process of representation" (Comaroff 1985:6) is a necessary premise to women's contestation of hegemonic constructions of their selves. In large part, the development of a public discourse on infertility has been achieved in Pemba through the dynamic interplay between local healing systems, one that legitimates the status of infertile women and encourages them to persist in their search for treatment. One suspects, however, that for individual women who perceive themselves to be infertile, the "ghosts in the machine" will persist until they envisage – and thus can contribute to – the making of a new order of gender and familial relations.

ACKNOWLEDGMENTS

The study on which this chapter is based was conducted in the course of an internship (October 1994 to January 1995) with the Deutsche Gesellschaft für Technische Zusammenarbeit (GTZ). I gratefully acknowledge the technical and advisory support of Dr. Richard Rohde,

Family Health Programme, Dar es Salaam, and Dr. Mohammed Zahran, Zonal Medical Officer, Pemba. Many thanks go to my research assistant, Sauda Subeit Ali, whose enthusiasm, dedication, and insight greatly benefited the study. For thoughtful comments on earlier versions of this chapter, I thank Connie Nathanson and the editors of this book.

NOTES

1 Although Zanzibar consists of Pemba and Unguja, it is the island of Unguja that is more familiar to Westerners under the name Zanzibar.
2 An exception is Craster's lengthy travel account, published in 1913.
3 The study was conducted in the context of a three-month field internship supported by the Deutsche Gesellschaft für Technische Zusammenarbeit (GTZ). Fieldwork in Pemba was carried out with permission from the Zanzibar Research Council and under the auspices of the Ministry of Health and the Family Health Programme (GTZ) in Pemba.
4 In countries that envisage growth rates below the social reproduction level, the problem of infertility has been highly medicalized. The quest for solutions in the realm of reproductive technologies has provoked debate on the very basic notions of human reproduction and mother/parenthood (Stanworth 1987; Ginsburg and Rapp 1992; Becker and Nachtigall 1994).
5 While the core level of infertility in sub-Saharan Africa lies around 5 percent, various estimates report exceptional rates of primary infertility within the so-called "infertility belt," an area stretching from Gabon in the west across to southwestern Sudan in the east. In East Africa, rates of infertility have been found to range from 3.9 percent in Burundi to 19.4 percent in Tanzania (Evina 1991). High rates of both primary and secondary infertility have been attributed to complications, bilateral tubal occlusion being the most common (WHO 1987), that result from elevated levels of STD (Wasserheit 1989:160), post-partum and post-abortion infections as well as endemic diseases and malnutrition (Mascie-Taylor 1992).
6 An overview of the literature on AIDS in sub-Saharan Africa, particularly in the early 1980s, reveals to what extent the paradigm of promiscuous sexuality guided both the early focus on sexual behavior and so-called high-risk groups including prostitutes (Packard and Epstein 1991; Kielmann 1993; 1997).
7 A recent volume compiled by leading demographers is prefaced by the assertion that "high levels of African fertility have cultural explanations and that particular combinations of the proximate determinants – nuptiality, abstinence, breastfeeding, sterility – find their origin in specific customs and institutions rather than in socioeconomic characteristics" (Ebigbola and van de Walle 1987:iii).
8 Examples include Greenhalgh (1994), Bledsoe (1990), Bledsoe *et al.* (1994), Handwerker (1986) and Fricke (1986).
9 Personal communication, Antje Becker, May 1995.
10 "The strike against bearing children is really the only political means that we

have . . . unemployment hangs like a threat over everybody: who will be next?" (Head of Saxon Women's Forum, cited in Atkinson 1995).

11 Ebin 1982; Katz and Katz 1984: Devisch 1993; Feldman-Savelsberg 1994; Inhorn 1994.

12 The study was carried out in three sites, chosen for their relative accessibility and representativeness of urbanized and rural settings. Wete, in the north-west of Pemba, is a small port town and the seat of one of the three hospitals on the island. Ole and Kiuyu are adjacent villages roughly 25 kilometres south of Wete. Each has a Primary Health Care (PHC) Unit staffed by a Maternal and Child Health (MCH) aid. Micheweni, a small town in the far north of the island, is the most rural and poorly accessible of the sites, but does have a relatively well-staffed cottage hospital.

13 This section is based on group discussions with women who were not infertile and interviews with practitioners (biomedical and local) at the three study sites.

14 In the past, there were initiation ceremonies to celebrate a girl's passage into womanhood (*unyago* or *sondo*); however, these had become very rare events at the time of my fieldwork, mainly because of increased cost and schooling since the 1940s.

15 Approximately US$ 20 to 200, according to December 1994 exchange rate.

16 Katapa (1994:77) refers to the Tanzanian daily newspapers' reporting of deaths occurring as a result of arranged marriages and abortions among teenagers.

17 According to Rose (1994:23), kinship in Pemba does not refer to biological or emotional relationships within families, but rather a sharing of bodily substances with others, including blood, womb, and semen.

18 For the neighboring island of Mafia, Caplan describes how potential violence generated by adultery cases is projected into the world of spirits: "Many exchanges between humans and spirits concern sexual relations: humans can seek the help of spirits to protect themselves from the sorcery of jealous spouses . . . or to make the husbands sick or impotent in order to gain favor with their wives" (1991:93; author's translation from the original French).

19 The syncretic *shetani* cult is found in most of the Swahili coastal regions that share Islamic faith. See Fuglesang (1994), Gray (1969), Caplan (1991), and Giles (1987) for discussion of spirits and spirit possession in Lamu (Kenya), mainland Tanzania, Mafia, Zanzibar, and Pemba.

20 Writing on women in Sudan and Malaysia respectively, Boddy (1988; 1989) and Ong (1988) point out that spirit possession is almost exclusively associated with married women and frequently connected to fertility problems (Boddy 1988:13).

21 Ong similarly points to cases of possession in Malaysia, where women are said to have been "penetrated by the devil" (1988:31).

22 This section is based on interviews with twenty-five women who perceived themselves to be infertile and interviews with practitioners (biomedical and local) at the three study sites. Most of the women were contacted through MCH-aids in the three settings and the majority of interviews (n = 20) were conducted either at the PHC units, or at Wete Hospital for reasons of convenience and confidentiality.

23 In demographic terms, infertility is measured as the percentage of women who remain childless at the end of their "reproductive careers." Hence, this number reflects neither the concerns of women who are unable to conceive between the ages of 15 and 49 years, nor of the many women who at any given point in time initiate treatment-seeking for infertility because they have been unable to fulfill the social expectations of conceiving within a year of marriage.

24 Although Pemba is less developed than Unguja, most people have very good access to primary health care, with the majority reportedly living within five kilometres of a PHC unit.

25 According to the Family Planning Coordinator at Masimoja Hospital, who supervises activities on both islands, family planning prevalence is estimated at 5 percent.

26 Bledsoe *et al.* suggest that technologies "undergo significant transformations in meaning in the process of being exported," drawing on the example of rural Gambian women who use the pill in conjunction with long-standing birth-spacing strategies to maintain long birth intervals (1994:105).

27 This term is somewhat misleading, as given the shortage of medical doctors, medical assistants have had to perform all tasks and minor operations regularly expected of a general practitioner.

28 Among the women I interviewed, almost two-thirds (n = 16) had never had a pregnancy, while over one-third (9) reported having an ectopic pregnancy or abortion.

29 Pelvic inflammatory disease often has its source in lower reproductive tract infections, such as gonorrhea and chlamydia. If left untreated, the organisms that cause these infections ascend into the upper tract causing salpingitis and bilateral tubal scarring (WHO 1987:968; Wasserheit 1989:145).

30 In discussions with women, the word *asherati* came up in connnection with adultery, prostitution, and divorce.

31 Craster notes in 1913 that "the natives of Pemba have a great reputation as magicians throughout East Africa" (1913:313) and Gray, over fifty years later, writes: "That island [Pemba] is highly respected by the Segeju as the home of the most skillful medicine men as well as the most ruthless witches" (1969:176).

32 A *mkunga* interviewed close to Micheweni recalled the case of a woman who came to her with abdominal pain accompanied by bleeding. When she examined the client by palpating the abdomen, she found the woman to have all signs of fertility yet a ruined abdomen (*tumbo bovu*) due to an "insect" (*mdudu*). She gave the woman some roots to relieve her pain, and advised her to consult a *mganga* in order to determine the basic cause of the problem before coming back.

33 *Hirinzi* are charms or amulets containing Koranic verses written on paper. They are either worn on the body, hung in the house or shop, or buried in the ground. *Kombe* are also Koranic verses, but are written with special ink on paper and burned, with the smoke driven toward the person, or written on a plate, after which the ink is washed with water and the infused water is given to the ailing person to drink.

34 Gray describes the hierarchy of these three practitioners among the Segeju

on the coast of Tanzania: "The *mganga* . . . has a rival for prestige in the village *mwalimu*, and, in a few villages, the *sheikh*. The *mganga* is generally more prosperous than the *mwalimu* (traditionally a poor man), but the *mwalimu* has moral ascendancy over the *mganga*" (1969:186).

35 The three cases were reconstructed on the basis of the information provided in the semi-structured interviews conducted with infertile women. All names are pseudonyms.

36 Overall, the reasons mentioned for infertility in the study included illnesses within the body (*mshipa*) (n = 9); possession by *mashetani* or *pepo* (n = 8); "God is not yet ready" (*Mungo hajamjalia*) (n = 7); complications resulting from hospital operations (*matatizo ya hospitali*) (n = 5); and sorcery (*urogaji*) (n = 3).

37 In theory, Form 3 corresponds to US Grade 11, that is, the third year of secondary schooling following eight years of primary school (Standard 1–8). In practice, it does not necessarily indicate a higher level of literacy as educational standards in Zanzibar dropped drastically after the enforcement of compulsory secondary schooling for girls in the 1960s.

38 Boddy suggests that a Hofriyati woman's illness is "reframed" by possession in such a way that "the precipitating behavior or event – for example infertility – becomes compatible with her self-image: she is fertile, for spirits have seen fit to usurp this most valuable asset" (1988:18).

REFERENCES

Abu-Lughod, L. 1990, "The romance of resistance: tracing transformations of power through Bedouin women," *American Ethnologist* 17:41–55.

Atkinson, R. 1995, "German unification lays heavy burden on Eastern working women," *The Washington Post*, March 29.

Barton, T. 1989, *Sexuality and Health in Sub-Saharan Africa: An Annotated Bibliography*, Berkeley: University of California Press.

Becker, G. and Nachtigall, R. D. 1994, "'Born to be a mother': the cultural construction of risk in infertility treatment in the US," *Social Science and Medicine* 39 (4):507–18.

Bergstrom, S. 1992, "Reproductive failure as a health priority in the Third World: a review," *East African Medical Journal* 69(4):174–80.

Bledsoe, C. 1990, "The politics of children: fosterage and the social management of fertility among the Mende," in P. Handwerker (ed.), *Births and Power: Social Change and the Politics of Reproduction*, Boulder, Colorado: Westview, pp. 81–100.

Bledsoe, C., Hill, A., D'Alessandro, U. and Langerock, P. 1994, "Constructing natural fertility: the use of Western contraceptive technologies in rural Gambia," *Population and Development Review* 20:81–113.

Boddy, J. 1988, "Spirits and selves in northern Sudan: the cultural therapeutics of possession and trance," *American Ethnologist* 15(1):4–27.

1989, *Wombs and Alien Spirits: Women, Men and the Zar Cult in Northern Sudan*, Madison: University of Wisconsin Press.

Bongaarts, J. 1991, "The KAP-gap and the unmet need for contraception," *Population and Development Review* 17(2): 293–313.

Caldwell, J., Caldwell, P. and Quiggin, P. 1989, "Disaster in an alternative civilization. The social dimension of AIDS in sub-saharan Africa," Health Transition Centre working paper no. 2, Canberra.

Caplan, P. 1991, "Un informateur swahili et son journal: esprits et sexe," in F. Le Guennec-Coppens and P. Caplan (eds.), *Les Swahili entre Afrique et Arabie*, Paris: Karthala, pp. 73–94.

Chintowa, P. 1991, "Spreading the word in Zanzibar," *Population* 17(8):3.

Craster, Captain J. 1913, *Pemba, the Spice Island of Zanzibar*, London: T. Fisher Unwin.

Comaroff, J. 1985, *Power and Body: Spirit of Resistance: The Culture and History of a South African People*, Chicago: University of Chicago Press.

Demographic and Health Surveys (DHS) 1993, *Tanzania Demographic and Health Survey 1991/1992*, Dar es Salaam: Bureau of Statistics, Planning Commission; Columbia, Maryland: Macro International Inc.

Devisch, R. 1993, *Weaving the Threads of Life: The Khita Gyn-Eco-Logical Healing Cult Among the Yaka*, Chicago: The University of Chicago Press.

Dixon-Mueller, R. 1993, "The sexuality connection in reproductive health," *Studies in Family Planning* 24(5):269–82.

Dixon-Mueller, R. and Wasserheit, J. 1991, *The Culture of Silence: Reproductive Tract Infections among Women in the Third World*, New York: International Women's Health Coalition.

Ebigbola, J. and van de Walle, E. 1987, "Preface," in *The Cultural Roots of African Fertility Regimes: Proceedings of the Ife Conference, February 25–March 1, 1987*, Ile-Ife, Migeria: Department of Demography and Social Statistics, Obafemi Awolowo University; Philadelphia: Population Studies Centre, University of Pennsylvania.

Ebin, V. 1982, "Interpretations of infertility: the Aowin people of southwest Ghana," in MacCormack, pp. 141–59.

Evina, A. 1991, "Effet des maladies sexuellement transmissibles sur la fécondité: l'infécondité en Afrique sub-saharienne," Unpublished manuscript.

Feldman-Savelsberg, P. 1994, "Plundered kitchens and empty wombs: fear of infertility in the Cameroonian grassfields," *Social Science and Medicine* 39(4):463–74.

Fisher, S. and Davis, K. 1993, *Negotiating at the Margins: The Gendered Discourses of Power and Resistance*, New Brunswick, New Jersey: Rutgers University Press.

Frank, O. 1983, "Infertility in sub-Saharan Africa: estimates and implications," *Population and Development Review* 9(1):137–44.

Fricke, T. 1986, *Himalayan Households: Tamang Demography and Domestic Processes*, Ann Arbor: University of Michigan Press.

Fuglesang, M. 1994, *Veils and Videos: Female Youth Culture on the Kenyan Coast*, Stockholm Studies in Social Anthropology, Stockholm: Gotab.

Giles, L. 1987, "Possession cults on the Swahili coast: a reexamination of theories of marginality," *Africa* 57(2):234–57.

Ginsburg, F. and Rapp, R. 1992, "The politics of reproduction," *Annual Reviews in Anthropology* 20:311–43.

Gray, R. 1969, "The shetani cult among the Segeju of Tanzania," in J. Beattie and J. Middleton (eds.), *Spirit Mediumship and Society in Africa*, London: Routledge and Kegan Paul, pp. 171–87.

Greenhalgh, S. 1994, "Anthropological contributions to fertility theory," The Population Council working paper no. 64.

Handwerker, P. 1986, *Culture and Reproduction: An Anthropological Critique of Demographic Transition Theory*, Boulder, Colorado: Westview.

Inhorn, M. 1994, "Kabsa (a.k.a. Mushahara) and threatened fertility in Egypt," *Social Science and Medicine* 39(4):487–505.

Katapa, R. S. 1994, "Arranged marriages," in Tumbo-Masabo and Liljestrom (eds.), pp. 76–95.

Katz, S. and Katz, S. H. 1984, "An evaluation of traditional therapy for barrenness," *Medical Anthropology Quarterly* 1(4):394–405.

Kielmann, K. 1993, "'Prostitution,' 'risk' and 'responsibility': paradigms of AIDS prevention and women's identities in Thika, Kenya," M.A. thesis, McGill University.

1997, "'Prostitution,' 'risk' and 'responsibility': paradigms of AIDS prevention and women's identities in Thika, Kenya," in M. Inhorn and P. Brown (eds.), *The Anthropology of Infectious Diseases*, Philadelphia: Gordon and Breach.

Lock, M. 1993, *Encounters with Aging: Mythologies of Menopause in Japan and North America*, Berkeley: University of California Press.

MacCormack, C. (ed.) 1982, *Ethnography of Fertility and Birth*, London: Academic Press.

MacLeod, A. E. 1991, *Accommodating Protest: Working Women, the New Veiling, and Change in Cairo*, New York: Columbia University Press.

Mahoney, M. and Yngvesson, B. 1992, "The construction of subjectivity and the paradox of resistance: reintegrating feminist anthropology and psychology," *Signs: Journal of Women and Culture* 18(1):45–73.

Maina-Ahlberg, B. 1991, *Women, Sexuality and the Changing Social Order: The Impact of Government Policies on Reproductive Behavior in Kenya*, Philadelphia: Gordon and Breach.

Mascie-Taylor, C. 1992, "Endemic disease, nutrition and fertility in developing countries," *Journal of Biosocial Science* 24(3):355–65.

Mazrui, A. M. and Shariff, I. N. 1994, *The Swahili: Idiom and Identity of an African People*, Trenton, New Jersey: Africa World Press.

Mbilinyi, M. 1985, "Struggles concerning sexuality among female youth," *Journal of Eastern African Research and Development* 15:111–23.

Mhloyi, M. 1987, "The proximate determinants and their socio-cultural determinants: the case of two rural settings in Zimbabwe," in *The Cultural Roots of African Fertility Regimes: Proceedings of the Ife Conference, February 25–March 1, 1987*.

Ministry of Health, Zanzibar 1988, *Mortality, Fertility and Contraception in Zanzibar*. Provisional Results of the 1988 Survey, Zanzibar: Department of Planning, Administration and Finance, Statistical Unit.

Moore, H. 1994 *A Passion for Difference: Essays in Anthropology and Gender*, Cambridge, UK: Polity Press.

Nathanson, C. and Hill, K. 1994, "The unmet need for meaningful measures in discussions of fertility policy," paper prepared for the SSRC African Fertility Workshop, Johns Hopkins University.

Ndosi, N. K. and Lema, R. S. 1992, "Phantom pregnancy at Muhimbili," *East African Medical Journal* 69(9): 539–41.

Neff, D. 1994, "The social construction of infertility: the case of the matrilineal Nayars in South India," *Social Science and Medicine* 39(4):475–85.

Nkounkou, J. 1989, "Elements for consideration for a population policy in areas of high infertility: the example of USEAC," in *Population Policy in Sub-Saharan Africa: Drawing on International Experience: Papers presented at IUSSP Committee, Kinshasa, Zaire.*

Ong, A. 1988, "The production of possession: spirits and the multinational corporation in Malaysia," *American Ethnologist* 15(1):28–42.

    1990, "State versus Islam: Malay families, women's bodies and the body politic in Malaysia," *American Ethnologist* 17:258–76.

Packard, R. and Epstein, P. 1991, "Epidemiologists, social scientists and the structure of medical research on AIDS in Africa," *Social Science and Medicine* 33(7):771–94.

Puja, G.K. and Kassimoto, T. 1994, "Girls in education and pregnancy at school," in Z. Tumbo-Masabo and R. Liljestrom, pp. 54–75.

Riedmann, A. 1993, *Science that Colonizes: A Critique of Fertility Studies in Africa*, Philadelphia: Temple University Press.

Rose, K. 1994, "Sickness and Malnutrition on Pemba: An Anthropological Study of the Social Relations of Food, Perceptions of Sickness, and Help-Seeking Behaviour," Unpublished report, Save the Children Fund, Pemba Island, Tanzania.

Sawicki, J. 1991, *Disciplining Foucault: Feminism, Power, and the Body*, New York: Routledge.

Scheper-Hughes, N. 1990, "The subversive body: illness and the micropolitics of resistance," *Anthropology UCLA*, Special issue, Winter, Essays in honor of Harry Hoijer, pp. 43–70.

Scheper-Hughes, N. and Lock, M. 1987, "The mindful body: a prolegomenon to future work in medical anthropology," *Medical Anthropology Quarterly* 1(1):6–41.

Sherbinin, A. de, Ashford, L. and Gelbard, A. 1994, "What I hear when you say 'population': interpretations of key population terms," paper presented at the Annual Meeting of the National Council for International Health.

Stanworth, M. 1987, *Reproductive Technologies: Gender, Motherhood and Medicine*, Minneapolis: University of Minnesota Press.

Swantz, M.-L. 1986, *Ritual and Symbol in Transitional Zaramo Society*, Uppsala, Sweden: Scandinavian Institute of African Studies.

Townshend, P. and McElroy, A. 1992, "Toward an ecology of women's reproductive health," *Medical Anthropology* 14:9–34.

Tumbo-Masabo, Z. and Liljestrom, R. (eds.) 1994, *Chelewa, Chelewa: The Dilemma of Teenage Girls*, Stockholm: The Scandinavian Institute of African Studies.

Udvardy, M. 1990, "*Kifudu*: a female fertility cult among the Giriama," in A. Jacobson-Widding and W. van Beek (eds.), *The Creative Communion:*

African Folk Models of Fertility and the Regeneration of Life, Uppsala: Almqvist and Wiksell International.

Wasserheit, J. 1989, "The significance and scope of reproductive tract infections among third world women," *International Journal of Gynecology and Obstetrics* 3:145–68.

Watkins, S. 1993, "If all we knew about women was what we read in *Demography*, what would we know?," *Demography* 30(4):551–76.

World Health Organization 1987, "Infections, pregnancies and infertility: perspectives on prevention," *Fertility and Sterility* 47(6):964–7.

Young, A. 1983, "The relevance of traditional medical cultures to modern primary health care," *Social Science and Medicine* 17(18):1205–11.

7   Wives, mothers, and lesbians: rethinking resistance in the US

Ellen Lewin

Feminist anthropologists long have tended to engage in what Lila Abu-Lughod (1990) has so eloquently described as a "romance of resistance," placing the effort to locate women's agency and refusal to submit quietly to domination at the heart of much of their work. The image of women's unquestioning subservience is hard for us as feminists to accept, both in examining ourselves and in interpreting the lives of those with whom we conduct research, and the discovery of evidence of even indirect or perhaps unconscious resistance, what James Scott (1985) has called "the weapons of the weak," seems to reassure us that we need not lose hope. But Abu-Lughod reminds us that vexing theoretical dilemmas arise from efforts to cast "everyday" behavior as resistance, dilemmas that require us to examine our notions of agency, consciousness, and politics.

Resistance, as we have come to know it in a literature that focuses largely on women's experience in the workplace and in health care settings, can be either conscious or unconscious, either carefully crafted or serendipitous, either direct and efficient in its impact or stymied by powerful forces beyond the control of the actors. Resistance can be physical and observable or may be imputed even to those who accede to the demands of the powerful while perhaps secretly harboring what seem to be subversive thoughts. "Resistance" is rapidly becoming a word that covers anything, defines itself, and may be said to exist because we insist that it do so. The more elusive forms of resistance, those which can be described as symbolic and which are discovered through interpretation, the forms that we as anthropologists find most engaging and which delight us in their subtlety, are perhaps those which are most amenable to distortion through the lens of whatever culture the interpreter brings to the task; it is these that we must subject to scrutiny.

It is most appropriate that the topic of resistance be taken up in the context of women's relations with biomedicine, as it has been in this volume. These interactions, along with those in the domain of work

(Lamphere 1987; Ong 1987), have provided a major context for feminist theorizing about resistance both because the dominant assumptions and goals of institutional medicine and those that motivate women are unlikely to correspond and because medical practices can impinge in such powerful ways on women's fundamental understandings of identity and personal integrity. Robbie Davis-Floyd (1992) and Emily Martin (1987), looking at women's reproductive health in the US, have been particularly concerned with these issues, characterizing women as needing to assert their own best interests through struggle against medical, i.e., male-dominated, hegemony. In contrast, Margaret Lock's comparative study of menopause in Japan and North America (1993) has called for a more nuanced application of the idea of resistance when examining how women understand the physical changes glossed as "menopause" in the West.

It is also particularly apt to launch a reevaluation of resistance in connection with an analysis of the changing shape of lesbian and gay life in the US today. In the wake of the gay liberation movement associated with the pivotal Stonewall riot of 1969 (Duberman 1993; Kennedy and Davis 1993), the increasing visibility of homosexuality that has been a consequence of the AIDS epidemic, and the queer movement that has followed and commented upon both of these developments, an acute concern with resistance, rebellion, and subversion has become a vital feature of the lesbian and gay political landscape (Escoffier and Bérubé 1991; Duggan 1992; Warner 1993). The queer sensibility, in particular, draws on a social constructionist perspective to question and denaturalize both gender and sexual orientation, not only rebelling against repression and discrimination but bringing into question the very validity of the categories on which such abuses are based. If dichotomous categories, such as male and female or gay and straight, are challenged, even common-sense notions of what they entail are thrown into uncertainty. Accordingly, many contemporary political agendas of resistance among lesbians and gay men focus on fundamental notions of constituency and definition, and aim at subverting the notion that people can be categorized according to gender or sexual orientation (or, by extension, race, nationality, or ethnicity) in an authoritative manner. Ironically, as we shall see below, the power of many of these subversive strategies depends upon accepting fixed definitions that constitute the essence of the very social institutions to be disrupted, such as parenthood and marriage.

The emergence of lesbian mothers

The surge of interest in motherhood and family formation that has come to be a significant part of lesbian and gay life in the US today is, apart from the AIDS epidemic and the debate over gay participation in the military, perhaps the most widely noted indicator of the increasing visibility of lesbians and gay men in our society. Further, because AIDS and participation in the military have been constructed as mainly men's issues (despite the sizeable presence of lesbians in the armed forces and the existence of lesbians with AIDS), these issues of "family values" tend to be most central to the growing public presence of lesbians in American life. While in the 1970s such family issues mainly concerned challenges to child custody for lesbians who had been married when they had their children, extensive coverage in the mass media has made donor, artificial, or assisted insemination – with the popular image of the "turkey baster" and the resulting "lesbian baby boom" – far more visible mechanisms for family formation than other pathways to reproduction for lesbians (Lewin 1993).

Whether more lesbians in fact become mothers through insemination than through more conventional reproductive methods cannot, of course, be determined; not only do relatively few lesbians make this information public, but, because there is much confusion on even how to define sexual orientation, exactly who counts as a lesbian mother is not easily agreed upon. In the wave of popular attention directed at "turkey baster moms" lesbian mothers who have been married or who became pregnant as a result of heterosexual liaisons arouse little interest. Their reproductive histories tend to be seen either as the passive outcomes of conformity in their younger years or as unintentional in some other way.

But becoming a lesbian mother through insemination seems to be all about intention, and by extension, resistance. Lesbians – women whose identity is commonly assumed to derive primarily from their sexual appetites, and who are thought to be self-indulgent, immature, and disconnected from traditional family values (if not from traditional families themselves) – demand, in a manner of speaking, access to the status of mother. To do so as a lesbian without engaging in heterosexual intercourse would seem to disengage sexuality from procreation, at the same time that it gives the lie to the notion that lesbian (or gay) relationships cannot lead to family formation in the traditional sense. Lesbians who become mothers in this way might be said to be *demanding* access to a source of value otherwise restricted to hetero-sexual women. We might anticipate, given the confrontation with heterosexism that lesbian motherhood seems to represent, that not only the fact of becoming a mother, but interaction with the institutions of reproductive health care might offer a context in which resistance would be most clearly undertaken and performed.

My work with lesbian mothers, and particularly with those who used donor insemination to achieve motherhood, suggests a more complicated picture, however. Insemination can be achieved in a number of ways. Choices individual lesbians make from among these options seem to have less to do with areas of specific agreement or disagreement with the values and assumptions promulgated by biomedicine than with individual efforts to establish a maternal identity in a way that meets particular cultural and personal goals. More specifically, lesbian mothers appear to use their encounters with the medical profession and with the reproductive technologies they employ to strengthen existing personal strategies and to make statements about themselves as people – and especially as women – that facilitate claims to aspects of feminine identity which confer value on the individual woman.

To illustrate this perspective, I'd like to cite four cases of donor insemination I collected during my research on lesbian mothers (Lewin 1985). But first, a few words about donor or artificial insemination. Artificial insemination is not one of the new reproductive technologies; it was developed originally for use in animal husbandry and has been around at least since the eighteenth century. Its use for human impregnation dates from the nineteenth century, and by the early years of the twentieth century physicians were using "donor" sperm to impregnate women whose husbands were sterile.

Throughout its history, artificial insemination has been regarded with some suspicion, for some because its use seems to imply a kind of adultery, for others because obtaining sperm donations depends upon sanctioning masturbation, and for still others, because it may stigmatize the sterile male who becomes the child's sociological father. For this latter reason, the use of donor insemination for married couples has tended to be shrouded in secrecy; many children who are born through the procedure are never told that their biological father is not the person they know as "father" but an anonymous donor. The fact that a large proportion of sperm donors tend to be drawn from the ranks of medical students seems to intensify the desire for secrecy, as fathers worry that evidence that their children had a "smart" progenitor might reflect poorly on them. Public awareness of the existence of artificial insemination and sperm banks seems to have paralleled the increasing visibility of lesbian mothers and the media attention given to the "lesbian baby boom" despite the fact that at least 10,000 babies are born in the

United States each year through artificial insemination, most of them to heterosexual married couples.

Insemination is, as I have indicated, a notably low-tech procedure. Sperm are obtained either frozen or fresh and introduced into or near the cervix with a plastic syringe. While it can be performed in a doctor's office and thereby invested with the mystique of modern technology, artificial insemination, similarly to what we used to think of as "natural" insemination, can easily be accomplished in a variety of settings, including the prospective mother's bed, or in any of the other classic non-clinical locations traditional in the lore of out-of-wedlock pregnancies.

Artificial insemination, now usually renamed "donor" insemination, "assisted" insemination, or just "insemination" by lesbians and some heterosexual single women who employ it, has obvious appeal for lesbians. Getting pregnant becomes a procedure not requiring a sexual or romantic relationship with the progenitor. This both relieves the prospective lesbian mother of the need to have sexual intercourse with a man, which may be a distasteful option, and offers a way to embark upon motherhood without potential interference from a "father" or his kin. The dismal history of lesbians and custody litigation, too complex to pursue here, gives us some idea of why lesbians might be concerned about the existence of a person who defines himself as the child's father (Lewin 1981; 1990). If there is no "father," discord is less likely to arise later over either custody or visitation, or disagreements over how the child is to be raised. Insemination offers lesbians the opportunity to be sole parents in the fullest sense of the word, or to share parenthood with a woman partner if they wish, although recent litigation over custody and visitation with non-biological mothers or co-parents shows that this may be more problematic than early predictions might have suggested (Gil de Lamadrid 1992; Lewin 1993).

The cases I will discuss here represent the different routes through the process of insemination taken by four different lesbian women I interviewed in the research I conducted in the San Francisco Bay area in the late 1970s and early 1980s. While the number of lesbians becoming pregnant in this way has increased dramatically since the time I did my fieldwork, recent popular writing about lesbian mothers makes it clear that, apart from instituting precautions to avoid HIV infection, these basic dynamics have not changed during the intervening years (Burke 1993; Martin 1993; Arnup 1995).

Not all of these cases draw their momentum from a conflict or interaction with the health care system, as such. Rather, what these examples illustrate is not only how some lesbians choose to relate to the medical system for assistance with reproduction, but how lesbians define their reproductive experience either in relation to or at some distance from what we would characterize as "biomedicine." For some lesbians, it is the very removal from biomedicine that constitutes their resistance, even if the terms of their actual interaction with health care providers indicates this less decisively.

Two of the women accomplished insemination with the assistance of mainstream medical practitioners, while two decided to go outside the medical establishment to obtain sperm privately and accomplish insemination on their own. These examples show how the medical establishment can be either accepted or circumvented, but suggest that the decision to undertake either route to motherhood may have less to do with resistance or accommodation to biomedicine specifically than with other objectives the women seek to achieve. In all of these cases, the women had to weigh alternatives that were imperfect in various ways, but manipulation of the conditions of insemination allowed them to avoid, or try to avoid, whatever threat they most feared.

For Joan, whose son was born after she was inseminated in her physician's office, using mainstream medicine seemed the best alternative. Financially secure, she felt that going through the medical establishment would assure some quality control; she assumed both that the sperm banks would screen for undesirable conditions and that the donors, being medical students, would be likely to have what she called "smarts." Most important to her was the anonymity that would accompany insemination in a medical setting; she was concerned that involving "some man on the street" might threaten the integrity of her family. "I wanted the total responsibility of the child," she said, "I guess I didn't want to take a chance of anybody trying to take him away from me."

Marilyn, who also chose insemination in a medical setting, like Joan, was concerned about anonymity, but also brought a desire to retain control of the procedure itself to her decision about insemination. Working through a local holistic clinic that was willing to act as an intermediary with a sperm bank, Marilyn planned a suitable date for her insemination based on her work schedule, her insurance coverage, and her estimate as to when her fertile period would occur. She saw herself as being in charge of the procedure, despite doing it in the clinic; she said that when she determined that she was ovulating she went to the clinic to inseminate herself. Once the insemination by an anonymous donor was successful, she departed from what she called the "established health care system," opting for a home birth. She decided not to enter "unknown" under "name of father" on the birth certificate, explaining that "writing 'unknown' sounds like you accidentally got pregnant or you don't know who the father is and I don't exactly know who the father is, but I do know how it came to be that I got pregnant." Marilyn insisted upon conditions that would offer her optimal control over the procedure; for insemination this meant using a clinic, while for the birth this meant home delivery.

Grace, who felt that no physician would be willing to inseminate a woman as openly and politically lesbian as herself, obtained sperm through a friend who acted as an intermediary between herself and an anonymous donor. While she valued anonymity because of fears that she could be vulnerable to a custody threat, she also hoped that the arrangement she had made might facilitate her daughter's later discovering the identity of her biological father, should she wish to do so. Using a physician or clinic and a sperm bank would permanently eliminate this alternative, she explained, and thus preclude her providing information she considered critical to her child's welfare.

Finally, Louise, a young, counter-culture woman whose economic position precluded using a physician or a sperm bank, approached a number of men and asked them if they would donate sperm; she finally found a man with whom she was slightly acquainted who was willing to assist. She carried out the insemination, which succeeded on the first attempt, alone in her room with candle light and soft music, envisioning a "perfect baby spirit" entering her. Although her delivery, which had to be moved under emergency conditions from her home to a large hospital, involved multiple interventions, she described the birth as a mystical experience: "It was about the best thing I ever experienced. I was totally amazed. The labor was like I had died . . . The minute she came out, I was born again. It was like we'd just been born together."

Louise broke off her acquaintance with the donor soon after she became pregnant, even moving to another city to avoid further contact. She sees herself as the sole parent of her child, and fears that any interaction with the donor might threaten her custody or her autonomy as a parent. While her desire to achieve motherhood through her own devices and her precarious financial status precluded use of the medical establishment for insemination, Louise was able to redefine even a highly medicalized delivery into the kind of intimate, mystical experience that met her need to be reborn as a mother. Her acceptance of a battery of obstetrical interventions indicated less an absorption into the powerful culture of medicine than an ability to construct her own interpretation of whatever was being done to her.

While all four of these women, like other lesbians who achieve motherhood through insemination, were on one level demanding entrance to a status ordinarily not available to them because of their sexual orientation, it is also clear that resistance to being excluded from motherhood does not necessarily entail a redefinition of motherhood itself. Lesbian mothers who inseminated, like lesbian mothers who had been married, and like heterosexual single mothers I also interviewed, used motherhood to make claims about their identities that suggested an acceptance of what we might see as the conventional attributes of maternal virtue. Being mothers offered access to sources of goodness and altruism not available to non-mothers, and wanting to be mothers, regardless of how the goal was accomplished, was viewed as a desire that grew out of deeply natural sources. These lesbian mothers either tended to describe their desires to be mothers as having been with them all their lives or as having arisen suddenly and without warning. As one woman put it, "It just kind of came over me . . . It was just a need." Both versions of what some called the "mother instinct" are grounded in a construction of motherhood as natural and beyond question, linking them with all women regardless of sexual orientation. Resistance was required to allow these lesbians to become mothers, but this resistance was grounded in strong beliefs in the dichotomous nature of gender and the existence of "natural" maternal urges in women.

Marriage as a site of resistance

The relationship of these four lesbians to the medical processes whereby they achieved motherhood resonates with another domain of lesbian and gay life in which resistance and conformity or accommodation intersect in complicated and often contradictory ways. Lesbians these days are not only demanding the right to be mothers, but also may be said to be claiming the status of "wife" through recent efforts to legalize lesbian and gay marriage, to establish the alternative legal status of domestic partner in the interim, and to use wedding rituals to solemnize and make public committed relationships.[1]

While on the one hand the increasing popularity of commitment ceremonies and gay weddings seems to suggest widespread acceptance of heterosexist standards for judging the validity of relationships, many lesbians who have such ceremonies tend to see the process surrounding them as a form of intense confrontation with the wider society and as an instance of pure resistance. Conformity, many argue convincingly, would consist in remaining in the closet, hiding their identities and using elaborate disguises to protect heterosexuals around them from having to recognize their existence. Getting married, they explain, involves a heightened form of "coming out," as not only family but other people with whom they come in contact must come to terms with the reality of their relationships. Even activities like selecting gifts at a bridal registry or picking out wedding rings or dresses may provide the occasion for confrontation and education. A lesbian bride who described a trip to register for gifts at Neiman-Marcus said,

It was a really nice feature I didn't expect, the coming out over and over, the assumption that there was a groom, the questions about "him," and my correcting it. And always the decision: Do I say something? I like the idea that we started some dialogue about it. The more straight people can see we're like them, the more we'll break the stereotype. (Sherman 1992:162)

At the same time, others who decide to hold wedding ceremonies argue that they should have access to this particular way of marking their relationships because they share the values of the wider society and wish to represent their similarities with the mainstream in a manner others can understand. For Rachel Goldberg and Nancy Weinstein, this sort of statement of belonging was central to the decision to have a wedding ceremony. Rachel explained,

You see, a lot of people see being gay as this really weird thing. I feel like just because I'm gay, that doesn't mean that all the other things that govern the world that I live in and the values that I have and the values that I grew up with and the society that we live in all of a sudden go out the window, just because my interest is in women.

Rachel and Nancy's ceremony was designed to be an exact replica of a heterosexual Jewish wedding, or, as Rachel explained, "an ordinary Jewish wedding," not to be confused with the newfangled concoction she disparagingly called a "commitment ceremony." The ritual followed Conservative Jewish liturgy to the letter, with the two women rejecting even slightly innovative reworkings of the traditional texts. Both Rachel and Nancy saw the ceremony as one that marked their establishment of a "Jewish home" and that sanctioned their desire to have children. They regarded marriages between Jews and non-Jews as truly reprehensible as such unions would lead, in their view, to the pollution and eventual erasure of Jewish heritage. But their marriage, between two Jews committed to the formation of a "Jewish home," and following the forms long used in Jewish wedding ceremonies, was, they explained, unequivocally part of Jewish culture. Since Conservative Judaism had not *explicitly* forbidden marriage between two women but had strict prohibitions on unions with non-Jews, they felt that their exclusion from the mainstream was in a way an oversight or technicality.

The heterosexual Conservative rabbi who officiated, in contrast, emphasized the elements of resistance to bigotry he saw as central to the ceremony. Since a marriage between two women was not, according to him, accepted by the wider Jewish community, his understanding of the event was not that it entailed conformity to existing standards, but that it represented a brave rebellion against the unjust and backward forces that would not sanction such a union. Because gays and lesbians are often accused of not maintaining stable or faithful relationships, he felt that not offering such supports as the religion could to those couples seeking to establish committed partnerships would be the height of hypocrisy. So despite his awareness of sanctions against rabbis who perform such ceremonies (though far less stringent than those imposed on those who perform, or even attend, interfaith weddings), he was willing to offer his services to this couple. But he was quite concerned about the repercussions that might result if his participation became widely known, so while not completely secretive about having taken part in this ceremony, he was adamant that I not reveal his identity to anyone else.

The only aspect of the wedding that disturbed and confused him was the clothing chosen by the participants. Members of the wedding party, including one of the "brides" – she jokingly called herself the "groom-ette" – dressed in tuxedos, while others wore long dresses, including the other "bride" who wore a white bridal gown and veil. This meant that, in addition to drawing on the liturgical elements associated with Jewish weddings, the ceremony "looked like" a traditional wedding. So conformity to community standards in this instance was achieved both through an effort to adhere to liturgical traditions and through the staging of a kind of drag performance, hardly a prescribed dimension of historical Judaism. While the wedding "drag" lacked the elements of satire and exaggeration key to such performances in other venues (Newton 1979; 1993), some of the heterosexual guests (not to mention the rabbi) clearly did not know what to make of this aspect of the ceremony.

In other instances, the wedding ritual may work both to encode conformity with some aspects of convention while also stimulating the celebrants to resist the invisibility politeness has long dictated for a lesbian couple. Margaret Barnes and Lisa Howard, who timed their ceremony to fall slightly before the tenth anniversary of their relationship, both saw the wedding as providing an opportunity to bring together their families and friends and as a context to make clear that their way of life did not differ significantly from those of their families. Both successful businesswomen from upper-middle-class backgrounds, Margaret observed in a letter to her parents,

Our lives are pretty much like that of our married friends – we work hard, we pay lots of taxes, we entertain some, we give as much time as we can to volunteer work, we're faithful to each other, and we take care of each other. Under the circumstances it is sometimes amazing to us to think that we can't be married legally; who could object to such a boring and conventional life?

Their wedding was held in a luxurious outdoor setting, a historic Victorian inn in California's wine country. The springtime ceremony was held on a verandah overlooking a formal garden, with both women wearing subdued pastel dresses in delicate shades of pink and green. A simple ritual officiated by a Unitarian minister was followed by dinner, dancing, and toasts to the couple. From the delicately engraved invitations, to the classic dresses they wore, to the food and music offered at the reception, everything about this wedding was calculated to be in good taste and compatible with family standards for such occasions, while also being intentionally discreet and low-key.

Conscious of the possibility that they might be asked to explain more than would be comfortable if they turned up at work wearing wedding bands, Margaret and Lisa carefully selected rings that they felt did not resemble conventional wedding rings, and they told very few people from their offices that they were planning the ceremony. Though Margaret's firm offers an extra week of vacation to employees who get married, Margaret did not request this time off, but took regular vacation time for the wedding and honeymoon.

When I visited Margaret and Lisa a month or so after their wedding, they described the public nature of the ceremony as having deepened their relationship in ways they had not anticipated. They had expected that the wedding would help them to feel more integrated into their families, more acknowledged as having achieved what their families had always wanted for them both professionally and personally. But after the ceremony, they were surprised to experience an intense desire to come out at work and to become much more public than they ever had about being gay. When Margaret returned to work after her week off, she responded to her colleagues' casual questions about her vacation by announcing that she and her partner of ten years had gotten married. And when the couple went to dinner with a heterosexual couple to mark the tenth anniversary of both couples having met, they found themselves demanding equal access to recognition as a married couple. Because the waiters had overheard talk of an "anniversary" while serving dinner, they decorated a small cake with a candle and presented it to the straight couple with effusive congratulations on their anniversary. Somewhat taken aback, the straight couple said, "But what about them?" pointing to Lisa and Margaret. The confused waiter said, "But they're not married." Margaret and Lisa immediately answered, "Yes, we are," holding out their left hands and displaying the very non-matching rings they had chosen so that they would not resemble wedding rings. The embarrassed staff immediately produced a second cake also bearing a candle.

The traditional style of Margaret and Lisa's wedding highlighted their desire to emphasize the values they shared with their families and, indeed, to mark their recognition of the ongoing significance of family ties. At the same time, however, the ritual worked to challenge their tendency to disguise their relationship and to allow them to present themselves as a married couple like any other. Thus, by making their relationship explicitly more like that of heterosexuals, they were freed to articulate their differentness, changes that were revealed both in Margaret's decision to come out at work and in the events that unfolded at the anniversary dinner.

Mothers and wives/resistance and accommodation

Lesbian mothers and wives both act to challenge traditional gender assumptions about how family and kinship systems should be con-stituted. They give the lie to the expectation that only heterosexual couples can reproduce or that procreation is intrinsically tied to heterosexuality. Conversely, they demonstrate that homosexuals can, in fact, reproduce and become parents. They further show that marriage as a representation of indefinite commitment, whether it leads to procreation or not, need not be limited to heterosexual couples.

At the same time, both lesbian motherhood and marriage also may be said to represent an accommodation to the basic shape of gender relations as represented in the institution of kinship. The wedding rituals, for example, whether they espouse explicitly confrontational or accommodationist philosophies, depend on reinscription of historical tradition and on making symbolic claims that lesbian marriage links a couple to the wider, that is, not exclusively gay, community. The rituals act to resolve paradox, to convince participants that, to use Barbara Myerhoff's words, "things are as they have been portrayed – proper, true, inevitable, natural" (Myerhoff 1992:161). Thus, the involvement of kin is considered highly desirable, and defections by key relatives are lamented and mourned.

An examination of the relationship between "resistance" and "accom-modation" for lesbian mothers and wives suggests that these two impulses are not in basic opposition to one another and that, in fact, they depend upon each other at every turn. Although a number of scholars (notably Abu-Lughod 1990) have noted that ambiguities abound in the opposition between resistance and accommodation, studies of biomedicine still tend to interpret women's behavior in health care settings in this light. While lesbian mothers and lesbian kinship arrangements are decidedly out of the mainstream, they enable us to look at oppositions between resistance and accommodation with more intense scrutiny, since these issues are more sharply delineated in a population that embarks on efforts in the domain of kinship and reproduction with more self-consciousness than do other women in our society.

NOTES

An earlier version of this chapter was presented at the annual meeting of the American Ethnological Society, April 1994, in Santa Monica, California. The paper benefited from discussion at the session and from comments by Margaret Lock and Patricia Kaufert.

1 The increasing visibility of this phenomenon is reflected in several recent and forthcoming publications. See Ayers and Brown 1994, for a popular guide to staging lesbian and gay weddings; Boswell 1994, for a highly specialized academic study of a related issue that received enormous public attention because of the political volatility of the gay marriage debate; Lewin 1996, for a discussion of the symbolic strategies employed in some lesbian wedding ceremonies; and Wolfson, 1994, for an analysis of the legal issues involved.

REFERENCES

Abu-Lughod, Lila 1990, "The romance of resistance: tracing transformations of power through Bedouin women," *American Ethnologist* 17(1):41–55.
Arnup, Katherine (ed.) 1995, *Lesbian Parenting: Living with Pride & Prejudice*, Charlottetown, Prince Edward Island: Gynergy.
Ayers, Tess and Brown, Paul 1994, *The Essential Guide to Lesbian and Gay Weddings*, San Francisco: HarperCollins.
Boswell, John 1994, *Same-Sex Unions in Premodern Europe*, New York: Villard.
Burke, Phyllis 1993, *Family Values: Two Moms and Their Son*, New York: Random House.
Davis-Floyd, Robbie 1992, *Birth as an American Rite of Passage*, Berkeley: University of California Press.
Duberman, Martin 1993, *Stonewall*, New York: Dutton.
Duggan, Lisa 1992, "Making it all perfectly queer," *Socialist Review* 22(1):11–31.
Escoffier, Jeffrey and Bérubé, Allan 1991, "Queer/Nation," *Out/Look* 11:14–16.
Gil de Lamadrid, Maria 1992, "Lesbians choosing motherhood: legal implications of co-parenting," in Dolores J. Maggiore (ed.), *Lesbians and Child Custody: A Casebook*, New York: Garland, pp. 195–218.
Kennedy, Elizabeth Lapovsky and Davis, Madeline D. 1993, *Boots of Leather, Slippers of Gold: The History of a Lesbian Community*, New York: Routledge.

Lamphere, Louise 1987, *From Working Daughters to Working Mothers*, Ithaca, New York: Cornell University Press.

Lewin, Ellen 1981, "Lesbianism and motherhood: implications for child custody," *Human Organization* 40(1):6–14.

1985, "By design: reproductive strategies and the meaning of motherhood," in Hilary Homans (ed.), *The Sexual Politics of Reproduction*, London: Gower, pp. 123–38.

1990, "Claims to motherhood: custody disputes and maternal strategies," in Faye Ginsburg and Anna Tsing (eds.), *Uncertain Terms: Negotiating Gender in American Culture*, Boston: Beacon Press, pp. 199–214.

1993, *Lesbian Mothers: Accounts of Gender in American Culture*, Ithaca, New York: Cornell University Press.

1996, 'Why in the world would you want to do that? Claiming community in lesbian commitment ceremonies," in Ellen Lewin (ed.), *Inventing Lesbian Cultures in America*, Boston: Beacon Press, pp. 105–30.

Lock, Margaret 1993, *Encounters with Aging: Mythologies of Menopause in Japan and North America*, Berkeley: University of California Press.

Martin, April 1993, *The Lesbian and Gay Parenting Handbook: Creating and Raising Our Families*, New York: HarperCollins.

Martin, Emily 1987, *The Woman in the Body: A Cultural Analysis of Reproduction*, Boston: Beacon Press.

Myerhoff, Barbara 1992, "A death in due time: conviction, order, continuity in ritual drama," in Marc Kaminsky (ed.), *Remembered Lives: The Work of Ritual, Storytelling, and Growing Older*, Ann Arbor: University of Michigan Press, pp. 159–90.

Newton, Esther 1979, *Mother Camp: Female Impersonators in America*, Chicago: University of Chicago Press.

1993, *Cherry Grove, Fire Island: Sixty Years in America's First Gay and Lesbian Town*, Boston: Beacon Press.

Ong, Aihwa 1987, *Spirits of Resistance and Capitalist Discipline: Factory Women in Malaysia*, Albany, New York: SUNY Press.

Scott, James 1985, *Weapons of the Weak: Everyday Forms of Peasant Resistance*, New Haven: Yale University Press.

Sherman, Suzanne (ed.) 1992, *Lesbian and Gay Marriage: Private Commitments, Public Ceremonies*, Philadelphia: Temple University Press.

Warner, Michael (ed.) 1993, *Fear of a Queer Planet: Queer Politics and Social Theory*, Minneapolis: University of Minnesota Press.

Wolfson, Evan 1994, "Crossing the threshold: equal marriage rights for lesbians and gay men and the intra-community critique," *New York University Review of Law and Social Change* 21(3):567–615.

The consequences of modernity for childless women in China: medicalization and resistance

Lisa Handwerker

Introduction

In China, the use of female bodies as symbols of modernity[1] and progress in nation-state building has resulted in numerous contradictions. These contradictions most clearly emerge in terms of women's reproductive and sexual choices; while overly (re)productive women (defined as giving birth to more than one child) must curtail their births, non-(re)producing women are stigmatized and encouraged to fulfill the one-child quota established by the Chinese government.

In March 1988 the media announced the birth of the first Chinese test-tube baby born to a 39-year-old peasant woman. While the announcement of this technological success appeared to be in strong contradiction to China's population reduction goal designed to counter the often cited population "crisis," the media attention given to this achievement was consistent with the Chinese Communist Party's (CCP) emphasis on technological innovation in science and medicine as a key symbol of modernity in the 1990s. The official birth announcement of this first test-tube baby was, in fact, presented in the media as a modern-day "success" story:

This healthy little girl 3900 gms. in weight and 53 cms. in height was born at Beijing Medical University at 8:56 a.m. She has a ruddy complexion. When Zou, a peasant from a rural southern province and father for the first time at 42, saw his lovely daughter, he clapped his hands and wiped his tears with joy. The twelve members of his family had already arrived in Beijing several days earlier to await this happy moment. Professor Zhang, the famous scientist and head of the in-vitro research program, took the baby in her arms and happily said, "I am a grandmother again." (*Beijing Review*, March 1988:11)

By 1993, Chinese doctors had produced fifty-one test-tube babies through the combined techniques of *in vitro* fertilization (IVF) and gamete intra-fallopian transfer (GIFT). Today, while newspaper articles and television programs continue to disseminate glowing success stories of test-tube babies and other reproductive technologies as a solution to infertility, an interview with one mother reveals that complex social issues are at stake, together with some unfulfilled dreams, and certainly no magical solutions:

I have been a primary school teacher all my life. I work with children daily and I love kids so I couldn't understand how this could have happened to me. You have no idea what a terrible disease this is, this infertility. It's the worst disease (*bing*) possible in China. I suffered so much in my life. My parents died when I was young so I was raised by my grandparents. After my grandmother died, my grandfather continued to take care of me and now he is in his eighties and my only surviving relative. I must care for him. When my husband and I married his family agreed to certain conditions due to my unusual family circumstances. First, rather than I move in with his family, he would move in with me and my grandfather. Second, our first child would be named after my grandfather and any subsequent children after his name. Who could have predicted I would be infertile? For ten years we tried every treatment in our area. We were poor and couldn't seek medical care in the larger cities. Then, in 1988, after we had already given up hope, my relative heard an interview with Professor Zhang on television and told me about the test-tube baby. At first, I didn't understand it – I thought you go and pick out a baby from a tube and bring it home. We saved our money, as it costs almost 2–3,000 yuan[2] to do the operation. Because of the economic reforms, my family is much wealthier now so it wasn't like before when we had no money. When I became pregnant, I was so happy. After the baby was born I named her after Professor Zhang and my grandfather. When my husband found out he was furious. Before this birth, even though I was infertile, he was always good to me but now he has started beating me. It is terrible and I don't know what to do. I came here to ask the doctor for a chance for a second baby and this time, I'll name the baby after him.

This narrative highlights tensions facing infertile couples and, in particular, infertile women. The transportation of reproductive technologies to China as part of larger emerging globalization processes intersects with local cultural practices and challenges women's accepted roles.

In this chapter, my aim is to document the complex issues highlighted in the stories told by infertile women. Challenges to gender norms, and specifically the position of women in society, have resulted in an increased medicalization of social problems, impacting on the definition and treatment of infertility, and attitudes toward childless women. I argue that the medicalization of infertile women does not merely reflect changing medical knowledge and practice but also political and popular sentiments that contribute to the way the female body is "seen" and interpreted (see, for example, Haraway 1989; Lock 1993; Terry and Urla 1995).

Specifically, I explore such practices as medical discourses, modern technoscientific practices, and local cultural beliefs that both enable and subjugate childless women. While childless women in China cannot always control the course of medicalization, they may at times choose among a range of medical and technological options and use them creatively to resist the very practices that seek to label them. An examination of both involuntary and voluntary childlessness reveals stigmatization and resistance processes. Ironically, discourses and behaviors suggesting resistance by childless women at times unwittingly extend and reinforce the very relations of gender domination they are opposing. Paradoxically, even women *choosing* to have no children, and thus challenging normative gender practices, may reinforce motherhood as a salient feature of womanhood in China. In other words, childless women, whether voluntarily or involuntarily so, are full-fledged social actors reproducing the complex set of contradictions which their social position signifies (Sawicki 1991).

Data collection

Even though infertile women are doubly and sometimes even triply exiled within their own culture – they are women, they are infertile, and sometimes they are poor – their critique of society is both eloquent and persuasive.   My chapter is based on an ethnographic study, the first comprehensive study of female infertility, conducted in 1990 among mainly Han Chinese. My study relies on anthropological methods for data collection including participant-observation in clinics, interviews with patients and doctors to elicit infertility beliefs, popular folklore expressions, and textual analysis of popular materials (such as magazine and newspaper articles and letters from patients to doctors) which highlight gender norms. This data contributes to an understanding of contemporary gender politics, including new micro practices for regulating women's bodies.

While single-locality studies do not permit one to draw conclusions about all of China, this study, conducted in Beijing, provides rich insights into mechanisms that are likely to operate in other areas as well (Greenhalgh *et al.* 1993:5). I selected Beijing as my primary research site because it is a city with numerous infertility clinics of both *xiyi* (Western) and *zhongyi* (traditional Chinese) medicine, and the birth-place of China's first test-tube baby. As the administrative capital from which family planning decisions disseminate, Beijing is an important place to observe some tensions between policies which discourage as well as those which unwittingly encourage pregnancy.

The one-child policy and its consequences for childless women

The idea of *renkou* (population) as a negative force to be managed, monitored, and surveilled is a modern concept linked to the emergence of Chinese socialist development policies. In 1949, the leaders of the People's Republic of China (PRC) believed that population problems would be solved through economic and social development. In 1954, with the first national census calculated, leaders voiced concern about their inability to meet the national development plans owing, in part, to a burgeoning population. Nevertheless, with the political and social disruptions caused by the Cultural Revolution, mandatory population measures would not be pursued for another twenty years.

In the late 1970s, demography, a field of inquiry to interpret population policies that was linked in China to the larger project of "scientism" and modernity, took firm hold (Kwok 1971; Wang 1988). In 1974, coinciding with the agenda of international health agencies, Chinese family planning became part of the overall national agenda and census data were routinely collected from this time (Wang 1988). Low birthrates became a symbol of modernity for developing countries in general and China in particular. When, in the 1970s, census surveys in China indicated the existence of 10 million women of childbearing age and a rapidly growing population the CCP became alarmed (Davin 1987:1). They shifted from an earlier reluctance to implement birth control measures to the Chinese socialist perspective of population growth as a problem requiring a compulsory one-child policy (See Croll *et al.* 1985; Greenhalgh 1986; 1990a; 1992; Banister 1987).

With the introduction of the one-child policy in 1979 and subsequent changes in birth policies such as a loosening of this policy to allow some families two children (Croll 1985; Greenhalgh 1990b), the most intimate realms of family life were opened up and made visible as objects of control within the panoptic gaze of the state (Foucault 1979; 1980; Anagnost 1988). Chinese citizens were made objects of public scrutiny through a system of sanctions and awards (Anagnost 1988; 1989). Briefly, those couples that agreed to follow the one-child policy were rewarded with job promotion, bonus money, better housing, or access to better childcare and educational facilities. Conversely, couples that refused to comply with the policy faced punitive measures such as large fines, house demolitions, and/or job transfers or demotions (e.g. Banister 1987; Croll *et al.* 1985; Greenhalgh and Bongaarts 1985; Kane 1987; Potter and Potter 1990). Various incentives and punitive measures are still in practice today.

Enforcement of the mandatory one-child policy led to unprecedented surveillance and regulation of the Chinese social body (population) in general and the female body in particular. The very act of the demographic survey designed to expose anomalies serves to impose a reproductive ideal through the circulation of statistics, and a standard of measurement against which work units, communities, individuals, and/ or households are judged (Anagnost 1988). While census statistics on men of childbearing age are rare, statistics on women's fertility and sexual and reproductive practices are gathered and widely circulated. Information is collected on the number of women of childbearing age, live births, miscarriages, abortions, pregnancies, and contraceptive use and knowledge. Furthermore, since the 1990s, semi-annual gynecological exams have been required for some married women of reproductive age. These examinations are designed to assist in the discovery of sexually transmitted and reproductive diseases, in the insertion of IUD's for women designated to use them, and in the detection of unplanned pregnancies (Greenhalgh 1993:32). Even before marriage, some women are required to undergo an examination to detect any visible structural problems with their reproductive organs and/or family history of genetic abnormalities which might lead to the birth of disabled children. When combined, this information becomes the means through which the state-party mobilizes social pressure to influence the reproductive and sexual practices of households/families (Anagnost 1988). This birth planning campaign and its results exemplify a "technology of normalization" (Foucault 1979) which systematically classifies, and controls anomalies in the social body.

While the CCP's attempt to control female reproduction through birth planning, new reproductive technologies, demographic surveys, and punitive actions has been, in many ways, an effective means of control and normalization, it paradoxically defines and reinforces infertile women as "Other." One woman, a Beijing resident, described this process to me:

I am sure the pressure to have children in China is greater than any other country. I especially feel a lot of pressure from my work unit. I think if I didn't work my pressure might be less. First, everyone in the *danwei* has children and they are always asking me if I had one. Second, June 1st is Children's Day in China and those couples with a child can take the day off. It would be helpful if I could have a vacation too. Finally, I feel so much pressure because of the birth certificate which gives me permission to have a child. I have had to turn in my certificate the last three years because I couldn't have a child. I felt terrible. Here they give you permission and then you can't even give birth. When I had to turn in my birth certificate the last three years in April, this created so much pressure for me. I feel so humiliated to have to get a new one each year. This

year I didn't even go to the birth planning authorities, they automatically gave
me a new one in April. (July 4, 1990)

Another woman, a 27-year-old *gongren* (worker) who had been
married for four years told me:

I feel so much pressure. If only I could have a child, I wouldn't complain about
anything and I would be willing to do anything. I want a child because if you
don't have a child you are different from everyone else – everyone else has a
child. I see everyone around me with one child. (*Biede ren dou you, ruoguo wo mei
you, bu xin*). Other people all have [a child], if I don't have [one], it's not alright.
(July 4, 1990)

Another woman worker said:

In the beginning I wasn't willing to let others know about my infertility problem
so I paid all the medical expenses myself. In that way, no one, not even my
colleagues, could find out. I have been to so many hospitals . . . For five years
the pressure was so great, I believe it is a natural thing for women to have babies.
Since I can't, I feel this kind of psychological pressure. (July 11, 1990)

Overall, there is the assumption that all women of reproductive age
will and should be fertile. Within the context of the population
reduction rhetoric one would anticipate that childless couples would be
rewarded for their contribution to the state. To the contrary, childless
couples complain that state policies actually perpetuate outright
discrimination against them. Childless women observe women with one
child receiving such benefits as better housing with more bedrooms,
monetary bonuses, childcare support, and a vacation on Children's
Day, while they receive no special rewards. They wonder why the
government, in seeking to reduce population, does not reward childless
couples as exemplars of population reduction goals. Even in the 1990s,
childlessness, whether voluntary or involuntary, is rarely an acceptable
option. As another woman in my study aptly summed it up, "the one
child policy is really the 'you must have one-child policy'" (Handwerker
1991:10; 1993).

Another consequence of pregnancy surveillance is that fewer babies
are available for adoption. While adoption was a relatively common
practice in ancient China (Waltner 1990), in the 1990s it has become
increasingly difficult. First, fewer babies, including girls, are available
for adoption. Demographic surveys indicate that 30 million Chinese
females are missing (Kristof 1991). Possible explanations include
female infanticide, formerly practiced in rural China, or the recent
trend of concealing the births of baby girls from authorities in rural
areas so that a couple can try for a baby boy in a second or third
pregnancy. Second, ultrasound testing has recently become widespread
in China. While Chinese laws prohibit doctors from telling prospective

parents the sex of the fetus, the prohibition simply seems to raise the cost of bribes to extricate the information from ultrasound technicians (Kristof 1991).

However, when couples do decide to adopt, it is usually girls who are available. In urban areas an infertile couple, on rare occasions, can adopt an abandoned girl or *sishengzi* (private or illegal birth) from an unmarried woman who has bypassed fertility surveillance.[3] Both the statistics on missing girls and the availability of baby girls and not baby boys for adoption point to a long-standing cultural bias against the birth of girls in Chinese society.[4] With adoption becoming increasingly difficult, and most couples still viewing it as an action of last resort, the demand for quality medical care and reproductive technologies increases in a culture that continues to value males more than females. Women continue to accrue value foremost as wives and mothers, and only secondarily as workers.

In sum, the modern Chinese surveillance technologies (including demographic surveys, birth policy regulations, and adoption practices) isolate childless women as "abnormal" or "deviant." Such women are controlled not by simple coercion but by reframing Confucian norms into a contemporary discourse which, with the availability of new reproductive technologies, has a major influence on women throughout their potential childbearing years.

The medicalization of infertility

The next section examines the distinct ways in which two major medical systems – traditional Chinese medicine (*zhongyi*) and "Western" biomedicine (*xiyi*), together with the way in which they are portrayed in popular culture – view infertile women in China.

Traditional Chinese medicine

Historically, the purpose of marriage in China, both in theory and practice, has been "to carry on the family line." In Confucian society a failure to have children, and especially sons, was a disgrace to ones' ancestors and a shameful act. The Confucian writer Mencius stated, "there are three things that are unfilial, and to have no posterity is the greatest of these" (Waltner 1990:13). Without a son there was no one to make ancestral sacrifices and to carry on the family line (Yuan 1991). While ancient classical Chinese medical texts acknowledge male as well as female infertility, in cultural terms infertility was a condition for which women were held culpable.

As Charlotte Furth has observed, historically, Chinese medicine had the important role of ensuring the continuity of the patrilineal family by guaranteeing women's reproductive health through a "female specialty" known as *fuke*. Medical theory taught that female disorders were commonplace, with menstruation, pregnancy, and childbirth subjecting women to serious blood loss, making them susceptible to *bing* or an imbalance of yin (feminine, dark, and cold) and yang (masculine, light, and hot). Because irregular menstruation is clearly indicated by the quantity, quality, and potency of the blood, it is made the focal point of female infertility problems in Chinese medicine (see Furth 1987; 1992; Flaws 1989; Zhang 1991). *Zhongyi* practitioners believe that fertility is an expression of a body full of the life force (*qi*) and an unobstructed blood flow.

In cases of infertility it is thought that the blood which collects and circulates in the uterus is either insufficient or blocked owing to two broad categories of *bing*. The first category is a congenital physiological deficiency. The *wu bu nu* (five not females) refers to five congenital anatomical abnormalities of the female genitalia associated with infertility. The second category of female infertility includes six basic patterns of disharmony which may combine to form complicated patterns including: kidney deficiency, liver depression and stagnant *qi*, blood deficiency, cold uterus, and phlegm dampness (Flaws 1989). Regardless of the cause, the primary goal of Chinese medicine is to restore order and balance to the female body. Only then is a pregnancy possible. According to Chinese medicine, a fetus is created when a man's sperm or "essence" (*jingzi*) unites with a woman's blood in her uterus (*zigong* or "palace or room of children"). The words for womb and sperm reflect Chinese cultural views about reproduction; while a woman's uterus serves as the vessel in which the child grows and is nourished, the man provides the essence or spirit of the child.

The diagnosis of a disorder is made using the recognized four methods: observation, interrogation, auscultation, and palpation. The doctor – the majority of them are female – asks the patient details about her menstrual cycle (color, timing, amount, pain), bowel movements, and urination. Less frequently, the doctor will inquire about specific sexual behavior including frequency, timing, and positions. Treatment of infertility uses a combination of techniques including herbs, acupuncture, massage, and moxibustion. Patients are encouraged to return to the clinic weekly for a minimum of four months.

Not only are patients prescribed herbal remedies, but they are provided with advice, some of which is overtly moralistic, about specific lifestyle choices including diet, sleep, emotions, family relations, career, and sexual behavior. The practice of Chinese medicine today both reflects and reinforces a long-standing belief: "childlessness is a consequence of exhausted virtue; it is a castration by heaven. It is a sign of heavenly disfavor and a punishment for moral and ritual transgressions" (Yuan 1991). Clearly, from this perspective, the failure to produce an heir was, and still is, a moral as well as a religious and social problem.

Today, in the traditional Chinese medicine (TCM) clinic women are taught about their moral vulnerability and shortcomings. Several doctors suggested to me that increased "sexual permissiveness" or "moral looseness" resulted in excess abortions leading to higher infertility rates. One doctor told me, "infertility is the result of too much sex leading to *shen* or kidney deficiency." She added, "previously young people did not usually have intercourse before marriage and during menstruation. Now they engage in premarital sex, and don't want to become pregnant. They have sex during menstruation because they believe it is a safe time." In her opinion, this was neither appropriate nor healthy behavior. It appears that some practitioners of Chinese medicine still echo the dangers of inappropriate sexual appetites present in "traditional" Confucian thinking. As Charlotte Furth has commented, "if family harmony is threatened by a woman who is lured away from her wifely duties, the vitality of a family's biological descent line is threatened by similar behavior" (1986; 1987).

Moreover, some of the patients' accounts about the causes of infertility converged with "traditional" medicine beliefs. Women suggested that their own actions which had defied cultural norms evident in traditional medical knowledge, such as engaging in sex during menstruation, actively participating in sports during menses, and drinking cold water, caused their infertility.

In popular journals, advertisements for Chinese medicine products also reflect and shape ideas about feminine morality and vulnerability:

Jie-Er Yin, natural Chinese herbal remedy for preventing sexually transmitted diseases and women's ailments. This medicine can prevent viral infection and is also a traditional Chinese remedy for uncomfortable and embarrassing female genital ailments . . . It has proven 95 percent effective in overcoming fungal, trichomonal, bacterial, gonococcal, viral and mixed bacterial infections as well as senile vaginitis, cervicitis, erosion of the cervix, eczema, and ringworm . . . It is also an excellent prophylactic for use before and after intercourse. (Zhong 1991)

The overall message suggests that the female body, especially the reproductive system, is extremely delicate and highly susceptible to disease (and possible moral transgressions).

Biomedicine

Only within the last ten years has infertility attracted the attention of biomedicine, the other major medical system in China. One Western-trained infertility specialist, a Chinese woman in her seventies, told me:

Before 1985, most hospitals [Western medicine] did not do much infertility investigation, even of simple procedures like hydrotubation or hysterosalpingo-gram. After the open [economic] policy, large amounts of work have started on family planning in collaboration with WHO. Although WHO suggested we begin infertility research – the other aspect of reproduction – not until 1985 did our government agree . . . Since then infertility clinics have begun throughout the whole country.

Today, doctors see no contradiction between aggressively assisting infertile women on the one hand, and enforcing strict birth control measures on the other hand. The founder of China's first *in vitro* clinic was asked, "Why should we [China] have test-tube babies when Chinese hospitals are busy with abortions in the context of population explosion?" She responded:

China has a huge population. Surely, there should be family planning which includes both contraception and abortion for control of birth rates and infertility treatment in some men and women. One may ask why treat infertility? With this logic, since China is overpopulated, why bother to treat diseases? Why help the disabled? Why cure the wounded and save the dying? Why set up hospitals? Why are we doctors needed? (translated version)

Infertility specialists also argue that they cannot ignore their patients' pleas for help. For example, one female patient, summarizing the sentiment of others, wrote the following letter to a doctor:

My family has had only one successor in three generations. As the only granddaughter-in-law, I have been sterile for ten years causing great unhappiness in the family. My family has lost its balance, its harmony and its hope. As I saw in myself, the imminent loss of the life chain, I thought of committing suicide three times to rid myself of the endless trouble and care . . . In my desperation you brought me a twilight of hope. I beg of you to help build a bridge for my family to survive.

There are distinct differences in the ways that TCM and Western "biomedicine" practitioners view prevention, diagnosis, and treatment in the clinics. While Chinese medicine, with its concern for balance, focuses on women's self-perceptions or "subjective" accounts of their illness, "western" medicine relies on technologically mediated tests and diagnostics to read the female body "objectively." Biomedical explanations for infertility include tubal obstruction, congenital abnormalities, endometriosis, and endocrinological dysfunctions.

There is a reliance on patient recall when a woman answers questions about her age, marital status, date of last menstrual period, number of previous pregnancies, miscarriages or births, history of childhood illness, and other non-specific aspects of her medical history. Ironically, there is a simultaneous mistrust by doctors, characteristic of biomedicine and its separation of mind, body, and spirit, of female patients' ability to "know" their own bodies. Rather than rely on patients' subjective symptom reporting, biomedical diagnoses for infertility rely on visualization through testing and dissecting of body parts to identify any anatomical irregularities and hormonal dysfunctions. The terminology used by biomedical doctors reveals a negative female body image, in which menarche is referred to as the *bu ganjing de shihou* (the unclean time), and lab tests and examinations (including HSG, laparoscopy, pap smear, endometrial biopsy) are scheduled in relation to one's menstrual cycle or according to "before the unclean time" or "after the unclean time." Also, because infertility now requires intense scrutiny by a physician and modern diagnostic tools, this necessarily produces an interpretation by women that their bodies require constant medical management.

Although Chinese and Western medicine "see" the infertile female body in distinct ways, both systems view a woman's health status as reflected primarily in her reproductive health with special focus given to regular menses, pregnancy, and childbirth as "normal" female functions. Standardized questions about reproduction and sexuality express normative feminine gender ideals against which an infertile woman is measured. Language, including the framing of questions, is powerful, in both shaping and reinforcing gender norms in both clinics. The narrow range of questions constructs women in reproductive terms by highlighting what "normal" female bodies can do, and by contrasting this with what infertile female bodies cannot do. The result is that both systems construe the fertile woman as normal and the infertile woman as abnormal. Practitioners of both medical systems believe it is natural for women in China to want a child. Ironically, this so called "natural" process is often accomplished through intense medical scrutiny and intervention in female bodies.

Male infertility

Despite the fact that treating female infertility is time-consuming, and an expensive and highly invasive technology, it was only in the 1980s that andrology (*nanke*) or the field of male reproductive science emerged in China (Yuan 1991:8). While previously it was assumed that the problem was mainly female in origin, many doctors, especially those trained in the West, now insist on an examination of the couple in an effort to avoid a practice common in the past: treating a woman for many years for infertility, only later to discover the problem was that of her husband.

While infertile men may also suffer from the stigma of infertility, they are ultimately protected from public ridicule in ways that women are not. First, some women continue to accept responsibility, seek risky medical procedures, and sometimes receive medical treatment even before a diagnosis of either male or female infertility has been made, as illustrated by the following comment:

I am sure I have some disease and the problem is mine. My husband hasn't had a check-up because I am sure the problem is mine. I always think something is wrong with me. Since my stomach often hurts during my periods, I am afraid I have endometriosis.

Second, in other instances, some women who know their partners have an infertility problem will protect them in ways that men do not protect infertile women. For example, a 36-year-old college graduate, while receiving her parents' support, feared the reaction of her larger community and lied about her husband's condition:

My husband and I married late because of the Cultural Revolution. When we married I was 31 years old and he was 45 . . . When we first married in 1985 we didn't want a child. Then we found out my husband had no sperm. The neighbors all think it is my problem. They tell me to go and get a check-up quickly and that I am old. My parents, both of whom are doctors, didn't believe me when I told them it was my problem. We only recently told them about our attempts to do AID. We came to Beijing from Zhejiang province because we didn't want anyone else from our hometown to find out that we are doing AID. (Fieldnotes, June 20, 1990)

The secrecy around male infertility is further perpetuated by the creation of government regulated sperm banks in the 1980s (Chao 1988) and the social stigma accompanying artificial insemination. A couple considering artificial insemination by husband (AIH) or by donor (AID) point to the female as the "problem" source. Assuming the woman conceives after undergoing AID or AIH, friends and family members can believe she was successfully treated, and furthermore they would never suspect a male infertility problem. Yet in one infamous case this backfired. A couple from Shanghai secretly underwent artificial insemination but after the birth the paternal grandparents became suspicious on the grounds that the child did not look like their son. Under pressure, the man admitted that he was infertile and that his wife had undergone AID. The parents, refusing to believe their son was sterile, pressured him until he both disowned the child and divorced.

There is another way in which women bear the stigma and social consequences of infertility. When a couple living in urban China decide to adopt a child, the *danwei* (work unit)[5] requires a medical certification of sterility, and only doctors have the authority to write them. While I did not observe any doctors of Chinese medicine writing these certificates, I did observe several biomedical practitioners writing certificates that read "female fallopian tubes blocked." They did this regardless of whether or not this was the actual cause of infertility, and regardless of whether or not a woman had a medical problem. They argued this was the only legitimate explanation accepted by the authorities at the *danwei*.

A lack of discussion about sexuality has, in addition, led to a misdiagnosis of, and contributed to, a male infertility problem. The consequences can be dramatic, as exemplified by the following story:

We had been married for ten years and only had sex one time. At the beginning of our marriage he went to see many doctors but they all said he had no problem – only his body was too "weak" (*shuairuo*). We first went to our neighborhood hospital and in 1986 we began coming to this hospital. He had to do the sperm test but he couldn't ejaculate. At the time he told the doctor he had no sperm for two or three years. They gave him prednisone but insisted nothing was wrong with him. While I was waiting to hear the results, an older woman said I shouldn't believe that there was nothing wrong and that the doctors were lying to me. I sneaked around the back to speak directly with the doctor. He assured me that nothing was wrong but then asked about our sex life and I told him. The doctor than asked my husband separately and he confirmed what I had said. The doctor learned that we did not move when we tried to have sex; my husband was on the top and I was on the bottom and we were absolutely still . . . Then the doctor taught us how to have sex. My husband told the doctor, "I am so stupid." The doctor responded that he was not stupid. He said, "many people, especially intellectuals (*zhishifenzi*) don't know about sex" . . . When we married there were no books to teach us this information. My husband reads all the time but not on this subject. Now he is able to ejaculate and even likes sex. Since sex has been successful we also have it more often. But my sister told me I should have a happy feeling [orgasm] and I have never had that. But after ten years I am now pregnant. (July 19, 1990)

While public discussions of female sexuality are rare, with a recent public acknowledgment that as many as 10 percent of Chinese men suffer from sexual dysfunction (Yuan 1991:10), discussions of male sexuality have become more common. However, because public opinion still conflates the existence of a male infertility problem with a male sexual problem, men are reluctant to seek an infertility check-up.

Furthermore, the lack of discussion about sexually transmitted diseases may inadvertently perpetuate infertility problems. While at least one source has suggested that the rate of STD's has tripled between 1982 to 1987 (Leonard 1995), I noticed while doing my research that STD's were rarely mentioned as a cause of infertility unless I directly asked the doctor. This was the case regardless of whether or not the patient was present.

Female infertility: a disease of moral transgression in a modern world

As I have illustrated, medicine operates within a larger social milieu, both reflecting and shaping gender norms. Doctors' knowledge and practice make female bodies into culpable objects of surveillance which ultimately construct infertile women as deviant. The treatment of female infertility reconsolidates specific cultural values, including Confucian thought, but also links these same values in new ways with the normative feminine gender identity and ideas about fertility present in modern China. Infertile women are increasingly perceived as culpable, bringing their "problem" upon themselves through modern lifestyles and choices. In China of the 1990s, there is a tendency to view a woman's body, and especially her reproductive capacity, as a direct index of conformity or non-conformity to appropriately gendered behavior. For example, in the clinic I learned the story of a young female graduate student who accidentally became pregnant several years earlier. Because pregnant women are not permitted to pursue graduate studies in China, she opted for an abortion. Now, having completed her studies, she attempted once again to become pregnant. I observed the doctor yelling at her when she sought infertility care because she had undergone an abortion and continued her studies, rather than fulfill her obligations to the state to have one child. While there is no evidence to suggest that sterility is more common among urban educated women, there is nevertheless an increasing perception in the 1990s that women's intellectual pursuits can potentially divert their energy away from reproduction.

Both practitioners and patients have increasingly constructed infertility as a disease, a disorder of civilization and modern living, involving acts for which women are held culpable. It seems that the childless female body embodies the anxiety and vulnerabilities of the larger social body. It appears that women's freedom to follow intellectual pursuits, and violate cultural norms about marriage, sexuality, and diet, is viewed as the source of both individual and social instability. These observations are made in public, as we will see in the next section, precisely as Chinese women gain more access to power, education, and lifestyle options. Accordingly, the disruption of the "natural" differences between masculine and feminine gender roles must be diagnosed, treated, and reinscribed to conform to social standards which are amenable to those currently in power.

Biomedicine adds to the Chinese medicine discourse in that in the biomedicine clinic infertility is considered a disorder of civilization and modern living, for which women are held culpable. We witness the medicalization of social problems while the underlying causes of infertility are never addressed. Why is it that in the 1990s infertile women are still subject to ridicule, beatings, or divorce? How is it that the state, the family, and the couple all maintain a veil of secrecy around male infertility, while female infertility is subjected to public scrutiny?

Popular culture

During the 1990s, childlessness, both voluntary and involuntary, has become the focus of an increasing number of television programs and dramas, and professional and popular books and articles (e.g. *Jiating ZaZhi*, *Jianlang Baozhi*, and *Zhongguo Funu*). The infertile person is often a tragic heroine embodied by a female character. This increase in materials suggests a level of anxiety about non-reproducing women in a time of changing gender norms, and leads to a belief that female infertility is greater than male infertility, despite the existence of some local statistics suggesting an equal proportion of male and female infertility problems. Comments about childless women circulating in one magazine include the following: "although she looks smart and healthy she is pitiably useless" or "her belly can't bring her a baby or win her credit" or "Keep a dog and it can watch the door, keep a cat and it can catch mice. But what's the use of such a wife?" (Chen 1990:53). Such remarks perpetuate the stigmatization of supposedly infertile women.

Additionally, in popular culture there is an emerging tendency to think of infertile women as afflicted by a disease of morality. A common perception perpetuated by popular materials is that peasant women are more fertile, and urban women are less fertile, especially fat women. Popular opinion attributes excess weight to laziness and "bourgeois decadence." These new explanations for female culpability are reflected in a modern variation of traditional folklore. The original folklore expression, "the hen that can't lay an egg," refers to a woman who cannot reproduce and is therefore proclaimed useless by society. In the 1990s, the new variation is "the fat hen that can't lay an egg."[6] Several women told me that they could tell, just by looking at a woman, whether or not she was infertile. When I asked how this was possible, they suggested that a person's physiognomy (including body shape and size, facial features) or personality type (angry or calm) revealed an infertile state. In the 1990s, it appears that infertility, a disease of morality, is now transparent.

Furthermore, popular sources disseminate glowing success stories about test-tube babies. Despite the fact that IVF is often used to address male infertility problems, these "miracle" babies are presented as the solution to female infertility. They are also presented as smarter than other babies. The *Beijing Review* reports on the first test-tube baby, now a 4-year-old child:

> Meng Zhu has never been sick. She was trained to brush her teeth and put on her clothes at the age of three. She is taller than children her age by half a head. Her intelligence is also higher than children of her age. At present, Meng Zhu has mastered 500 Chinese words, can recite 20 poems, sing 10 songs, and perform 10 dances.

When infertile couples desperately want a child, baby-making is especially vulnerable to market forces and public opinion. Overall, popular media images both reflect and perpetuate infertility as a culpable female problem in the 1990s.

Resistance to gender conformity and medicalization

While the normalizing machinery in the clinics and in popular culture attempts to recirculate and (re)produce normative feminine gender ideals about marriage, heterosexuality, and reproduction, gender images are in flux in China in the 1990s. As a result, "in a multitude of ways women assert their alternative view of their bodies, react against their accustomed social roles, reject denigrating scientific models, and in general struggle to achieve dignity and autonomy" (Strathern 1992:67). Even while popular media, population experts, and medical practitioners attempt to reascribe reproduction to the realm of the "natural," I observed considerable challenges from diverse women.

For example, in *The Ark*, a popular novella written by Zhang Jie, one of the main characters is a childless divorcee; she had one pregnancy that ended in abortion, contributing to her husband's hostility and eventually to her divorce (Prazniak 1989:274). Zhang Jie believes that the legal and economic achievements of women under socialism are insufficient for their full emancipation. Through her characters' lives she argues not only against the official government position which states women are not oppressed under socialism but also for a female consciousness about their condition. One of her characters proclaims:

Women's liberation is not only a matter of economic and political rights, but includes the recognition by women themselves, as well as by all of society, that we have our own value and significance. Women are people, not merely objects of sex, wives, and mothers. But there are many people, women among them, who think that their sole purpose in life is to satisfy the desires of men. (Prazniak 1989:278)

According to Prazniak, "Zhang suggests that women must mature beyond motherhood and wifedom as part of their essential journey to self-awareness – not necessarily by abandoning the roles of mother and wife but by choosing them under conditions that support their self-confidence and awareness as full social beings."[7] Despite women's oppression under socialism, Zhang Jie puts forth a view that Chinese women have a potential consciousness about their situation and therefore the possibility to change.

In the clinics, despite attempts to move toward standardized medical definitions and treatment schedules, there remains considerable variation among labeling practices. Definitions by individual practitioners, many of whom are urban educated, and patients' self-definitions do not always concur, because infertility takes on different meanings according to women's life circumstances. Some women reject the infertility label outright, as in the case of one woman who had not conceived in five years but nevertheless would not consider herself infertile. By accepting the infertility label this woman also must acknowledge the potential social implications of the label (including stigma, ridicule, beatings, and divorce).

For others, the label offered hope for treatment, as in the case of one informant, a peasant woman and mother of four young girls, who had an infected fallopian tube.[8] According to her, the doctors had refused treatment arguing that she was not infertile and furthermore had already exceeded her birth quota. But because of her inability to conceive a son, she considered herself infertile. She protested that her reproductive task as a woman was incomplete. The urban doctors, on the other hand, had previously refused to recognize her medical condition as infertility and labeled her desire for a son as "feudalistic."

There are also considerable differences among women as to when they first seek medical treatment. Some women, especially peasant women or women who married late, who had not conceived within the first few months of marriage and were feeling anxious, sought treatment early.[9] But many other women delayed treatment, expressing ambivalence about their desire for a child. These women had come to the clinic only upon the insistence of their husband or another family member, often a mother or mother-in-law. Several patients even admitted they had little or no desire for a child. One woman said, "no I don't feel sorry for not being able to have a child. Why should I feel sorry toward my husband?" When I asked doctors about the possibility of some women not wanting a child they told me it was "natural" (*ziran*) for every Chinese woman to want a child. They strongly suggested to me that I should not believe any woman who said she does not want a child because, in their opinion, she only said this when she did not have the ability to have one. For these doctors, the possibility that someone would choose not to have a child did not exist.

When infertile women seek care, they shop around for doctors. One 28-year-old female worker told me:

When we first married I used an IUD from September 1987 to June 1988. In February 1989 I was told my tubes were not patent. In 1986 I had tuberculosis of the lungs. I don't remember ever being told the TB had spread to my uterus. Since I didn't agree with the diagnosis and don't believe I have TB, I came to this hospital to get another opinion. (Fieldnotes 1990)

If a diagnosis did not conform to a woman's explanatory model, she would often seek out another health practitioner until she found one whose beliefs coincided with her own. Also, most peasant women admitted to seeking out services and engaging in practices that are considered "feudalistic" or superstitious by the CCP such as practicing *feng shui*, praying to *Kuan Yin*, the Goddess of Mercy, and/or eating dyed red eggs at a wedding to increase fertility. Such practices represent a challenge to the party-state that equates science with truth. Anagnost (1988) suggests that infertile women's reliance on a number of systems may be viewed as counter-hegemonic, reflecting competing moralities that persist between individuals and the state. In contemporary Chinese political culture, the advances of scientific-medical practices presuppose a disenchanted world in which magical belief appears to be a misguided understanding of reality (Anagnost 1988), with which clearly not all women agree.

My data suggest that poor peasant women in China may be able to challenge the scientific-medical model in ways that urban educated women cannot. Their lack of immersion in scientific paradigms may work to their advantage (cf. Martin 1987; Sawicki 1991). Because peasant women are often labeled as "backward" by many urban doctors, they have nothing to lose by rejecting biomedical explanatory models. However, rather than view different treatments as competing forces, most infertile women, but especially peasant women, openly rely on many different kinds of treatment methods. Biomedical constructions do not usually displace indigenous logic, but rather increase reliance on a broad range of treatment (see Kleinman 1980; Lock 1980; Leslie and Young 1992).

Furthermore, women use medical services to meet their own personal needs, whether or not their expectations are met. One peasant woman said:

> I spent a total of 5–6,000 *yuan* on Chinese medicine. I ate a *fu* [a measurement equivalent to one bag of herbs] daily which cost 3 *yuan* and in one year I spent 900 *yuan*. Furthermore, this money all came from my family; my mother-in-law did not contribute one *yuan* because she thought the treatment was useless. She wanted her son to divorce me. But I kept on eating all the medicine. I ate so much medicine all those years and sometimes I felt so nauseous but still I kept on eating it. I believed if only I kept on taking the medicine I could become pregnant.

This next story exemplifies how women can manipulate the system even when they have given up hope of having a baby. One woman, a nurse in her late thirties, told me:

> Since I was a teenager I have suffered from painful menstrual periods because of endometriosis. I am unable to conceive and after seeking all kinds of medical treatment over the years, I decided it was best to have a partial hysterectomy now. Although I was unable to have a child, I felt luckier than most other infertile women, because I knew my husband loved me and would not divorce me. But recently I gave up all hope of having a baby and did not want to suffer anymore from endometriosis. My womb is useless (*Wode zigong mei you yong*). And I don't want to have so much pain every month. Why keep suffering when I already know I can't have a child? . . . Now I have good *guanxi* (social relations) through work and I can be assured I will receive good care. I can even pick the best doctor to operate on me, and receive 100 percent medical coverage for the operation . . . In the future I have no such guarantee.

Some doctors also resist the hegemonic medical models. For example, one well-known endocrinologist refused to open an IVF clinic, pointing to the need for prevention services in a country with limited resources. Another doctor deliberately misrepresented the age of her patient, a 40-year-old woman who would, otherwise, have been unable to undergo IVF. As a 39-year-old woman she was still eligible. Another doctor, practicing in a Western medical clinic, encouraged her patients to visit traditional Chinese medicine practitioners.

While infertile women and their doctors are active at times in resisting dominant meanings of infertility in the context of their diverse lives, resistance takes place as part of a social world that defines normative womanhood in terms of motherhood. As such, even challenges to specific medical practices do not remove dominant social expectations that all women should be fertile. When I asked doctors about the option of remaining childless, they said that all Chinese women want a child.

They also told me not to believe any woman who said she did not want a child. While manifested in distinct ways, it appears that in China, as in other countries, women are still not fully in possession of the power of self-definition.

Voluntary childlessness: an act of resistance?

Women who choose to remain childless still represent a small percentage of the population. Nevertheless, recent articles in the media highlight the increasing number of urban women who choose this option. The attention given to this new "problem" in the popular media points to the ways in which the dominant ideology continues to emphasize women's reproductive role. One article appearing in the magazine *Nexus* illustrates this point:

After accidentally becoming pregnant, one woman who did not want a child sought an abortion. The doctor, at the clinic, discovering that she had no children after being married for several years, refused to perform the abortion. The woman insisted and after two or three hours of unsuccessfully trying to convince her of the advantages of having a child, the male doctor relented. She was told, "You can have an abortion but first you need a document signed by your husband."

At her *danwei* her supervisor provided her with the document adding, "You were someone we were planning to promote. What a pity you have such serious bourgeois ideas. You are not willing to carry out your duties to society. All you want is to seek pleasure for yourself." After her abortion her promotion was delayed for two years. Not only did she suffer negative consequences from the abortion at work but she also received criticism from her family. Her mother-in-law angrily said, "You marry to have children. If you knew this why did you get married and bring us misfortune?" Even her own mother expressed anger, "How could you have been so silly as to do such an evil thing? And how will I be able to look at people in the face?" The woman was really perplexed. She wondered, "What have I done to offend so many people? All of a sudden I decided not to have a child and I am guilty of all sorts of crimes."

Her husband had agreed with her decision but nevertheless all repercussions were directed at her and not him. Fortunately, she had like-minded friends who considered her a forerunner of women's liberation. Over time her reputation also improved at work. After hearing that she had no child some co-workers presented her with a doll that had the ability to cry. The doll only stops crying when a feeding bottle is thrust into its mouth. She thanked them for the gift but was not the least bit interested herself. Instead, she presented it to her mother-in-law to satisfy her cravings for a grandchild. (Lin 1991)

This story is illustrative of several important points. How is it that abortion, which is promoted among women with one or more children, is stigmatized especially among urban educated women? This restriction on abortion reveals that childless women, who have not yet fulfilled the one-child quota, are discouraged from experiencing sex which does not result in a pregnancy. Stigmatizing childless women is one way to attempt to restrict women's sexual autonomy by tying it back to heterosexual reproduction. A childless woman ruptures the long-standing association between reproduction and sexuality which dates back to the Ming dynasty. Childlessness means that a couple are potentially engaging in intercourse without the intent of making babies. Medicine not only serves to restrict women's ability to make their own reproductive choices that may fall outside of cultural norms, but also attempts to control sexuality by defining its terms (Petchesky 1984).

Despite social pressure to have a child, the woman in the above example forces a challenge to childbirth as "natural" and inevitable. Her decision not to become a mother questions a cultural norm which binds a woman to a man as the medium of lineage continuity, or, even more strikingly, the "traditional" tie between the woman and her husband's family symbolized by the mother-in-law and daughter-in-law relationship. It is significant that abortion, which is often encouraged by the state, in this case is seen as self-indulgent, presumably because it separates reproduction from sexuality. Another woman was also accused of shortsightedness: "All you do is reap pleasure now. When you get old, you will reap whatever you have sown and suffer greatly" (Lin 1991).

Even in the China of the 1990s, there appears no normative identity for women who are not mothers. The idea of sex as pleasurable for women is something the CCP defines as decadent or immoral. They claim that the influence of Western culture has led to the moral and spiritual disruption of the family in modern socialist China during the 1990s (cf. Lock 1993 for Japan).

This story further reveals ongoing class struggles around reproductive norms in China. Who are these women choosing a childless lifestyle? According to a recent survey, those couples choosing childlessness have a higher socioeconomic status, higher education level, and a more prestigious family background compared to those couples who have at least one child (Lin 1991). More than 73 percent of childless couples are intellectuals or cadres. The childless couples in this survey provided several reasons for their decision not to have a child or become a parent. These included the desire to have a more relaxed life style than their parents who devoted themselves to raising children, a fear that a child would jeopardize their career mobility or lower their standard of living, a strong aversion to a traditional lifestyle, husbands' desire to spare their wives the pain of childbirth, and the fear that a child may result in the loss of affection from a spouse. One person even admitted that, after the Tiananmen Square massacre, he had little hope for the future of China and therefore for the future of his potential child.

Finally, childless couples sometimes expressed a hope to contribute to the solution to China's population problems. One person said: "The government has tried very hard to publicize its family planning policy amongst Chinese citizens. By choosing not to have a child, I want to foster population control in China" (Lin 1991:4). While couples hope that their decision to remain childless will be acknowledged as a contribution to the state family planning policy, this has not been the case.

The increasing numbers of educated women choosing to remain unmarried and child-free signal contradictory ideologies. On the one hand, this is applauded by some Chinese as a sign of the "modern," something that occurs in industrialized countries. Not having children may be considered a sign of modernity because *"Waiguo mei you women ye mei you"* ("Foreigners don't have; we also don't have"). On the other hand, the decision not to have a child, I argue, has created anxiety among some leaders because it is perceived as an act of rebellion against the significant role of mother assigned to women in normative culture.

With more educated women opting for childlessness there is a fear on the part of the government that (re)producing the common class will result in the denigration of the Chinese state. One childless couple was told by their CCP boss: "Both of you are talented and good-looking. If you don't give birth you will bring a disadvantage to the development of a high quality population. What a pity" (Lin 1991). Furthermore, as rates of "abnormal" births increase, Chinese leaders, including public health officials, are concerned about improving China's population quality. In December 1993, China's Minister of Public Health, Chen Minzhang, proposed national legislation to stop "abnormal" births through abortions and sterilizations if necessary (Tyler 1993). He cited statistics showing that China now has more than 10 million disabled persons who could have been prevented through better controls. This proposed new legislation would, in effect, require even tighter surveillance of pregnant women, for any woman diagnosed as carrying an infectious disease or an abnormal fetus would be advised to terminate the pregnancy. Five years earlier, in northwestern Gansu province, legislation was passed to prevent those people labeled as mentally retarded from having any children (Tyler 1993).

In China it appears that different classes of women, assumed to have different intellectual capacities, are called upon to serve the Chinese nation in distinct ways. While a poor female peasant or worker has the duty to restrict her fertility, a female intellectual or cadre is now encouraged to fulfill her one-child quota. Normative procreative values are reinforced to the extent that if individuals are not educated and do not have children, it is assumed they are not good socialists, in that they aren't contributing to the (re)production of the modern Chinese nation-state. Furthermore, non-reproductive female sexuality registers a suspicion of sexual practices as non-economic and driven by pleasure. Female sexuality for its own sake, unproductive of babies, is considered unproductive of social and economic efficiency. It also challenges ideas about female chastity, female virtue, and heterosexuality.

Despite new challenges to the normative ideology linking feminine roles to procreative ability, such ideas persist in the 1990s. Couples, but especially women without children, encounter hostility and prejudice. Most of them face potential ridicule from friends, colleagues, neighbors, and family for their failure to conform to the social prescriptions to reproduce. Ironically, in their attempt to defy norms, childless women are most concerned that they will mistakenly be accused of being sterile. One woman remarked, resentfully, that although she was capable of bearing a child (she had aborted an earlier pregnancy), even if she was really sterile this wouldn't be anything to be ashamed of. "How strong traditional ideas are," she sighed (Lin 1991).

The decisions and plights of childless couples exemplify the perplexing contradictory nature of resistance to reproductive policies and practices in China. I have illustrated ways in which some Chinese women resist gender norms and the role of resistance in individual and social reproduction. Yet, rebellion itself may lead to the reproduction of the very ideas it seeks to challenge – namely, normative Chinese feminine gender prescriptions in the 1990s. Resistance has the paradoxical ability to feed directly into dominant social expectations while apparently subverting authority. This sometimes cancels out the power of the refusal, in that childless women highlight the very role – woman as mother – that they are challenging in a society where women with children are the norm. These women in a very literal way confront the task of separating reproductive capacity from female identity (Ireland 1993:19). A woman choosing to remain childless may be saying to the world that she is on a personal quest in which motherhood plays no part (Ireland 1993:71). Paradoxically, the childless woman highlights reproduction as a salient feature of normative gender identity (Ireland 1993:42). In contemporary China, the challenge is how to expand a "childless" woman's place in society beyond the realm of "deviant." Only then will she be able to choose freely from an array of reproductive choices, including the choice not to be a mother.

ACKNOWLEDGMENTS

This chapter is based on twelve months of research conducted in China in 1990, generously supported by a joint grant from the Fulbright-Hays Doctoral Dissertation Award and the Committee on Scholarly Communication with the People's Republic of China. Assistance was also provided by the Wenner-Gren Anthropological Association Dissertation Fund, a National Science Foundation Doctoral Dissertation Improvement Grant (No. BNS89–13347), and the Association for Women in Science. Additionally, the Soroptomist International Award and the University of California San Francisco Humanities Award provided dissertation writing support. Also, Stanford's Institute for Research on Women and Gender provided me with important writing time and support. Thanks to Ann Anagnost for comments on an earlier version of this chapter. I appreciate the insightful editorial comments and the encouragement provided by Pat Kaufert and Margaret Lock. My work has benefited from comments at earlier stages by J. Ablon, G. Becker, T. Gold, A. Ong, J. Urla, and J. Terry. For their support, I thank Dr. Zhang Li Zhu and Drs. Zuo, Chai, Gao, and Lu, M. Hardie, the Handwerkers, and Y. Verdoner. I am warmly indebted to Dr. Yuan Hong without whom this project could not have been completed. I also thank Meera Jaffrey for my initiation to China. The above persons bear no responsibility for my data results or interpretations.

NOTES

1 According to Anthony Giddens, modernity refers to the modes of social life or organization which emerged in Europe from about the seventeenth century onward and which subsequently became a more worldwide phenomenon (Giddens 1990:1). He argues that the modes of life brought about by modernity have swept us away from many traditional types of social order. While there are continuities between the "modern" and the "traditional," the changes occurring have been dramatic. Modern social institutions are distinguished from traditional ones in the pace and scope of their change, and the form of institutions.

2 A *yuan* is the Chinese monetary unit. In 1990, at the time of my research, 5 or 6 *yuan* were the equivalent of 1 US dollar.

3 In my visit to an orphanage in China, the only boys available for adoption either had Down syndrome or severe cases of cleft palate.

4 While most families, especially peasant families, in China still prefer a son for lineage continuity, I observed an increasing trend among urban women toward a preference for girls. They argued that baby girls were more dependable and more likely to take care of them in their old age. Women also believe they can have a closer relationship with girls.

5 The state *danwei* or "work unit" is an elaborate social institution in urban China

which potentially can manage every aspect of state employees' daily life, including food, health care, housing, money, education, childcare, and pension. See Henderson and Cohen (1984) for an excellent description of the *danwei*.

6 Another interesting variation of this folk expression appeared in the new film, *Ermo*, directed by Zhou Xiaowen. The story depicts tensions between modernity and female morality in a plot focused on keeping up with the Joneses. *Ermo*, the main female actress, is determined to purchase a color television which is bigger than her neighbor's. Her determination leads to her affair with the neighbor's husband, selling vast quantities of her blood to earn money, and starting her own noodle business. But she must contend with her old-fashioned husband, who repeats that he wants a new house instead of a television, stating "A television is an egg. A house is a hen" (Caryn James, *New York Times*, May 15, 1995).

7 Zhang is critical of the party for dismissing the increased rates of divorce as "bourgeois ideology" instead of looking seriously into the causes (1989:281–2). While challenging many gender norms, according to Prazniak, "Zhang may fail to understand the different material and psychic needs of women from different classes" (1989:279).

8 When I asked her how she was able to have four children, she told me that she wasn't allowed to but that she had circumvented the state policy. After the one-child quota, she had a different strategy to hide each subsequent birth: during her second birth she went to a hospital in another village, after her third birth she hid the baby in her mother's home, and for the fourth birth she had told local authorities that the baby had died during a homebirth. Hiding the number of births is an increasingly common phenomenon and may contribute to the missing statistics on girls in China.

9 Couples' beliefs about conception also determined when they sought care. Some women believed that they would become pregnant after only one act of sexual intercourse. Another couple engaged in frequent and vigorous sexual intercourse because they believed that conception occurred over a one month period and not during any one act of intercourse.

REFERENCES

Anagnost, Ann 1988, "Family violence and magical violence: woman as victim in China's one-child family policy," *Women and Language* 11(2):16–22.
    1989, "Transformations of gender in modern China," in Sandra Morgen (ed.), *Gender and Anthropology*, Washington, D.C.: American Anthropological Association, pp. 313–42.
Banister, Judith 1987, *China's Changing Population*, Stanford: Stanford University Press.
Beijing Review 1988, "First test-tube baby on mainland," 31(12):11. (Chinese announcement appeared in the *Renmin Ribao*, March 1988.)
Chao, Jingshen 1988, "More than three hundred women in Tianjin have received artifical insemination," *Renmin Ribao* (overseas edition), October 24.
Chen, Huihe 1990, "China's childless couples," *Nexus: China in Focus*, Autumn, 52–5.

Croll, Elizabeth, Davin, Delia and Kane, Penny (eds.) 1985, *China's One-Child Family Policy*, London: Macmillan Press.

Davin, Delia 1987, "Gender and population in the People's Republic of China," in H. Afshar (ed.), *Women, State, and Ideology*, New York: State University of New York Press, p. 1.

Flaws, Bob 1989, *Endometriosis, Infertility and Traditional Chinese Medicine: A Laywoman's Guide*, Boulder, Colorado: Blue Poppy Press.

Foucault, Michel 1979, *Discipline and Punish*, New York: Vintage.

1980, *The History of Sexuality*, Vol. 1, *An Introduction*, New York: Vintage.

Furth, Charlotte 1986, "Blood, body and gender: medical images of the female condition in China 1600–1850," *Chinese Science* 7:43–66.

1987, "Concepts of pregnancy, childbirth, and infancy in Ch'ing dynasty China," *Journal of Asian Studies* 46(1):7–35.

1992, "Chinese medicine and the anthropology of menstruation in contemporary Taiwan," *Journal of Medical Anthropology Quarterly* 6(1):27–48.

Giddens, Anthony 1990, *The Consequences of Modernity*, Stanford: Stanford University Press.

Greenhalgh, Susan 1986, "Shifts in China's population policy, 1984–86: views from the central, provincial, and local levels," *Population and Development Review* 12(3):491–515.

1990a, "The evolution of the one-child policy in Shanxi 1979–1988," *The China Quarterly* 122:191–229.

1990b, "The peasantization of population policy in Shanxi: cadre mediation of the state-society conflict," Population Council working paper no. 21, New York

1992, "Negotiating birth control in village China," Population Council working paper no. 38, pp. 1–46, New York.

1993, "The peasantization of the one-child policy in Shaanxi: negotiating birth control in China," in Deborah Davis and Steven Harrell (eds.), *Chinese Families in the Post-Mao Era*, Berkeley: University of California Press, pp. 219–50.

Greenhalgh, Susan and Bongaarts, J. 1985, "An alternative to the one-child policy in China," *Population and Development Review* 11(4):585–617.

Greenhalgh, Susan, Zhu Chuzhu and Li Nan 1993, "Restraining population growth in three Chinese villages:1988–1993," Population Council working paper no. 55, pp. 1–48, New York.

Handwerker, Lisa 1991, "The hen that can't lay an egg: preliminary thoughts on infertility research in China," paper presented at the University of California Berkeley Center for Chinese Studies.

1993, "The hen that can't lay an egg (*Bu Xia Dan de Mu Ji*): the stigmatization of female infertility in late twentieth century People's Republic of China," Ph.D. dissertation, University of California, San Francisco and Berkeley.

1995, "The hen that can't lay an egg (*Bu Xia Dan de Mu Ji*): conceptions of female infertility in modern China," in Jennifer Terry and Jacqueline Urla (eds.), *Deviant Bodies: Critical Perspectives on Difference in Science and Popular Culture*, Bloomington: Indiana University Press, pp. 358–79.

Haraway, Donna 1989, *Primate Visions: Gender, Race, and Nature in Science and Medicine between the Eighteenth and Twentieth Centuries*, Madison: University of Wisconsin Press.

Henderson, Gail E. and Cohen, Myron S. 1984, *The Chinese Socialist Work Unit*, New Haven: Yale University Press.

Ireland, Mardy S. 1993, *Reconceiving Women: Separating Motherhood from Female Identity*, New York: Guilford Press.

James, Caryn 1995, "A film review of *Ermo*." *New York Times*, The Living Arts Section B, May 15.

Kane, Penny 1987, *The Second Billion: Population and Family Planning in China*, London: Penguin Books.

Kleinman, Arthur 1980, *Patients and Healers in the Context of Culture: An Exploration of the Borderland between Anthropology, Medicine, and Psychiatry*, Berkeley: University of California Press.

Kristof, Nicholas D. 1991, "Stark data on women:100 million are missing," *New York Times*, November 5, A1.

Kwok, Daniel W. Y. 1971, *Scienticism in Chinese Thought 1900–1950*, New York: Biblo and Tannen.

Leonard, Andrew 1995, "Review of *China Pop* by Zha Jianying," *New York Review of Books*.

Leslie, Charles and Young, Allan (eds.) 1992, *Paths of Asian Medical Knowledge*, Berkeley: University of California Press.

Lin, Yihe 1991, "A recent survey of couples who choose not to have a child," *Nexus* December.

Lock, Margaret 1980, *East Asian Medicine in Urban Japan*, Berkeley: University of California Press.

  1993, *Encounters with Aging: Mythologies of Menopause in Japan and North America*, Berkeley: University of California Press.

Martin, Emily 1987, *The Woman in the Body: A Cultural Analysis of Reproduction*, Boston: Beacon Press.

Petchesky, Rosalind 1984, *Abortion and Women's Choice: The State, Sexuality and Reproductive Freedom*, Boston: Northeastern University Press.

Potter, Sulamith Heins and Potter, Jack M. 1990, *China's Peasants: The Anthropology of a Revolution*, Cambridge: Cambridge University Press.

Prazniak, Roxanne 1989, "Feminist humanism: socialism and neofeminism in the writings of Zhang Jie," in Arif Dirlik and Maurice Meisner (eds.), *Marxism and the Chinese Experience*, New York: M. E. Sharpe, pp. 269–94.

Robinson, Jean C. 1985, "Of women and washing machines: employment, housework, and the reproduction of motherhood in socialist China," *China Quarterly* 101:32–57.

Sandelowski, Margaret J. 1990, "Failures of volition: female agency and infertility in historical perspective," *Signs* 15(3):475–99.

Sawicki, Jana 1991, *Disciplining Foucault: Feminism, Power and the Body*, London: Routledge Press.

Strathern, Marilyn 1992, *Reproducing the Future: Anthropology, Kinship, and New Reproductive Technologies*, New York: Routledge Press.

Terry, Jennifer and Urla, Jacqueline (eds.) 1995, "Introduction," in *Deviant*

Bodies: Critical Perspectives on Difference in Science and Popular Culture, Bloomington: Indiana University Press, pp. 1–19.

Tyler, Patrick E. 1993, "China weighs using sterilization and abortions to stop 'abnormal' births," *New York Times*, December 22.

Waltner, Ann 1990, *Getting an Heir: Adoption and the Construction of Kinship in Late Imperial China*, Hawaii: University of Hawaii Press.

Wang, Feng 1988, "Historical demography in China," *Review and Perspective* 236:53–69 (Hawaii: East-West Population Institute).

Yuan, Lili 1991, "Reproduction and happiness," *Women of China* February:8–10.

Zhang, Ting-liang 1991, *A Handbook of Traditional Chinese Gynecology*. (Compiled by Song Guang-ji and Yu Xiao-zhen of the Zhejiang College of Traditional Chinese Medicine. Edited and annotated by Bob Flaws) (*Zhong Yi Fu Ke Shou Ce*). Original publication date 1984 (1985 edition used for translation).

Zhong, Lu 1991, "Relieving women's genital ailments," *Women of China* November.

9 Perfecting society: reproductive technologies, genetic testing, and the planned family in Japan

Margaret Lock

Reproductive technologies and genetic testing are often touted as medical services that fulfill a desire not only to reproduce, but to reproduce healthy offspring full of promise to become successful human beings. In order for this to happen, where infertility is assumed to be the source of the problem, this condition must be conceptualized as a disease-like state subject to amelioration through medical intervention. Before genetic testing can be instigated, the embryo and fetus come to be visualized as patient-like entities entirely or largely independent of the mother's body. However, without the desire of "consumers" to cooperate, reproductive technologies and genetic testing would remain confined to the research laboratory. That they do not, suggests that certain knowledge about the "worth" of individual reproduction and of the production of healthy offspring is in circulation in which, at least to some extent, health care professionals and their clients alike participate.

Although research is as yet scant, it is clear that not all women are willing to avail themselves of these new technologies, even when labeled as infertile or "at risk" for carrying a fetus with a major genetic disorder (Beeson and Doksum forthcoming). That there are those who apparently resist technological intervention suggests that competing ideologies and practices, contradictions and inconsistencies must be at work. It is at the "intersection of discourses" (Yanagisako and Delaney 1995), particularly when decisions have to be made with grave consequences for the lives of involved individuals and their families, that we can gain some valuable insights about medicalization and its reception – insights, not only with respect to individual responses to distress, but also into the way in which medicalization and its acceptance or rejection by women and involved others reflects conflicting views about the appropriateness of technological intervention into reproduction.

Moreover, since reproduction is never simply procreation, but inevitably has significance for society at large, the potential impact of reproductive and genetic technologies on gender, kin, family, and community relations is also of concern. Possible disruption of what are assumed to be the "natural" human relations basic to moral order in any given society may not pose much of a problem for individuals, but without doubt create national concern (Franklin 1995; Strathern 1995). Thus, although governments may, for utilitarian reasons, encourage the production of offspring who are unlikely to become a "financial burden" to society, at the same time a certain ambivalence can be detected about a possible threat to the moral order which the new technologies can pose if not rigorously regulated.

Strathern has pointed out that technology "enables." Paradoxically, its artifice facilitates control over what is taken as "natural" (1992) and unruly, capricious nature is tamed into producing that which culture deems appropriate. Thus we would expect to find some significant societal variation in the reception and application of reproductive technologies, revealing not only differing attitudes about the control and manipulation of the individual bodies of women but, more profoundly, about what is perceived to be natural and morally appropriate in connection with the reproduction of society.

Medicalization of reproduction exhibits a coalescence of the two poles of biopower articulated by Foucault. At one pole the human body, usually the female body, is made into an object for the enactment of technologies of control – a site to be manipulated. Women (and their partners) who subject themselves to such manipulation do so, it is assumed, because they have been "disciplined" into an ideology in which individual reproduction is considered both a "natural" outcome of a committed relationship and essential to a fulfilled life. At the other pole, where the control of populations is located, political concern about reproductive outcomes ensures that medicalization is simply neither a personal nor a medical matter (although it is almost always billed this way in clinical settings). For example, the "greying" of society is a major concern for many governments today, with the result that in Japan women are actively encouraged to produce more children in order to compensate for the spiraling numbers of economically "non-productive" elderly, as well as eventually being available to provide care for them (Lock 1992). Similarly, because health care costs are a concern for the majority of governments today, women are increasingly encouraged to submit to genetic screening and other technologies in order to produce "healthy" children with no medical liabilities, while aborting those fetuses deemed undesirable (Nelkin 1995).

The concept of biopower, while providing valuable insights, has been faulted by certain anthropologists, feminists, and philosophers in similar ways (see, for example, Hartsock 1990; Lock and Scheper-Hughes 1996). Although Foucault acknowledged the heterogeneity of the social, and the importance of the micropolitics of power relations, little attention was given by him to body praxis as it is enacted by those whom power objectifies. Foucault insisted that individuals are not wholly determined by those in powerful positions; nevertheless, his attention was focused on the mechanisms of repression and stimulation created by those in power. In contrast, many feminist anthropologists and philosophers, rather than highlighting subjugated knowledge and the work of repression, take the accounts and experiences of women as primary (cf. Hartsock 1990). Agency becomes focal and constitutive of reality as it is enacted and experienced in daily life. Such an approach makes problematic the usual interpretation of the relationship among knowledge, power, and practice created by many followers of Foucault. Responses of individuals are not simply those of either compliance or resistance; indeed they need not be *responses* at all. Rather, there is abundant evidence of pragmatism in action. A pragmatism that, although it is confined by social circumstances, nevertheless is often initiated and orchestrated by individuals, rather than simply being the effects of repression. Most important of all, individuals often juggle strategically to their own advantage among networks of power. Alternatively, as Paul Willis has shown for British youth, they many retain a cynical distance (1977).

I am less concerned in this chapter, therefore, with the medical manipulation of individual bodies, and the outcomes of such manipulations, than I am with the accounts given about reproductive technologies and genetic testing as told to me by women of reproductive age living in Tokyo.[1] Their active interest in, or alternatively their resistance to and/or vacillation in connection with, medical services to assist reproduction is a provocative starting point for examining the question of whether or not biopower is indeed "naturalized." Do technological interventions appear as logical and inevitable resolutions to reproductive dilemmas?

The body is clearly a site where power is enacted and negotiated, as Foucault argued, but body praxis must be contextualized in specific histories and social contexts. Knowledge and actions are inevitably shaped by non-discursive formations, by the "thick tissue" of the "background of intelligibility" (Dreyfus and Rabinow 1982:58). In his later work, Foucault argued that discourse is both dependent upon and also feeds back into and influences the non-discursive practices it "serves." In this chapter, therefore, not only must ideas about Japanese gender relations be considered, but also the recent history and transformation of family relations in Japan, attitudes toward children and their worth, attitudes toward technology and the "mastery" of nature, and struggles with cultural identity, particularly as it is debated with respect to the alterity of "the West." This is the social milieu within which the government, medical professionals, and individual women produce knowledge and make judgments about reproductive behavior. Of course, in a society such as contemporary Japan, much of this knowledge is tacit and hegemonic; once made explicit, it is open to dispute. Among other things I will discuss how Japanese feminists struggle with the contradictions they experience both among themselves and in society at large when trying to produce appropriate reactions to assisted reproduction.

Much of the research to date on the subject of reproductive technologies has been limited to arguments about the risks to which women's bodies are put in their application (Overall 1987). There has also been commentary to the effect that the decisions which women are expected to make about the termination or otherwise of pregnancies do not constitute a straightforward "choice," as is so often suggested (Rebick 1993). I am in full agreement with much of this literature, but seek to push the discussion in a new direction – one which moves beyond black and white arguments of oppressive paternalism and vulnerable women. Discussion about reproductive activities, in any society, must not only consider political and professional discourse about the construction and manipulation of individual female bodies, but also articulate the range of responses of women from various walks of life to such discourse, while taking into account the larger social context in which these transactions take place.

Following one case study, I will present the non-discursive background which influences reproductive behavior in Japan today, and then embark on a discussion of the interview results. Japanese women are exposed to similar "risks" and "choices" in connection with reproduction as are women in North America, but their accounts about and responses to the new technologies are significantly different. By contextualizing these interview data, the concepts of biopower, medicalization, and resistance will, in concluding the chapter, be critically revisited.

Protecting the family from nature's mistakes

Yamada-san (let us call her), has two boys under the age of $2\frac{1}{2}$, the elder of whom, Kenji, unmistakably has Down syndrome. She lives in a rather spacious house, by Tokyo standards, with her husband, parents-in-law, unmarried brother-in-law, and mother-in-law's mother. The young Yamada couple occupy two rooms on the second floor where all the activities of their daily life take place, except for the relatively rare occasions when the entire family engages in some activity together. Yamada-san's husband was out at work when I visited their home at her invitation, proffered when I met her at a routine clinic visit in connection with Kenji's health. She sat and talked to me in the confined space which serves as both kitchen and living room. An enormous television set, the sound turned down as we talked, dominated the scene, but it failed for the most part to distract the youngsters as intended, who worked very hard at capturing their mother's attention, using the entire gamut of tactics available to children with an as yet limited verbal capacity. Yamada-san, 28 at the time of her first pregnancy, had been assured that everything was "normal," and she experienced a rather easy and uneventful birth, although the baby was rather small, and was kept in hospital for a couple of weeks. It was only four or five months later that, together with her husband, she was informed that Kenji had Down syndrome. Yamada-san insists that she did not suspect that anything was wrong prior to hearing the doctor's diagnosis, but in retrospect she feels certain that the medical staff were aware of the problem soon after the birth. Yamada-san and her husband debated as to who should be told about the diagnosis. After consulting with their doctor, who agreed with them that nobody other than themselves *need* know, they decided not to tell even members of their extended family who to this day *apparently* are unaware of any major difficulty. The family has been told only that Kenji is a little slow in developing, and that is all.

The interpretation given by the ten or more Japanese acquaintances to whom I have talked about this case, is that Yamada-san's brother-in-law can expect great difficulty in securing a marriage partner if it is publicly known that there is Down syndrome "in the family." Further-more, it is too painful for the "elders" to have to confront directly such "shameful" knowledge, namely that there are "poor" genes in their lineage. (The assumption that this condition is inherited is, of course, mistaken. The chromosomal abnormality which results in Down syndrome occurs *in utero*.) It is agreed that in all probability the grandparents have surmised what is wrong with their grandchild. However, that which is not verbalized does not exist, even if visual evidence works to the contrary.

Not all Japanese families would, of course, deal with the situation in similar fashion, but this particular family is living out a dominant ideology of long standing (equally evident in many other societies), namely that it is understandable that no one would want to marry into a family where there is clear evidence for genetic disability (even if it is not an inheritable disability) or madness in the progeny. Hence the affected child and his mother must be isolated, hidden, lied about, in order that the family as a unit can be protected. Before the war a child like Kenji might well have been kept as a virtual prisoner in the house. Today many institutions in Japanese society – support groups, the medical world, the school system – provide some assistance. Nevertheless, behind closed doors of the family residence, women are often confined with their offending children to an inconspicuous corner from where they must reach out secretly, as does Yamada-san, to obtain what communal help there is.

My reading of why Yamada-san asked me to come and visit the family is that she wished her plight to be known and talked about, no doubt in order that others might become more aware of the constraints on women in her situation. Yamada-san did not hesitate for a moment to undergo amniocentesis during her second pregnancy, and she would have had an abortion if an anomaly had been detected. She states that she could not possibly have cared for two children with Down syndrome given the circumstances in which she finds herself. However, Yamada-san does not believe that one should use technology to create the "perfect" baby, nor would she have submitted herself to amniocentesis if it had been offered to her during her first pregnancy. Although she could not manage two affected infants, Yamada-san has reacted, as do many women in her position, in that the birth of her first child, Kenji, made her fully alert to the prejudice inherent in Japanese society toward those citizens labeled as "deficient." She loves and is devoted to her child, and seeks to protect him from stigma, but Yamada-san occasionally detects feelings of ambivalence in herself, since she admits that at times she longs for Kenji to be "normal." This is in spite of the fact that their current doctor has encouraged the Yamadas to think of Kenji not as abnormal or diseased but simply as having a particular body constitution – a body "type" – similar to someone with an allergic predisposition or a tendency to put on weight. Yamada-san remains conflicted about the abortion of fetuses in which an "abnormality" is detected, not because she is against abortion or testing in principle, but because she fears (as do many people around the globe concerned about the rights of the disabled) that there will be a backlash against children such as her son, so that even the limited progress made to date in Japan to integrate such children fully into society will be undone, and the prejudice they often experience continue unchallenged.

Yamada-san's case gives us a glimpse into the pressure placed on Japanese women with respect to reproduction, pressure which one would predict might drive them to cooperate willingly with the medicalization of their bodies. Pregnancy and childbirth are not the affair of an individual, or even in most cases of a couple. In Japan they remain, as was the case historically, the intimate concern of the extended family, even when the family no longer resides under one roof (Miyaji and Lock 1994). The extended family should be protected at all costs, the "standing of the family" (*iegara*) must be maintained, and, although public campaigns and media exposure have worked to reduce the stigma associated with disability of all kinds, people with psychiatric diagnoses, for example, are still at times abandoned by their relatives in institutions, as are babies born with deformities, or unwanted infants. Although many of the physically impaired are more publicly visible than formerly, others pass their lives secreted away from public view. Concern about genetic anomalies has also meant that those people exposed to atomic bomb radiation, together with their offspring, have found it exceedingly difficult to get married, except among themselves. The Japanese are not alone, of course, in responses such as these to sick and marginalized people.

Yamada-san and her husband, like virtually all Japanese except the very old, understand simple Mendelian inheritance. They are cognizant of what so many people fail to recognize, even when primed about genetics in general, namely that Down syndrome is not transmitted through family lines. Perhaps because this is the case, Yamada-san's husband has suggested that Kenji's problem may have resulted from something his wife did during pregnancy. Such an attitude is common in Japan, and stems in part from an awareness shared by most educated people that the genotype rarely, if ever, determines phenotypic expression, even in the case of inheritable diseases. Yamada-san has gone over her memories of the nine months before the birth of her son, for she too is fearful that her behavior may have influenced the fate of her child. Genetic explanations, although apparently providing rational accounts about the way in which certain diseases are beyond human control, do not necessarily rule out multicausality in the minds of those seeking answers as to why their particular family is afflicted. Nor do they necessarily relieve the family, especially the mother, of moral responsibility. This is particularly so in societies, such as Japan, which have never been enamored with explanations grounded in biological determinism.

Protecting culture from technology

Contemporary Japanese attitudes toward science and its associated technologies are difficult to pin down because the expansion of technology is intimately linked to a wide-spread ambivalence about the more general process of Japanese modernization. Moreover, Japanese attitudes toward modernization cannot be understood in isolation from ever-changing interpretations, given both inside and outside the country, about the relationship of Japan to the West. The form that current debate takes about body technologies – the feasibility of tinkering with the margins between culture and nature, and the very creation of those margins – reflects in part concerns about the condition of Japanese society and the ever-present fear among powerful conservative forces, and indeed also among many liberal-minded thinkers, about yet more "Westernization."

In Japan throughout the late nineteenth century an eager quest for Western science and technology "was grounded in [a] sense of cultural certitude" (Najita 1989), an awareness that the "core" – the bass note (koso) of Japanese culture – would remain unaffected. Technology, self-consciously aligned with the Other, was placed in opposition to culture in this discourse, and epitomized by the platitudes *wakon yōsai* (Japanese spirit and Western technology), and *tōyō dōtoku, seiyō gijutsu* (Eastern morality, Western technology). Najita and other historians have shown how this confidence in the endurance of culture was gradually eroded. Early this century and again particularly after the Second World War, internal tension erupted over Japan's increasing technological sophistication and internationalization (Najita 1989). Fears about an imminent collapse of the nation's cultural heritage became commonplace, and one reaction was a reassertion of cultural essentialism (Harootunian 1989). Throughout these transitions, although Japan was obviously geographically part of Asia, it nevertheless thought of itself as fundamentally different from other Asian countries, in particular because, until relatively recently, it was the only Asian country to have successfully trodden a capitalistic path to modernization. Japan, therefore, has consistently and self-consciously set itself off from other nations, and continues to be regarded in turn by many outsiders as culturally impenetrable and different.

Perhaps the dominant theme in the internal Japanese cultural debate over the past forty years, among policy makers and intellectuals alike, has been the extent to which it is possible or appropriate to continue to cultivate this sense of uniqueness, of "natural" difference from all other peoples. Not surprisingly, it is usually those of a conservative persuasion who vociferously insist that Japan is inherently unlike the Other of both the West and Asia. Reactionary historical reconstructions argue that the Japanese continue to be, as they have been from mythological times, "naturally" bonded together as a moral, social, and linguistic unit (Yoshino 1992). The majority of Japanese take strong exception to the extreme form of this rhetoric, which slips easily into racism and xenophobia, but it is evident that such a powerful discourse, at times explicitly supported by the government (Pyle 1987; Gluck 1993) and inflamed by trade wars, whaling and international peace-keeping disputes, cannot easily be dismissed *in toto* (Kalland and Moeran 1992; Cummings 1993).

Inherent to this sense of difference is an oft-repeated rhetoric that the Japanese are closer to nature than are Westerners. People recall the traditional medico/philosophical system, made wide use of today, derived largely from Taoist thought, in which the microcosm of the individual is conceptualized as being in harmony with the macrocosm of the natural world and the universe. When an imbalance is detected in this relationship, as when seeking to restore individual health, no effort is made to overcome the natural order. On the contrary, individual bodies are adjusted to the unique specifics of the macrocosm of their environment (Lock 1980). Japanese informants also bring up for discussion the indigenous religion of Shinto, frequently described as animistic. The idea that deities inhabit rocks and trees is recalled, but usually dismissed again quite quickly as a nostalgic return to the past, although popular Shinto is at present undergoing a revival (Hardacre 1994). The Buddhist philosophy of non-interference – of taking inspiration from the contemplation of nature, and of resigning oneself to that in nature which is beyond human control – is also central to the Japanese heritage, a heritage in which many people take active pride. Lower rates of hysterectomies, cesarean sections, and other invasive technologies, as compared to North America, is in part testimony to medical practice which does not resort to major interventions in haste (Ikegami 1989). In short, a rhetoric of being at one with nature and of gaining insight from its contemplation, product of a syncretic philosophical heritage, is pervasive in Japan, and infuses daily life. Moreover, this rhetoric is self-consciously poised against the rational and mechanistic bent of the West.

On the other hand, of course, no one can deny that the Japanese are adept at technological innovation, a by-product of which is enormous pollution and destruction of the natural environment. Those in Japan who have fought legal battles to obtain compensation for victims of industrial pollution usually argue not against technological development in principle, however, nor against the application of technology to ease human suffering, but against its misappropriation, and particularly against a lack of public responsibility about the uses to which technology is put. There are, I think, fewer narratives in Japan about technology gone wild, no Frankenstein, and no widely read accounts of dystopias such as that of George Orwell, although there are endless stories and TV programmes about the magical worlds one can enter by means of technology.

Technology can be used effectively for the good of all, it is assumed, for building the economy, and for better health care for the entire population. It can also be used as an entrée into the realm of fantasy – an escape from the shackles of routine Japanese life and culture (in this sense it parallels the uses to which meditation has traditionally been put). But technology should not be used to transform the "core" of Japanese culture, the continuance of which is often, as we will see, likened to the cultivation of nature; such a use of technology leads to potential anarchy and decadence. Attempts to apply those technologies perceived to threaten the moral order, particularly in connection with human relationships, including transplant technology (Lock 1995) and certain of the reproductive technologies, produce vociferous and unresolved nation-wide debate.

After the defeat in the Second World War, an industry grew up which enabled the female body in Japan to become Westernized – the eyes were "rounded," the breasts made larger, the hair was curled. That enterprise has virtually collapsed over the past fifteen years, and in its place an influential movement in the world of fashion cultivates the classical Japanese body in which eyelids with only "one fold" are accentuated. This reassertion of the "true" Japanese body is reflected in many other aspects of culture and, together with the characteristic transformation or "Japanization" (*nihonka*) of knowledge absorbed from the "outside," indicates a self-assurance in which an aping of the Other is neither appropriate nor necessary. Japanese responses to the application of reproductive technologies take place in this multifaceted cultural milieu.

Innovative techniques are not in themselves threatening or "foreign"; on the contrary, sex selection technology, for example, was invented and first applied in Japan. Technology is assumed to be, as has been the case for more than a century, culturally autonomous. What is of concern is its appropriate application and any ensuing consequences which may disrupt the moral order. With negative societal outcomes in mind, the West is eyed from afar, as a place where rampant individualism and selfishness dominate the social order at tremendous cost, it is assumed, to all concerned. When technology is appropriated with individual gain, or even the attainment of individual rights in mind, then more often than not this is construed as a threat to social stability and order as it is understood in Japan, and must therefore be guarded against. Allusions to this kind of thinking were present in the responses of the women who were interviewed about reproductive technologies and will be elaborated on below.

Nature as model for the planned family

It is widely agreed that the dominant gender ideology in Japan today is one in which women are expected to enter into marriage and to produce two children, preferably one of each sex, for whose health and well being the mother is held to be primarily responsible. It is also recognized by a good number of Japanese cultural commentators that this is a postwar ideology, a hardening of more flexible prewar conceptions about women's roles in the family (Wakita and Hanley 1994). Until well into this century, the majority of Japanese women were valued above all for their economic contribution to the household. If no offspring were forthcoming from a marriage, or if the children were unable for whatever reason to carry on the family business, then a suitable substitute could be adopted quite easily into the extended household, either as a child or as an adult (Bachnik 1983; Lebra 1993). Prior to the Second World War economic pragmatism was the rule, and if blood ties (*chi no tsunagari*) were not effective in keeping the household competitive, then kin-related or even non-kin adoptees would do as substitutes. Of course, fertility was of concern; women were described at times as a "borrowed womb," or a "household utensil" or "tool" until the end of the nineteenth century, and those who did not produce children within a year or little more after marriage were labeled as "stone women." Women could on occasion be sent back to their natal families if they failed to conceive; nevertheless in many households their physical labor and management skills were equally as if not more important than fertility. After the Meiji Restoration of 1867, women were also valued highly as educators of their children, particularly in connection with morals, community, and national objectives. Motherhood and the raising of children rather than fertility was invested with prestige, so much so that Japanese feminists have described the Meiji government literature designed to invest worth in mothering as *boseiron* (treatises on motherhood) (Mitsuda 1985).

The planned family was a key concept used by the Japanese state founded at the Meiji Restoration of 1867, but it has been argued that something akin to family planning has a history which commenced long before the nineteenth century (Hanley 1985). La Fleur notes the evidence that infanticide was practiced from at least medieval times in Japan. Nevertheless, by 1725, the population had swelled to approximately 30 million and Edo (now Tokyo), at 1 million, was the most densely populated city in the world at that time, followed closely by Osaka and Kyoto. There is very reliable historical evidence, however, from both temple and government records which show that for at least one hundred years, from the mid-eighteenth century, population growth leveled off, in strong contrast to China and Korea, and also, as far as can be ascertained, to the rest of the world at that time (La Fleur 1992).

Malthus's thesis was that a reduction in the growth of a population could be attributed only to famine, war, or epidemics, since the majority of individuals would not exert control over their own reproductive behavior. La Fleur creates a more sophisticated argument. He suggests that in Japan, in areas ravaged by poverty and food shortage, high infant mortality existed, probably exacerbated by the practice of infanticide. However, in central Honshū, where, in the eighteenth century, there was considerable prosperity, reduction in family size can be largely attributed to human volition. The explicit objective was to create small, healthy, and economically productive families. It is of note that official government policy of the time strongly encouraged population growth, because the shogunate wished to increase its income through taxation based on the number of individuals in family units. Despite government edicts concerning the increase in family size, sufficient people chose to enhance the quality of their family life by exerting control over unwanted pregnancies and births, producing an effect on the size of the entire population. Although abortion and infanticide were common practices, apparently no sex selected disposal of newborn babies took place (La Fleur 1992).

Recently, Cornell has produced an argument more finely tuned than that of La Fleur in which, using the methods of comparative micro-analysis on fertility and mortality rates, she concludes that deliberate fertility control through infanticide was not as systematic or as carefully planned on a long-term basis as the idea of the "planned family" might suggest. She concludes that the most important factors that contributed to a low fertility rate in early modern Japan were the cultural practices of prolonged lactation and out-migration of married men in order to work. She notes in addition that considerable variation existed among villages, variation that can only be accounted for through the use of carefully nuanced contextual analyses. Furthermore, Cornell argues that infant mortality rates from infectious disease, although they fluctuated, remained high during this period, and therefore families could not feel secure until a child had matured, a situation that it seems reasonable to assume would not encourage infanticide practices.

Cornell insists, however, that multiple components were at work, and she does not deny that people made active choices in connection with reproduction. The data show that in the village of Yokouchi, for example, over a 200-year period from 1671 to 1871, in each of one hundred households, five children survived to age one. All of these households experienced one death of an infant before age one from disease or other causes, and in addition, it appears that, in one in every three of those households, one infant was deliberately killed. These findings suggest to Cornell that short-term choices were being made about family size and infanticide was one form of fertility control which was made use of by a good number of people (Cornell 1996). It is highly likely that deformed or obviously impaired infants would be among those who were killed.

The term for infanticide, *mabiki,* is a euphemism whose prime referent is to rice cultivation, and specifically to the culling of seedlings. It was well established among Japanese farmers of the time that thinning of seedlings, particularly the weaker ones, would yield the best crop, and an analogy was explicitly made to the cultivation of human families. Perhaps the continual likening of social arrangements to the natural order in connection with virtually all social life, basic to philosophic thinking of the time, encouraged use of the term *mabiki* in connection with the manipulation of human life. Infanticide was relatively easily justified as a "natural" but necessary human intrusion into reproduction, and was performed in spite of government policy to the contrary. This reconstruction of the historical record tells us nothing, of course, about the suffering of those people directly involved in such practices. The fact that infanticide was likened to the cultivation of crops and was carried out, usually by midwives, for the "benefit" of the family, should not be read as an indication that there was little or no individual remorse.

From the time of the Meiji Restoration, systematic planning of the population was nationally orchestrated, and a self-conscious attempt to encourage "human development" was part of this program (Garon 1993) in which planned families played a central role. Although abortion was tacitly accepted prior to the Meiji Restoration, after 1880, it was assumed that economic growth could not be sustained without population growth, and abortion was made a criminal act. By the late nineteenth century virtually all women received some schooling. Less emphasis was placed on the Confucian edicts of chastity, obedience, patience, and devotion – the essentials of "good wives and wise mothers" – and women were now educated more broadly, with a focus on moral education and hygiene. According to government tracts of the time, the masses were to be educated to rationalize their lives in the name of progress; Japan had to "catch up" with the West, and the "habits" of the people must therefore be reformed through "moral suasion" (*kyōka*) (Garon 1993). Family units were explicitly likened to the family of the Emperor, conflating the macrocosm of the nation state with the microcosm of the family. Families, like the state, were in theory to be harmonious units in which, with the exception of certain ritual occasions, individual desire was suppressed for the sake of social and moral order.

Since power was for the first time legally assigned to the male head of the extended family, the government representative "naturally" present in every household (Sievers 1983), women were made more vulnerable than had formerly been the case. However, there is evidence of resistance on the part of a good number of women to the economic dependence foisted on them by the Meiji government. By the early part of the twentieth century at least 2,000 local women's groups existed in which matters relating to health and reproduction were given priority as discussion topics. Regional and national women's movements also began to coalesce at this time, but their objectives of gender equality and independence for women, stimulated by similar activities in Europe, were firmly quashed.

The Taisho era of 1912 to 1926 saw the routinization of a systematic collection of vital statistics, and public health interventions were set in place throughout the country. Despite the continuing widespread belief that *mabiki* was beneficial to society – that it was, in effect, a humanely instituted means of perfecting Darwinian natural selection – efforts were made to eliminate this practice, and to reduce the infant mortality rate. At the time, public concern was evident, however, because it was thought that encouraging the survival of every baby would simply increase the presence of "weak" people in society (Miyaji and Lock 1994). By 1940, when human bodies were in great demand for military service, those couples who raised more than ten healthy children were given awards, a policy not unlike those of Europe and North America of the time. Although a high birthrate was actively encouraged, at the same time, shortly before Germany introduced a similar ruling, the abortion law was amended and renamed the National Eugenic Law. Abortion was now legally permitted for eugenic and medical reasons, which meant in practice that those women designated as unfit to be mothers would forcibly undergo abortions. Many Japanese women remain aware of these war-time policies, and a lingering resentment is evident at any effort on the part of contemporary Japanese governments to intrude into reproductive matters (see below).

Individual desire as a threat to the natural order

The formal extended family, the *ie*, with its national obligations and patriarchal power base, was officially abolished as a result of postwar reforms. Sixty percent of Japanese people now live in a nuclear family. However, in addition to those 40 percent officially designated as extended households, many people spend much of their lives in a loosely affiliated vertically extended family where elderly relatives live close by, and a sense of obligation and familial ties remain strong (Lock 1993). Although usually described as a secular society, the ancestors central to the *ie*, and keepers of moral order, continue to play a visible role in Japanese life today (Robert Smith, ms). However, most women are quick to point out that rather than for the entire patriarchal lineage, as was formerly the case, it is simply in memory of the deceased parents and grandparents of their spouse that rituals are performed today. In addition, a good number venerate the memory of their own parents, even though women no longer officially belong to their natal lineage once married. These ritual activities, usually described simply as part of daily life and not as religious belief, testify to the importance of family continuity, and to the hold past generations have over the living.

Although there is evidence that many people actively uphold extended family ideals, albeit in modified form, a dominant ideology exists that the values commonly associated with nuclear households have swept through Japan. Because these values are associated with individualism and private, rather than communal or national interests, they cause the government considerable discomfort (Lock 1993). Paradoxically, it is evident that nuclear household living, while it liberates women from reproducing the patriarchal *ie* (both in economic terms and as the next generation), leaves them increasingly vulnerable to the foibles of the current Japanese labor market with its built-in discrimination against women (Brinton 1993). With the exception only of those small but increasing number of women who choose to remain single, and can today adequately support themselves economically, the financial security of most women has in effect been diminished in recent years, and their function remade from that of a major contributor to an extended household economy into one in which full dependence on spousal support is often the case. Thus while women today, in contrast to Meiji times, have legal rights, they now suffer a pernicious form of economic discrimination which was less evident formerly. An exception to this is to be found among women who, from the beginning of this century, were placed with increasing frequency in blue-collar jobs where exploitation of all kinds was often brutal (Tsurumi 1990).

The production and socialization of two healthy children today is expected to occupy women fully, together with the care and nurturance of husbands and elderly relatives. Despite the fact that nearly 70 percent of Japanese women are currently in the labor force (most designated as part-time workers and with no security, but working full-time at low wages), the "professional" housewife is assumed by virtually everyone to be representative of contemporary Japanese women. Those numerous women who work, almost without exception, also manage the household and raise their children virtually single handedly. Under these conditions, a child with a disability places an enormous burden on its mother, particularly so because institutionalized social support is minimal. Because a woman's financial contribution to the household is often assumed to be simply for luxury items (quite erroneously in the majority of cases), the expectation is that, should a child need special attention, a mother will relinquish her job to provide this service. Because women are also made fully responsible for the care of dependent parents-in-law, the combination of economic deprivation together with the physical burden of family care and nursing duties can easily become insupportable.

Despite official fears, given continuing gender discrimination in the workforce, life in a nuclear family provides relatively little opportunity to foster individualism and independence among women. Current family law, despite its proclaimed concern about equality and dignity, adds further restrictions to female independence (Toshitani 1994). Nevertheless, the rhetoric about family life in Japan, influenced by what are thought to be "modern" and "Western" ideals, has shifted markedly in the past twenty years to one of individual rights and choice, and independence for young couples. Nevertheless, implicit in this "modern" discourse remains the assumption that all women will "naturally" embrace the tasks of reproduction, together with the nurturing of family members.

Until as recently as ten years ago, 98 percent of Japanese women married. Today this number has dropped to 88 percent, and the divorce rate is increasing, but remains low, at 1.45 per thousand, much lower than in North America. Until very recently, virtually all women married in their mid-twenties and produced the required two children within a very narrow time span of the ensuing five or six years. Families were usually completed in size when the mother was aged 34 or younger.

Women who remained unmarried at 25 were described as *urenoki* (unsold merchandise) or *tō ga tatsu* (overripe fruit). Nevertheless, the average age of marriage has in the past few years increased to 27, but the basic pattern remains in place. Virtually all children are born to married couples (99 percent of women who gave birth in 1992 were married or in committed common law arrangements, a figure which has been stable for three decades), and the majority of women stop working once pregnant for the first time (many of them are in effect forced to leave their place of employment as it is believed that women cannot work effectively with young children in the household). Desired birth spacing and family completion is accomplished by a combination of contraception (the condom is the preferred technique) and abortion. As is well known, abortion plays a major role in current family planning in Japan, although in recent years, with more effective use of contraception, the numbers have decreased so that figures are now lower than in America, this in spite of the fact that the Pill remains unavailable for contraceptive purposes (Lock 1993).

The Eugenic Protection Law of 1948, designed to pave the way for relatively easy legal abortion in order to control population size and quality, remains in place today with a few modifications. Japanese feminists continue to be concerned that the legality of abortion was decreed from above by those in power as a national policy, rather than being the result of activism on the part of women (Hara 1996). In theory most abortions are carried out because of economic hardship, and, although abortion among young unmarried women is on the increase, the majority are performed on women who have completed their planned family of two children.

There is at present a national panic because so many young women are apparently postponing or even avoiding marriage entirely. The birthrate has hit an all time low of 1.5, making the burden of the "greying society" seem all the worse, because there will be few devoted daughters-in-law to look after aging parents and relieve the government of responsibility for welfare of the elderly. The government is once again actively encouraging young women to have more children, and it is not surprising, given these circumstances, that it has informally supported the development and application of reproductive technologies (although the low success rate of these technologies and the relatively small number of infertile women overall means that national demography is unlikely to be affected).

The government and the Japanese medical profession have both published guidelines for the application of reproductive technologies which make clear that as far as they are concerned current family relationships should remain essentially inviolate. Technology may be used for the production of the "correct" family should married couples need assistance with parenting, but it should not be used *simply* to fulfill individual desire.

It is estimated that infertility rates are about the same in Japan as those reported for North America. Japan has a socialized health care system, but reproductive technologies do not come under its umbrella. Available for the most part at private clinics, and at one or two teaching hospitals, the technology is expensive and therefore not accessible to everyone, although prices are not prohibitive for the majority of Japanese. The rhetoric which accompanies its use is one in which individual desire predominates – if a woman's greatest wish is to have a baby, then the clinic will do its best to "make" a baby for her. Implicit in this rhetoric is the assumption that the woman is married, and therefore the desire to have offspring is "natural," and the experience of pregnancy an essential part of motherhood. Both artificial insemination and *in vitro* fertilization are readily available, but only for married couples. The first Japanese "test-tube" baby was born in 1983; approximately 150 institutions perform IVF, and more than 3,000 Japanese babies have been born using this technique. Failure rates at infertility clinics are high, about the same as in North America (that is, between 85 and 90 percent), and couples are offered repeated attempts on an unlimited basis at approximately $4,000 a time.

Insemination by donated sperm is strongly opposed, as is surrogacy, and both government and medical guidelines adamantly discourage such practices. Nevertheless, at least one well-known clinic quietly makes use of sperm donors (donors are said to be medical students, but no one I have talked to will confirm or deny this). Women who make use of this technique cannot be traced, and keep their identities hidden. So too do the few women who have resorted to the use of surrogate mothers, the majority of whom contact American surrogates of Asian descent through one of two agencies set up in Tokyo expressly for this purpose. One woman I was told about had faked a pregnancy, so that when she returned from the United States with a baby everyone would think she had herself given birth. I heard about this case because the woman had asked a friend of mine, a female gynecologist, to falsify the official documents so that it would appear that the baby had been born to her in Japan. Although it is becoming increasingly difficult, contents of family registries can be made available for public scrutiny in Japan, and families making use of reproductive technologies are very concerned, because any child other than those sired by the social father will be classified as adopted, clearly labeled as such for perpetuity, and not therefore automatically eligible for full inheritance rights (a father must first specifically acknowledge a child which is not genetically related as having full inheritance rights). Thus reproduction achieved through technology where biological and social parenting do not correspond remain of concern for a lifetime, and furthermore are available in perpetuity for public scrutiny.

Abortion for the purposes of sex selection is officially discouraged in Japan with the sole exception of eliminating those very few male fetuses with major sex-linked malformations. However, everyone knows the technique is available at several major hospitals, and that if a woman insists, particularly if she hands a suitably valued gift over to the physician, she can have an abortion solely on the basis of the sex of the fetus. It is usually claimed that today in Japan it is male fetuses which will be eliminated because couples want to ensure that they have a girl to look after them in their old age (this is also borne out by adoption practices in which girl babies under one year old are preferred, although adoption is not usual in Japan today [Roger Goodman, ms]). There is, however, no reason for concern at present that the sex ratio of the Japanese population could be skewed through the application of sex-selected abortions.

Although adoption has been widely accepted in the past in Japan, this practice has usually been carried out with the pragmatic purpose of making an extended family economically viable, where none or very few offspring were born. Surrogate mothers were extensively used until the end of the last century, particularly among the samurai class (Shimazu 1994). Concubines were most often household servants whose male children could be officially adopted, written into the family registry, and sometimes treated as equals to biologically related children, while their birth mothers retained the status of servants. Children were rarely adopted as babies, however, because their "potential" as economic contributors to the household had first to be established. Alternatively, "spare" children of relatives would be adopted once their "worth" was clear (Lebra 1993).

In contrast to the "controlled" rational selection of concubines as surrogates, and child adoptees for economic ends, insemination by donor and contract surrogacy with a stranger raise moral concerns and anxieties in contemporary Japan. Principal among them are two: if only one parent (in particular the mother) is the biological parent, then it is usually assumed that such a family will not be "harmonious." People are explicit that a non-biological parent (especially a father) is unlikely to find himself able to love and care appropriately for a child created through semen donation (Shirai 1992) Moreover there is a chance that he may not officially acknowledge (*ninchi*) the child, which will then have a diminished status as a citizen. Secondly, there is concern because the donor is anonymous and one cannot, in effect, "control" the "quality" of the outcome. Goodman (ms) notes the same reservation about adoption and cites a Japanese adage: *doko no uma no hone ka wakaranai* (you can't tell from which horse the bone comes). As noted above, a few Japanese families seek out Japanese Americans as surrogate mothers (if necessary Chinese Americans are acceptable as substitutes), but this is reported in the media as desperate and unsuitable behavior, in which the financial transaction adds a considerable burden to an already distasteful act.

Almost every woman interviewed in this study, often without being asked, expressed surprise and a certain repugnance at what they understand to be a common desire among "Western" women to adopt "foreign" babies, especially when the external features of the child are different from those of the parents. Even though exotic facial features have a certain fascination there is, evidently, an overriding concern about both the appropriateness of physical features and the human "qualities" of an adopted child for successful integration into Japanese society. Offspring in which "difference" is clearly apparent, whether it be that of "race," disability, or behavior will, it is assumed, encounter discrimination. Accounts of returnee Japanese children raised abroad clearly indicate that such a concern is justified (Goodman 1990).

Reproductive praxis and the Other

A dominant conservative ideology today, known as *aidagarashūgi*, argues that the nation can best be understood, as it was earlier this century, as one large harmonious family. The historian Harootunian has characterized this rhetoric as a "social constellation held together by fundamental and culturally irreducible relationships which determine how one is to behave with reference to others within the confines of Japanese society." Included is an assumption of a "national subjectivity devoid of regional, class, or even gender distinctions," the basic form of which has remained unchanged, it is claimed, throughout history (1989).

Women are bombarded daily with advice and stories about how to create and produce healthy families, but much of this information is explicitly "Western" in origin. Reflective women have to deal ceaselessly with the conflict inherent in accepting an ideology of being above all else Japanese, and hence essentially different from all non-Japanese, or of being first and foremost a woman who is subjected, like other women, to a male-dominated value system, in this particular instance that of contemporary Japanese-style patriarchy. Women's responses to the body politics of reproductive technologies, and their attitudes about the "correct" family, should be interpreted in light of this conflicted discourse about self and Other, Japan and the West, tradition and modernity, and technology and nature. A distinct ambivalence on the part of a good number of women, including many vocal feminists, can be detected about whether what happens in the "West" can or should be taken as a model for Japan. This ambivalence is present in the responses of the majority of women interviewed, and ensures that no simple hankering after freedom from the acknowledged constraints of Japanese society, nor a desire to emulate the West, emerges in the attitudes of women when discussing reproductive technologies.

To summarize thus far, throughout the history of the planned family in Japan, women and their partners have at times actively resisted government intrusion into their sexual activities, at other times they have apparently cooperated. It is not as yet clear how much resistance, if any, took place during the war years, when women were explicitly made into "mothers of the war effort," but, as the interview data to be discussed below suggest, there is a somewhat mixed reception today in connection with the dominant ideology of reproducing the "correct" family. Many women of all ages are sensitive about government intrusions in the past into what is now thought of as their private family life (a concept which barely existed in prewar years). The majority have some awareness of the government and military propaganda broadcast in connection with reproduction during the war years, and resent it. It is not surprising that the rhetoric of today's government, to produce more children, is greeted with a mixture of cynicism and outright dismissal. By contrast, although there is some dissent, the majority of women *appear* to participate with little hesitation in a dominant ideology, also fostered by the government, with respect to the production of a healthy, "normal" family in which a married woman is placed at the hub as the principle nurturer.

It is not government communications which directly affect the ideas and behavior of women, however, but tacit knowledge, shared by the majority, about what kind of human relations and family arrangements are best for the creation and raising of children who will "fit" successfully into society. Whereas in the past the potential economic contribution of children was of overriding importance, today there is room for sentiments such as individual happiness, pleasure, and even untrammeled desire on the part of parents in connection with their offspring. Provided, that is, these aspirations remain contained within the structure of the conventional family, and do not in the long run disrupt the dominant social and moral order.

Until the recent past it was customary to investigate potential marriage partners in connection with their character and health. Such inquiries covered not only "inherited" diseases, including "mental" illness, but also tuberculosis and cancer. Today these investigations are not as intensive as used to be the case, but continue to take place, particularly in connection with those marriages arranged by the extended family. A large number of middle-aged and older people remain uncomfortable about so-called "love marriages" in which in theory individuals may freely choose their partners – it is thought that a match created out of the capricious fancy of sexual attraction is unlikely to weather the stresses of full participation in Japanese society. Just as it is acceptable to have the making of a marriage overseen (even if discreetly) it is also thought by many, both young couples and the older generation alike, to be a sensible move to make use of technology where necessary in order to create the next generation as desired. Of particular concern is the health and well-being of unborn children, because it is widely believed that any child who "sticks out" is likely to lead an unhappy and unfulfilled life owing to the stigma and prejudice present in Japanese society. Given this environment, technologically assisted reproduction of a healthy child is an attractive option for many, but any wish to resort to technology is frequently countered by another widely shared belief, namely that intrusive technologies are unnatural, contrary to Japanese custom, and dangerous to both individuals and society.

Planned families and the language of individual rights

No nostalgia was apparent for the formal extended family of the past in the interviews I conducted, at least not with respect to its hegemony over female reproduction. Several women stated explicitly that a woman's body should not be used "like a tool" in the service of the family, as had been the experience of many of the mothers of the women interviewed (Lock 1993). However, none of the fifty women, whose ages range from 19 to 44, is unequivocally opposed to technological interventions into reproduction. Without exception they find the use of contraceptives acceptable, and all but one are unopposed to abortion. Abortion among young unmarried women, most respondents agreed, is a sign of irresponsible behavior on their part (the male contribution to pregnancies is almost always ignored in this type of discussion [see also Hardacre 1997]). However, within marriage, when used to keep the family at the desired size of two children (usually determined it is claimed, as in the past, by family economics), abortion is considered to be a sad event, but an unavoidable outcome of "human nature." One woman stated explicitly that if the government gave more assistance for child support then there would be fewer abortions (see also Shirai 1989). Like every other woman interviewed, she believes strongly that children should be actively desired, and that there should be sufficient resources for nurturance and education through to university level. Several women stated that it is unfair to bring children into the world who cannot be given a good chance in life. Nevertheless, more than half the women regard abortion as "a kind of murder" because they accept that human life commences at conception. Half of the women have made use of, or would if the occasion arose make use of, a ritualized ceremony designed to placate the soul of an aborted fetus (*mizuko kūyo*) (see also Hardacre 1997).

The majority of those interviewed are explicit that availability of the Pill would ensure fewer overall unwanted pregnancies among Japanese women, but nevertheless, none wishes to use it personally because of a fear of iatrogenesis. Several women stated spontaneously that Japanese men are not "ready for the Pill," meaning that Japanese men do not usually take responsibility for their part in reproduction, and if women had access to the Pill then men could be promiscuous with even less concern than they apparently exhibit at present. It is possible that because the Pill is essentially a "fool proof" contraceptive, its rejection is not simply because of iatrogenesis, nor even because of the supposed irresponsibility of men, but because its use means that women too would, of course, be free to disentangle sexual life from reproduction. Rather few Japanese women *apparently* want this freedom, suggesting that for many the responsibilities associated with reproduction take priority over sexuality. Nevertheless, in principle, use of technology to achieve the planned family is very acceptable. For most women, the simple technology of the condom is considered sufficient, although if contraception fails, abortion is available when it is believed that a pregnancy would result in a child who could not be fully loved and provided for.

Women comply willingly with technologies which in their view are non-invasive. Ultrasound, for example, is given routinely three or four times during each pregnancy and up to seven or eight times at certain institutions ensuring, women report, that they feel "safe." The interviews revealed that women often regard pregnancy as a dangerous time. It was clear that the possibility of giving birth to a baby with an "abnormality" creates considerable anxiety, and that women feel personally implicated, as did Yamada-san, if a child is born who is less than perfect. Even the remote chance of a neonate having "minor" aberrations such as six fingers or toes was frequently cited as a reason for undergoing repeated ultrasound examinations and cooperating with medical interventions.

The majority of women are cautious about all types of reproductive technologies deemed as invasive: nevertheless there is a widely shared sentiment that if nature can be perfected through technology, then there is nothing inherently wrong with its use (Shirai [1993] found that infertile women feel more strongly about this than do others). Even when reminded that powerful chemical stimulation is involved in all technologies used in connection with infertility, any fear of iatrogenesis is, it seems, outweighed by the desire to have children. This is a paradoxical response given that the Pill is rejected by women themselves on grounds of iatrogenesis, nevertheless forty-six people responded that if a woman really desired a child, then IVF is acceptable. However, most of these same women went on to add that they themselves hoped that they could avoid such an unpleasant dilemma (although several of them were visiting the gynecologist because of a fear that they were unable to conceive). The technology should be available as a service for judicious use in times of distress. Those few interviewees completely opposed to IVF stated explicitly that women and their families should be educated into realizing that life can be fulfilled in many ways, and that child-bearing should not be the unquestioned goal of every woman.

Although IVF is acceptable to most, the thought of its use by unmarried or gay couples makes most Japanese women uncomfortable, although lesbian couples are regarded more favorably. Once again, nurturance of the child in a legally recognized family, and society's negative reaction to any child not raised appropriately, is uppermost in people's minds when they give these responses. Artificial insemination by donor (AID) and surrogate motherhood are considered acceptable by only five women, who agreed that if someone believes her life to be completely without meaning unless she has a child to care for, then she should make use of technological assistance. However, the majority are very concerned that a child conceived by these means would not be loved or cared for adequately; most believe strongly that biological and social parenting should coincide, and that if they do not then the child may suffer. Tsuge has found that Japanese gynecologists hold similar opinions (1993).

All but six women are opposed to adoption, and among those six only one would adopt a child of foreign parentage. Nearly everyone agreed that today "blood ties" are important and, in effect, going outside the family is "risky," biologically speaking. Women also suggested that the child might not be cared for as would a genetically related offspring. However, several women stated that if their husbands wanted to adopt a child then they would acquiesce. Adoption is explicitly associated by most women with the patriarchal extended family and even with concubinage, and so is shunned. Nearly half of the women were clear that if IVF failed (as they well know is often the case), they would rather not have a child at all than adopt one. Once again, the well-being of the child was stated as a concern, because without exception everyone agreed that children who are "different" have a hard time growing up in Japan. Resort to the artifice of technology to achieve the planned family, one where the biological and social parentage coincide, is better, it seems, than transgressing categories of self and other, Japanese and foreigner, even though by so doing one could avoid the "unnatural" use of invasive medical technologies. Under the circumstances it is perhaps not so surprising that, despite the exceptional invasiveness of the procedure, for more than half the women interviewed, an artificially induced postmenopausal pregnancy would be acceptable, if this was the only means by which a woman could achieve the family size she desired.

Given that the economic unit of the *ie* – the formal extended family – is no longer recognized, a planned family deliberately created with economic purposes primarily in mind has fallen into disrepute and "smells" of the old patriarchal order. Nevertheless, the planned family remains as a dominant ideology in contemporary Japan, but it is one composed of two children in which biological and social parentage coincide, where the welfare of the children rather than the family is uppermost in people's minds. When necessary, it is acceptable to use technology, whatever the involved risks, to achieve this laudable desire. The justification for careful planning remains in part economic, because most people believe that they cannot afford to raise and provide advanced education for more than two children. However, very few people expect that their children's lives should ultimately be devoted to the family economy, as was the situation in the past (although farmers and craftspeople often hope that this might in the end be the case). Children, no longer under the jurisdiction of the *ie,* are expected to become economically independent and "make their own lives," although many middle-aged and older people wish to be cared for by their children, when they themselves become very elderly. Thus some obligations and assumptions present in the prewar planned family remain in place as ideals to be emulated.

Resort to IVF and other reproductive technologies is usually couched in the language of individual rights – the rights of a woman to have a child – but further questioning reveals that this rhetoric is quite superficial. All the women interviewed consult with their husbands about reproductive decisions, and the majority indicate that husbands usually have the final word in most families. Despite the fact that everyone agreed that discussions about reproduction are no longer appropriate or necessary among the extended family, two young pregnant women whom I interviewed had been brought to the clinic by their mothers-in-law for genetic testing. It was quite evident, in spite of the doctor's efforts to keep the older women out of the clinical encounter, that it would be they who would make decisions on behalf of the younger women, both of whom had received very little education by Japanese standards. In my previous work I have come across cases where women were forcefully urged to have abortions at the insistence of their mothers-in-law, on the grounds that the older woman would not act as a baby minder as was expected given the family circumstances (Lock 1993). The ideal today is one of freedom from the extended family, but reality does not always bear this out, particularly when grandparents form part of the household. Sometimes, as in the case of the Yamada family, secrets may have to be kept, causing severe limitations on aspirations for independence.

It has been argued that Japanese women are becoming increasingly autonomous (Iwao 1993), but I want to suggest that at the same time the majority participate fully in what has been described as a "community-based family type" where the principles of authority and equality are *both* recognized (Todd 1995). Thus, even if residence is that of a nuclear family, individual rights and liberty do not necessarily take priority. On the contrary, fulfilling community and extended family values tends to take precedence over individual desire. Similarly, communities and families often expect to influence reproductive decisions made by young couples, and explicitly censure what are deemed as inappropriate behaviors. Japanese feminists are concerned that these values drive women toward an uncritical acceptance of reproductive technologies, and increasingly to genetic testing, for the sake of the family, even when individual women may themselves be opposed to their use (Aoki and Marumoto 1992). At the same time many feminists are equally critical of an unfettered individualism that they associate with America.

Earlier I considered the "naturalization" of biomedical technologies, but as Raymond Williams has shown, nature is an extraordinarily condensed concept with many possible interpretations (1986). Space does not permit a deconstruction of the development and usage of the Japanese term *shizen*, glossed as nature, but it is equally complex as its English counterpart. For a minority of women, as we have seen, intrusive therapeutic interventions are deemed "unnatural" (*fushizen*) and likely to cause iatrogenesis. Many of these women are suspicious of much that biomedicine offers, and find East Asian medicine with its reliance on herbal medicine more appropriate. But the idea of nature can also be used to create a powerful argument for acceptance of reproductive technologies. As noted above, metaphors from cultivated nature – from agriculture – have long been used as analogies for social arrangements in Japan. As with the perfection of agriculture through technology, similarly technology can and should be used to perfect the social order. Only the most conservative of commentators are explicit in their use of tropes about Japanese moral order based on the controlled cultivation of rice. However, increasingly evident are arguments from commentators living both inside and beyond the Japanese borders, that in common with most other Asian societies, Japan, despite long exposure to Euro-American modernization, retains a "collectivist" vision. This vision is of a community living in harmony – a *Gemeinschaft* bonded historically through cooperative agricultural practices (Beller 1995). Of course, this is ideology, a vision in which individuals, especially women, were and are expected to suppress individual aspirations for the sake of group harmony. A powerful nostalgia for the past supports such a rhetoric (Kelly 1986; Ivy 1995), and there is plenty of evidence that in daily life people continue to be indirectly exploited by such a vision (Lock 1993; Roberts 1994).

The responses of women in this study reveal the tension inherent in the rhetoric of individualism and freedom on the one hand (intrusions from Euro-America which pervade almost every aspect of Japanese society today), and an unavoidable immersion in and obligation toward the family on the other hand, which brings considerable satisfaction for most women (particularly when contrasted with media images of the violence and hedonism associated with the West). At the present time this tension veers toward resolution in favor of the collectivity, but a striving for increased autonomy on the part of women may well be on the increase. Thus far, however, reproductive behavior in which a known genetic heritage is cultivated through careful planning and socialization to create, as far as is possible, desired and healthy children who will "fit" with society, remains rock-like at the center of the collectivity, giving it a remarkable stability. Thus, rationalized through the fostering of happiness, health, and the well-being of children, the two poles of biopower tend to coalesce, concealing contradictions and tensions between the public and private domains, individuals and the collectivity. This rigorous normalization of the planned family means that a heavy price is paid by those women and children who are socially marginalized for whatever reason, whether they be single women,

women who are unable to bear children for whatever reason, or children who are perceived to be disadvantaged in any way (Goodman, ms; Miyaji and Lock 1994; Shimazu 1994).

Biopower revisited

Although Foucault explicitly recognized the heterogeneity of power, nevertheless explication of the medicalization of reproduction by social scientists has, probably because of its focus on the clinical encounter, tended to create an oversimplified picture of physician domination. Furthermore, where resistance to medicalization on the part of women has been noted, it is often interpreted in feminist literature as a situation of marked conflict in which women find themselves entirely opposed to the health care professions (Rothman 1989). Alternatively they must battle faceless bureaucracies. The Japanese data suggest a more complex situation, in which family members play a powerful role, often in support of medicalization, one which is sometimes contested by individual women, feminists, and even physicians. Nevertheless, the majority of women in this study self-consciously support the use of reproductive technologies, however intrusive, if they believe it will bring a woman the satisfaction she seeks in her daily life (as indeed do many women in other corners of the world). However, satisfaction for Japanese women by no means coincides in any simple way with individual desire.

Certain critical theorists may be moved to label such behavior as derived from false consciousness, but I have discussed the historical and cultural context of reproductive behavior in Japan at length in order that this temptation might be dispelled. Any simple dismissal of communitarian values as self-deception tends to leave the language of autonomy and individual rights unscathed, firmly in place as the only route to equity and justice. I am not suggesting an uncritical acceptance of cultural relativism as a solution; I am deeply disturbed that people such as Yamada-san together with her husband and children are made to suffer as they do in contemporary Japan. What I *am* arguing for is a stance which does not make uncritical use of dominant language and practices facilely adopted from a Western philosophical tradition as the basis for commentary on women's behavior wherever they reside.

Perhaps because a good number of Japanese women are aware that they form the Other as seen from the West, many are sensitive these days to cultural imperialisms arising not only from within but also outside of Japan (as are other women beyond the Euro-American axis when they reflect upon their respective societies). This situation helps to make some women exceedingly alert to the complexities and contradictions in the praxis of reproductive technologies. With this in mind one eminent research group in Japan composed largely of feminist social scientists has called for a reexamination of the idea that technological developments of all kinds possess uncontestable "virtue" (Ochanomizu Jōshidaigaku Seimei Rinri Kenkyūkai 1992). At the same time this same group extends a sympathetic understanding to those women who choose to use technology to bring nature onside with respect to individual aspirations and familial demands.

Japanese women are in a position to, and for the most part do, resist fully any obvious intrusion on the part of government into their reproductive lives. They remain, however, much more ambivalent about questioning medical authority. Many women are equally ambivalent or actually unable, without severe penalty, to resist authority exerted directly over their fertility by husbands or close family members who are senior to them. However, other women who participated in this study reported that they live in largely satisfying, cooperative family environments, whether that of a nuclear or an extended household, where they believe that their opinions and interests are given due consideration.

Biotechnologies will only escape from the laboratory, with its particular forms of debate, and be naturalized if a good number of the public actively supports their use, if their artifice is judged as facilitating individual and familial aspirations in connection with reproduction without causing untoward harm. However, whether instigated primarily by the interest of individual women, or by willing participation in familial objectives, or through coercion of individuals by family members or medical interests, if the outcomes of the application of reproductive technologies do not coincide rather closely with widely shared societal values, they may well be judged as disruptive to the moral order, no matter how well packaged and promoted. At present, the Japanese government can turn a blind eye to a small number of sex-selected pregnancies, and a few babies produced through artificial insemination by donor or through surrogacy, provided these behaviors are not openly institutionalized, even though such practices contradict moral order in Japan. The government can rest assured that the majority of Japanese do not support such practices. At the same time it can actively support closely allied technological practices when used to reproduce the ideal family. Such support is indirect and mediated through the medicalization of reproduction.

Among the small number of Tokyo women who were interviewed, cooperation with the use of biomedical technologies is pragmatically expedient and usually arouses feelings of ambivalence. Given the shortage of social support for physically disadvantaged children, and the persistent stigma they experience, together with the ready availability of abortion, this pragmatism may well drive the rapid proliferation of genetic testing and screening as this technology develops. Should this be the case, Japanese feminists and other critics commenting on these technologies will no doubt increasingly create arguments which move beyond questions of agency and coercion, self and other, individualism and collectivity, and focus instead on the specter of the perfect society and the possible application of the new eugenics now at our fingertips in its creation. The mixing of a language of needs and interests, whether individual or collective, with poorly understood, highly invasive technologies, subject at present to repeated failure in practice, is a dangerous brew. This is especially so if the application of technology is unhesitatingly naturalized and marketed as in the best interest of individuals, something to which they are rightfully entitled, especially when hegemonic interests are at the same time concealed in their practice. Biomedical technology only enables when it delivers what it promises with little or no iatrogenic effects, is not used capriciously or with coercion, and is applied with equity in mind. Appropriate regulation is a major stumbling block; so too is an accurate assessment of both the outcomes and dangers inherent to the technology itself, which, of course, is constantly changing. The biggest problems lie, however, with tacit knowledge, with the unexamined assumptions on the part of both individuals and collectivities, whether they have access to considerable power or not, as to what constitutes justice and moral order, how this should relate to that which individuals and families perceive to be in their best interest, and who should be designated to make decisions in this arena.

ACKNOWLEDGMENT

This research was funded by the Wenner-Gren Foundation for Anthropological Research Inc., grant number 5533.

NOTES

1 This research was conducted in 1994 with fifty women attending gynecological and genetic counselling clinics in Tokyo. The women are aged between 19 and 44 years of age and all but two have received at least a high-school education. Fifteen gynecologists, a planned parenthood executive, and four Japanese sociologists and anthropologists working on related research were also interviewed.

REFERENCES

Aoki, Yayoi and Marumoto, Yuriko 1992, *Watashi rashisa de uma, umanai* (Being Myself: To Give Birth or Not), Tokyo: Nōsan Gyoson Bunka Kyōkai.

Bachnik, Jane 1983, "Recruitment strategies for household succession: rethinking Japanese household organization," *Man* (n.s.) 18:160–82.

Beeson, Diane and Doksum, Teresa, forthcoming, "Genetic testing and family values," in B. Hoffmaster (ed.), *Ethnography and Bioethics*.

Beller, Steven 1995, "Postscript to the postscript: the continuing battle between rival ideas of modernism," *Times Literary Supplement* 4811:10–11.

Brinton, Mary C. 1993, *Women and the Economic Miracle: Gender and Work in Postwar Japan*, Berkeley: University of California Press.

Cornell, Laurel 1996, "Infanticide in early modern Japan? Demography, culture and population growth," *Journal of Asian Studies* 55:22–50.

Cummings, Bruce 1993, "Japan's position in the world system," in A. Gordon (ed.), *Postwar Japan as History*, Berkeley: University of California Press, pp. 34–63.

Dreyfus, Hubert L. and Rabinow, Paul 1982, *Michel Foucault: Beyond Structuralism and Hermeneutics*, 2nd edn, Chicago: University of Chicago Press.

Franklin, Sarah 1995, "Postmodern procreation: a cultural account of assisted reproduction," in Faye Ginsburg and Rayna Rapp (eds.), *Conceiving the New World Order: The Global Politics of Reproduction*, Berkeley: University of California Press, pp. 323–45.

Garon, Sheldon 1993, "Women's groups and the Japanese State: contending approaches to political integration, 1890–1945," *Journal of Japanese Studies* 19:5–41.

Gluck, Carol 1993, "The past in the present," in A. Gordon (ed.), *Postwar Japan as History*, Berkeley: University of California Press, pp. 64–95.

Goodman Roger 1990, "Deconstructing an anthropological text: a 'moving' account of returnee school children in contemporary Japan," in E. Ben-Ari, B. Moeran and J. Valentine (eds.), *Unwrapping Japan*, Honolulu: University of Hawaii Press, pp 163–87.

ms, "'You don't know from which horse the bone came': adoption and fostering in Japan."

Hanley, Susan 1985, "Family and fertility in four Tokugawa villages," in S. B. Hanley and A. P. Wolf (eds.), *Family and Population in East Asian History*, Stanford: Stanford University Press, pp. 196–228.

Hara, Hiroko 1996, "Translating the English term 'reproductive health-rights' into Japanese: images of women and mothers in Japan's social policy today," *Proceedings of the 1996 Asian Women's Conference "The Rise of Feminist Consciousness Against the Asian Patriarchy,"* Ewha Women's University, Korea: Asian Center for Women's Studies.

Hardacre, Helen 1994, "Response of Buddhism and Shinto to the issue of brain death and organ transplant," *Cambridge Quarterly of Healthcare Ethics* 3:585–601.

1997, *Marketing the Menacing Fetus in Japan*, Berkeley: University of California Press.

Harootunian, H. D. 1989, "Visible discourses/invisible ideologies," in M. Miyoshi and H. D. Harootunian (eds.), *Postmodernism and Japan*, Durham, North Carolina: Duke University Press, pp. 63–92.

Hartsock, Nancy 1990, "Foucault on power: a theory for women?," in L. J. Nicholson (ed.), *Feminism/Postmodernism*, New York: Routledge, pp. 157–76.

Ikegami, Naoki 1989, "Health technology development in Japan," *International Journal of Technology Assessment in Health Care* 4:239–54.

Ivy, Marilyn 1995, *Discourses of the Vanishing: Modernity, Phantasm, Japan*, Chicago: University of Chicago Press.

Iwao, Sumiko 1993, *The Japanese Woman: Traditional Image and Changing Reality*, New York: The Free Press.

Kalland, Arne and Moeran, Brian 1992, *Japanese Whaling: End of an Era?* London: Curzon Press.

Kelly, William 1986, "Rationalization and nostalgia: cultural dynamics of new middle-class Japan," *American Ethnologist* 13:603–18.

Kosaku, Yoshino 1992, *Cultural Nationalism in Contemporary Japan: A Sociological Inquiry*, London: Routledge.

La Fleur, William 1992, *Liquid Life: Abortion and Buddhism in Japan*, Princeton: Princeton University Press.

Lebra, Takie 1993, *Above the Clouds: Status Culture of the Modern Japanese Nobility*, Berkeley, University of California Press.

Lock, Margaret 1980, *East Asian Medicine in Urban Japan: Varieties of Medical Experience*, Berkeley: University of California Press.

1992, "Ideology, female mid life and the greying of Japan," *Journal of Japanese Studies* 19:43–78.

1993, *Encounters with Aging: Mythologies of Menopause in Japan and North America*, Berkeley: University of California Press.

1995, "Contesting the natural in Japan: moral dilemmas and technologies of dying," *Culture, Medicine and Psychiatry* 19:1–38.

Lock, Margaret and Scheper-Hughes, Nancy 1996, "A critical-interpretive approach in medical anthropology: rituals and routines of discipline and dissent," in Thomas Johnson and Carolyn Sargent (eds.), *Medical Anthropology: A Handbook of Theory and Method*, 2nd rev. edn., New York: Greenwood Press, pp. 41–70.

Mitsuda, Kyko 1985, "Kindaiteki boseikan no juyō to kenkei: kyōiku suru hahaoya kara ryōsai kenbo e (The importance and transformation of the condition of modern motherhood: from education mother to good wife and wise mother)," in H. Wakita (ed.), *Bosei o tou* (What is motherhood?), Kyoto: Jinbunshoin, pp. 100–29.

Miyaji, Naoko and Lock, Margaret 1994, "Social and historical aspects of maternal and child health in Japan," *Daedalus* 123(4):87–112.

Najita, Tetsuo 1989, "On culture and technology in postmodern Japan," in M. Miyoshi and H. D. Harootunian (eds.), *Postmodernism and Japan*, Durham, North Carolina: Duke University Press, pp. 3–20.

Nelkin, Dorothy 1995, *The DNA Mystique: The Gene as a Cultural Icon*, New York: Freeman.

Ochanomizu Jōshidaigaku Seimei Rinri Kenkyūkai 1992, *Funin to yureru onna tachi: seishoku gijûtsu no genzai to jōsei no seishokuken* (Infertility and Women's Agony: The Current Situation in Connection with Reproductive Technologies and Women's Rights), Tokyo: Gakuyō shobō.

Overall, Christine 1987, *Ethics and Human Reproduction: A Feminist Analysis*, Boston: Allen and Unwin.

Pyle, Kenneth 1987, "In pursuit of a grand design: Nakasone betwixt the past and future," *Journal of Japanese Studies* 13:243–70.

Rebick, Judy 1993, "Is the issue choice?," in Gwynne Basen, Margrit Eichler and Abby Lippman (eds.), *Misconceptions: The Social Construction of Choice and the New Reproductive and Genetic Technologies*, Hull, Quebec: Voyageur Publishing, pp. 87–9.

Roberts, Glenda 1994, *Staying on the Line: Blue-Collar Women in Contemporary Japan*, Honolulu: University of Hawaii Press.

Rothman, Barbara Katz 1989, *Recreating Motherhood: Ideology and Technology in a Patriarchal Society*, New York: W. W. Norton and Company.

Shimazu, Yoshiko 1994, "Unmarried mothers and their children in Japan," *US–Japan Women's Journal* 6:83–110.

Shirai, Yasuko 1989, *Japanese Women's Attitudes toward Selective Abortion: A Pilot Study in Aichi Prefecture*, Studies in Humanities, no. 23, Shinshu University, Faculty of Arts.

   1992, "Japanese attitudes towards assisted procreation," *The Journal of Law, Medicine and Ethics* 21:43–52.

Sievers, Sharon 1983, *Flowers in Salt: The Beginnings of Feminist Consciousness in Modern Japan*, Palo Alto: Stanford University Press.

Smith, Robert, ms, "The ancestors from veneration to memorialism." Paper presented to the Council on East Asian Studies, Yale University.

Strathern, Marilyn 1992, *Reproducing the Future: Anthropology, Kinship and the New Reproductive Technologies*, New York: Routledge.

   1995, "Displacing knowledge: technology and the consequences for kinship," in Faye Ginsburg and Rayna Rapp (eds.), *Conceiving the New World Order: The Global Politics of Reproduction*, Berkeley: University of California Press, pp. 346–63.

Todd, Emmanuel 1995, *The Explanation of Ideology: Family Structures and Social Systems*, Oxford: Basil Blackwell.

Toshitani, Nobuyoshi 1994, "The reform of Japanese family law and changes in the family system," *US–Japan Women's Journal* 6:66–82.

Tsuge, Azumi 1993, "The situation of restriction for infertility treatment and gynecologists' stance towards the new reproductive technologies in Japan" (nihon ni okeru "funin chiryō" gijutsu no kisei jokyō to sanfujinkai no taido), *Japan Journal for Science, Technology and Society* 2:51–74.

Tsurumi, Patricia E. 1990, *Factory Girls: Women in the Thread Mills of Meiji Japan*, Princeton: Princeton University Press.

Wakita, H. and Hanley, S. (eds.) 1994, *Kindai to Gendai Nihon to Josei*, Tokyo: University of Tokyo Press.

Williams, Raymond 1986, *Keywords: A Vocabulary of Culture and Society*, London: Fontana Press.

Willis, Paul 1977, *Learning to Labour*, Westmead, London: Saxon House.

Yanagisako, Sylvia and Delaney, Carol 1995, *Naturalizing Power: Essays in Feminist Cultural Analysis*, New York: Routledge.
Yoshino, Kosaku 1992, *Cultural Nationalism in Contemporary Japan*, London: Routledge.

10   An ethnography of the medicalization of Puerto Rican women's reproduction

Iris Lopez

This chapter explores the relationship between sterilization developed within eugenic ideology as a method of population control and the medicalization of Puerto Rican women's reproduction. Although technically sterilization is birth control in its most extreme form, a distinction must be made between tubal ligation and other forms of contraception based not only on their different consequences for a woman's fertility in the long term, but also on the way each is used as a tool of population policy (Lopez 1993). The key issue is not sterilization relative to other forms of contraceptive technology *per se*, but the way in which sterilization is defined, translated, and implemented within the framework of public policy.

Sterilization is seen by some researchers as an individual choice (Stycos *et al.* 1959; Schrimshaw 1970; Presser 1973), but has been defined by others as an act of state-imposed domination of the individual (Mass 1976; Henderson 1976; Rodriguez-Trias 1978). Based on my research with women from Puerto Rico living in New York, I will argue that sterilization needs to be seen from the perspective of the individual woman, but must also be understood from within the framework of state policy. When used to curtail the rate of population growth among a particular class or ethnic group because they are considered, in eugenic terms, a social burden, and therefore deemed unworthy of procreation (Hartman 1987), then sterilization can more easily be seen as a matter of state policy imposed not only on women but on the wider community of the poor. The role of the state is far less visible when women appear to choose sterilization over other forms of fertility control, but is usually still present, if differently expressed.

My main focus is on the intersection between gender, race, and class in relation to the forces that maintain and perpetuate the high rate of sterilization among Puerto Rican women in New York City. These forces are not the same as those encountered by an earlier generation of women living in Puerto Rico in the 1930s, when the use of sterilization as an instrument of state power was at its height. Yet, current practices are clearly rooted in this colonial history and, therefore, in the relationship between Puerto Rico and the United States. The geographical shift from Puerto Rico to New York, and the historical shift from one generation of women to another, has changed the political and economic context of *la operacion*. Determining the reasons for the persistence of sterilization as women have moved from Puerto Rico to New York requires a reexamination of the meaning of agency, resistance, accommodation, and constraint within this new setting and time.

Given the economic and social conditions within which Puerto Rican women must survive in New York, issues of choice and their ability to control their own fertility have now quite different implications for these women than for their grandmothers, yet understanding this history is still relevant. Therefore, prior to turning to a discussion of the forces that maintain and perpetuate the high rate of tubal ligation among Puerto Rican women in New York City, I will examine the rise of sterilization in Puerto Rico and briefly discuss how this process led to the medicalization of Puerto Rican women's reproduction several decades later.

Colonialism, the eugenic movement and the commodification of family planning in Puerto Rico

In Puerto Rico state policies such as sterilization developed within a social and historical context of colonialism. Prior to 1898 the Puerto Rican community had developed a communal system of birth control beliefs and other social mothering practices which worked fairly effectively. In 1898 a new political economy, the presence of North American imperialism, created a different political and economic dynamic, one which excluded the Puerto Rican people and attributed poverty and underdevelopment to overpopulation.

This new political economy reorganized Puerto Rican society as a whole and Puerto Rican women's reproduction specifically by infusing the medicalization of women's reproduction into the culture through the commodification of family planning. This was implemented through the rise of a cadre of medical specialists, whose primary goal was to sterilize Puerto Rican women.

These family planning specialists began to appear in Puerto Rico as early as 1934. Between 1935 and 1936, sixty-seven maternal clinics were opened around the island (Ramirez de Arellano and Seipp 1983). In 1937 sterilization was transferred to Puerto Rico as part of the larger eugenic movement that had been in effect in the USA since 1924. The goal of the sterilization campaign was to sterilize individuals considered genetically or intellectually inferior. This xenophobic and social Darwinist campaign, which took place within the broader social context of the Big Depression in the United States, was based on the belief that crime, alcoholism, and imbecility were inherited. Although the Puerto Rican people initially rejected sterilization on the basis of economic reasons, they accepted it for health purposes (Lopez 1993). Whereas the church originally opposed tubal ligation, many of the family planning specialists as well as doctors adhered to the eugenic ideology that these poor women were either too ignorant, too promiscuous, or both to control their own fertility and thus sterilization was the best solution.

In Puerto Rico clinics offering temporary methods of birth control opened and closed depending on the political and religious climate. For example, the position of Puerto Rican politicians toward contraceptives varied with and depended on the attitudes of the President of the United States, or who was running for office (Ramirez de Arellano and Seipp 1983). Consequently, temporary methods of birth control were not always available because most of these clinics did not have proper funding, personnel, or birth control merchandise to stay open. An important reason why these clinics opened and closed haphazardly was that federal funds for contraceptives did not become available island-wide in Puerto Rico until 1968. In contrast, tubal ligation was consistently available, free of charge or moderately priced since 1937. In addition, it is important to keep in mind that although the Catholic Church opposed *la operacion*, it was also adamantly against abortion. Abortion did not become legal until 1973. Therefore, for many women the "choice" was between sterilization, which was performed before pregnancy, or abortion that took place after conception. Many women "chose" *la operacion* as the lesser of the two evils.

Ironically, although quite in congruence with their history of colonialism, Puerto Rican women were used as subjects to test the birth control pill, the IUD, and Emko contraceptive foam in the 1950s (Henderson 1976). Given this history of population control, it is not far fetched to consider that Puerto Rican women may have also been used as experimental subjects for sterilization technology because this technology was implemented in Puerto Rico as early as 1937 and refined there before it was marketed in the United States and other parts of the world as birth control.

In summary a large proportion of Puerto Rican women either accepted or opted for sterilization in Puerto Rico between 1937 and the 1950s because it was presented as the solution to the overpopulation problem, which would lead to greater individual and national prosperity. It was also condoned by government officials and most physicians, made consistently available, free of charge or moderately priced, while temporary methods of birth control were difficult to obtain, expensive, and inconvenient. Within this framework, Puerto Rican women were used as subjects for the testing of birth control and sterilization technology. Moreover, because federal funding for temporary methods of birth control did not become an option island-wide until 1968 there was an unequal distribution of tubal ligation versus contraceptives. For example, while sterilization was persistently obtainable for thirty-one years, contraceptives were only haphazardly attainable. Finally, abortion did not become an option until 1973, and there was and still is a stigma associated with it. Thus, in the framework of a long-standing colonial relationship, Puerto Rican women became predisposed to sterilization because of its widespread availability and convenience, social acceptance, and overall lack of viable options. Thus, the current popularity of sterilization in the United States obfuscates the complex reality of Puerto Rican women's fertility histories and experiences as colonial/neo-colonial women of color.

In essence, the state undermines Puerto Rican women's community practices by substituting state and professional practices. The state's objective was not just cutting fallopian tubes, its goal was to cut some of the social ties that made existing community practices viable. Once Puerto Rican women's reproductive decision-making is medicalized, they lose the ability to control their own fertility. They come to depend more and more on doctors and less on their family and friends, because only a physician can perform a tubal ligation. The medicalization of women's reproductive behavior infused and gave medical and state authority more control over the alleged "population problem" and subverted many other community practices, transforming women's social and cultural practices through the larger process of colonialism.

The commodification of family planning is not unique to Puerto Rico: this is a Western capitalist process which has occurred worldwide. What is unique is the medicalization of Puerto Rican women's reproduction. In 1982, a Puerto Rican demographer, Vasquez-Calzada, found that 39 percent of Puerto Rico's female population between the ages of 15 and 45 were surgically sterilized (Vasquez-Calzada 1982). Today the rate of sterilization among Puerto Rican women on the island and in New York City continues to grow.

Let us now turn to the present situation of Puerto Rican women in New York. This part of the chapter focuses on the personal and individual forces that shape, constrain, maintain, and perpetuate *la operacion* among the Puerto Rican community I worked with in New York City. It highlights the diversity of Puerto Rican women's fertility experiences and explores the meaning of agency, resistance, accommodation, and social constraints.

The reproduction and perpetuation of *la operacion* in New York City

Puerto Rican women migrating to New York City in the 1950s were already familiar with *la operacion* because of its extensive use in Puerto Rico. The high rate of sterilization on the island was then reproduced in New York through poverty, social policies, racism, the state apparatus, and women's cultural ideologies. For example, in New York City, where this research took place, Latinas have a rate of sterilization seven times greater than that of Euro-American women and almost twice that of African American women (New York City Health and Hospital Corporation 1982). The following woman's statement illustrates how pervasive and culturally acceptable sterilization has become among the Puerto Rican community at the present.

When I decided to get sterilized I didn't give it a lot of thought mostly because almost everyone I knew had done it, and no one ever suggested that I should do anything else. My mother is sterilized, and so are two of my sisters. My father has two sisters and one of them is sterilized. My mother-in-law is operated on and so are all three of her daughters. My sister was also sterilized. On my father's side I have six brothers; three of their wives are sterilized. The majority of the women where I work are sterilized. The doctor thought I should do it too, so after my second child, I was operated on not to have any more children.

In discussing the experiences that Puerto Rican women have had with sterilization, it is important to recognize the cultural dimensions of *la operacion* in the Puerto Rican community. Given Puerto Rico's history of colonialism and population control, this is a delicate subject, particularly for individuals who adhere to a class, race, and gender analysis because of the fear of having their data misinterpreted and/or quoted out of context, or being accused of being a cultural reductionist. In part, this is an overreaction to the culture of poverty thesis era which blamed everything on the victim. A lot can be gained by examining the dialectical process between culture, history, and social structure. Consequently, this section of the chapter hopes to illustrate the ways in which a population policy that medicalized the reproductive practices of Puerto Rican women is transformed over time on the individual level and takes on a multiplicity of cultural nuances – part of which manifests itself as an element of resistance. It is in the context of women's lives –

in their neighborhoods – as they grapple with their daily problems that we can begin to understand and appreciate how women perceive *la operacion* and how they also use it, to the best of their ability, to solve their problems. In order to understand the forces that constrain and shape individual Puerto Rican women's reproductive options, I will consider the individual players within their community ensconced in their sociohistorical context. Prior to presenting a socioeconomic and demographic overview of the Puerto Rican women in the neighborhood I worked in, I will present a brief synopsis of how I collected the data.

Methods

My methodological approach focuses on the relationship of the individual to the larger social, cultural, and historical fabric and examines how these forces operate simultaneously to shape and actively guide the fertility options of the Puerto Rican women in one neighborhood in Brooklyn, New York. This outlook entails the reinterpretation of the individual as unit of analysis within the larger context of societal pressures that constrain individual options.

The ethnographic methods used to collect the data for this study are participant observation, oral histories, and an in-depth survey of a selected sample of Puerto Rican women. After spending two months in the field doing participant observation, I developed an in-depth question guide to help me document the similarities and differences between women. This questionnaire, which was the main tool of the survey, contained 200 open-ended and closed questions, and was administered by three local women and myself in Spanish and English. In this survey intensive interviews were conducted with 128 Puerto Rican women, ninety-six of whom were sterilized.

Although quantitative data are important in providing information about women's socioeconomic backgrounds and demographic characteristics – and this technique enabled me to document the pervasiveness of *la operacion* among the women in this neighborhood – it is my experience that in and of itself, survey data are too static to shed light on the complexity of people's lives. The multifaceted strategies used to collect the data illustrate the power of women's testimonies and the strength of the ethnographic method when combined with survey techniques in urban areas.

After the survey, I continued doing participant observation and collecting oral histories from a select number of women whose life histories represented different situations that lead women to either accept or opt for sterilization. In addition to the in-depth survey interviews, I also collected oral histories from seven families on an intergenerational basis. This approach permitted me to compare the perceptions, experiences, and knowledge of sterilization of mothers, daughters, and grandmothers from the same families.

The following section concentrates on the results and analysis of this study. It describes the general conditions that frame women's reproductive decisions. The percentages are drawn from the survey data and the women's voices are selected from the oral history material. The oral history data are not presented on an intergenerational basis.

There is an old saying in Puerto Rico. Where one child eats, ten can eat. The problem is what are they going to eat?

As the above subtitle suggests, the folk wisdom of the Puerto Rican community is changing to reflect the hard economic reality of the 1990s. The folk belief that where one eats, ten can eat, is rooted in an old folk philosophy of an agricultural era. In this ethnography, poverty is not just another variable that has equal weight to other factors – it is one of the most important components that permeates every level of women's lives.

While most lower-income women experience difficult socioeconomic situations, households headed by female single parents fare even worse (Abramovitz 1988; Perales and Young 1988). Sixty-six percent of the women in this study are heads of households. Almost all of the women in this study stated that they had been married at least once, though 53.1 percent said that they were separated, divorced, or widowed. Almost three-quarters (70 percent) receive either supplementary or full assistance from Aid to Dependent Children. The mean annual income in 1981 was $7,000 or less. This income supports a mean of 3.4 children, the woman herself, and usually a husband/companion or sometimes a female relative. With this money, women support themselves and their children, buy food and clothing, and pay the rent.

In 1981, more than three-quarters of the women in this study were not working, although 12.5 percent were looking for jobs. Only 31.3 percent had husbands who were working and 15.6 percent had husbands who were unemployed at the time. The relatively small group of women who were working when they participated in the study were employed as low-wage workers with little job stability, generally in tedious jobs and often under difficult conditions. In addition to their wage labor, when these women left their place of work they went home to start a second shift as mothers and housewives. Housework and childcare frequently consumed most, if not all, of their evenings and weekends. Most did not work outside the home, not only because of the difficulties of coordinating a job and running a household but also because it did not make sense for them to work only to spend the majority of their wages on a baby-sitter. The lack of low-cost and good-quality childcare services is another factor that forced many to stay home. As one of the women stated:

Salaries are so low that all of a woman's money would go into the baby-sitting expenses. See when someone takes care of your children not only do you have to pay them, but you have to buy them the food they will eat that day. After I had my third child, I stayed home so that I could rear them myself. If I had continued working, I would have worked just to pay the sitter. It didn't make sense.

Eighty percent of the women in this study claimed that their economic circumstances had a direct or indirect effect on their decision to get sterilized. Forty-four percent felt that if their economic conditions had been better, they would not have undergone surgery. Nilda is one of these women:

If I had the necessary money to raise more children, I would not have been sterilized. When you can't afford it, you just can't afford it. Girl, I wish that I could have lived in a house where each of them had their own room, nice clothing, enough food, and everything else that they needed. But what's the sense of having a whole bunch of kids if when dinner time rolls around all you can serve them is soup made of milk or cod fish because there is nothing else. Or when you are going to take them out, one wears a new pair of shoes while the other one has to wear hand-me-downs because you could only afford one pair of shoes. That's depressing. If I had another child, we would not have been able to survive. There's an old saying in Puerto Rico: where one child eats, ten can eat. The question is what will they eat.

Other problems women face daily that affect their fertility decisions are the physical environment and material conditions in which they live. For example, one of the major complaints of the women in this neighborhood is the lack of hot water and adequate heat in the dilapidated tenements in which they live. Moreover, mothers constantly worry about the adverse effect that the run-down environment of their block and the surrounding area might have on their children. It was my experience that mothers are afraid to let their children play outdoors because they fear that the children may get involved with the wrong friends. In order to protect them, mothers try and keep their children indoors for as long as they can. This is a problem, especially during the summer, because of the relative lack of space in the apartments, the heat, and the noise level of kids playing indoors. Mothers often claimed they were sterilized because they could not tolerate having children in such a dangerous environment and/or because they simply could not handle more children than they already had under the conditions in which they lived.

Although it is important to note that women do not reduce their reasons for getting sterilized strictly to economic considerations, another way that poverty impinges on their daily lives is through the high rate of crime and drugs in their neighborhood. Because of this condition, a recurrent theme in their conversations pivoted around their concern about leaving their apartments alone for an extended period of time for fear of being burgled. Bobbie's oral history is a powerful testimony of the way that poverty pervades poor women's lives.

Like I was robbed a few months ago. Ever since the burglary I stay home more. I came home one evening after work and they were here. I had a fight with him and I got cut. He got away. I'll fight anybody, especially for something I worked so hard for. They cleaned me out of jewelry, mine and the kids, money – my rent . . . *Eran pinceros*, they were lock pickers, that's what got me mad. My mother was downstairs too. I heard something, a footstep which is *verry* strange. I was sitting at the table. I was just about to have dinner. My mother watches her *novelas*, soap operas, really loud so I screamed to her "mom *baha eso*," lower that. "*Quien esta arriba*? Who's upstairs?" I said, "Mommy no body's upstairs, I just walked in. I came to eat." So we got into the hallway and I was gonna go for something but I saw my mother leave the door first. God . . . so I ran after her. I came up with nothing in my hands to protect myself. Then this guy is coming down the stairs. They had just finished, you know, and he's got my record player. I got that piece back because in the other burglary they cleaned me out completely again. He's coming down the stairs and mommy says, "*a quien vd. Esta buscando*?" Who are you looking for? The guy says, "*yo estoy vendiendo una radiola senora*." I'm selling a record player madame. I said, "ooohhh, let me see." So the guy opens the bag and shows me my record player. He says, "I bought this off this guy but I need some money and wanna sell it." I says, "you ain't selling shit cause that's mine!" He said, "nahhh nahhh I just bought this off this black dude, I wanna sell it you know." I said, "well if it's yours lets go up to my apartment and check my living room." He says, "*noo noo es mia*", no no it's mine. So I said, "well, let's go upstairs" . . . so I grabbed him and he dropped it there and Mommy picked it up. She backed off and I shoved him into the wall. Big guy too. Mommy let out a yell and he pulled out the knife. He got me on my hand. If Mommy hadn't yelled he might have gotten me in the chest. In this neighborhood you live with this tension, you live with this shit.

Women's perceptions of their bodies and reproductive rights

In unraveling the complicated subject of the interplay between agency, resistance, constraints, and accommodation, I began with an examination of the ways that women exert agency. This is best illustrated through women's perceptions of their bodies and who should control them, as well as through the circumstances that have led some of the women to use sterilization as an element of resistance to patriarchy and female subordination. The elements of resistance occur as each woman's individual struggle to gain some control over her body and life – which sometimes includes confronting and fighting sexism – versus any kind of a collective sociopolitical or gender struggle to change the individual and social constraints that have led women to get sterilized. In other words there are elements of resistance in women's decisions to get sterilized as well as a degree of accommodation. That is, women resist to the degree that they can and also acquiesce to the multiple forces constraining their options.

Women get sterilized because of a myriad of forces operating simultaneously to limit and constrain their options. Angie's story is compelling because it stresses how women's responsibility for and difficulty with birth control, child rearing, and domestic work in conjunction with financial problems, marital strife, and a desire to do other things with their lives in addition to having children constrains their fertility options. Her story also illustrates how strongly most women feel about being able to make the decision to get sterilized.

Women get operated on for a combination of reasons. It's not just money, it's everything combined. If you're alone that has a lot to do with it. If you're with somebody, the kind of relationship you have has a lot to do with it. You know it's combined. It has to do with mental anguish. The mental thing can come if you're frustrated 'cause you don't have enough money to get what you want or to live comfortable anyway. Or you have problems with one kid, or you have problems with your old man – all these things combined. It puts your mind like wanting to do it. That's what happened to me. All this bullshit. I can't afford to have another kid because money-wise it was tight. The kids were giving me a hazel. I wanted to become somebody and I couldn't if I would have had more kids. I don't want to have one dangling on top of the other because that would be rough all around. My situation with my old man wasn't good. My husband helps a little but it's the kids who really help the most. That's why I think women should have the final decisions about whether or not she gets sterilized. Because the woman, she's the one that's going to go through the changes. She's the one that is going to bring them up. Men go to work and bring in the bread but there are few men who help out altogether. They might help here and there but it's the woman who has to deal with everything. All the burden of the housework. We have a twenty-four-hour job. That's why the decision to get operated is my decision because men aren't always around to help. My job doesn't stop when he comes home from work. He lays down and he relaxes. I don't say I'm a slave but if you come down to it, I have a twenty-four-hour job that I don't even get paid for. So as far as men are concerned, why should it be their decision to say no when we're the ones who have to deal with all the ups and downs.

With the exception of those women who were openly victims of sterilization abuse, most women in the Brooklyn neighborhood adamantly shared the view that to be sterilized was their decision because "it was their body and they would do with it as they pleased." As Tati's story illustrates many women also felt that sterilization was the first step in their being able to do anything productive with their lives.

I want to do something for myself, go back to school, a training, anything. My financial situation has everything to do with my decision to get sterilized. If I have a kid then I can't go to work. Just as long as I know that I'm not going to get pregnant again I can do it. It's too difficult to get a baby-sitter and then they almost cost your entire salary. Even if you pay them the minimum fifty dollars a week. If you have more than one child, there goes your pay check. I don't want to be dependent on welfare for anything. There's nothing holding down this kid. *Me opero*, I'll get operated on, and then I get to take it from there. Then I'll go register for school, get my GED. First, I have to get the operation before I can do anything. *Eso me tiene la mente que* (that has my mind that) I can't concentrate in school. I can't because I'm terrified of the operation. I'm also taking my chances now. What if I get pregnant. Once I get operated I feel that's when I'm going to begin to live again. When my mother was young they didn't have all of these operations. All they had was the IUD. If they had this operation when I was younger, my mom says, I only would have had one kid, or maybe none. What she says is true. My mother was a working woman. She always worked. Having kids really got in her way. My mother had six kids altogether. One died. My mother is the one who nags me the most . . . "are you avoiding kids?" My mother wanted me to get sterilized when I was nineteen. She got very mad at me because I didn't do it. She still tells me if I had done it, I wouldn't be going through everything I'm going through now. She didn't think I was too young at nineteen to be operated on because I already had two kids. She said that was the best time to do it, when you're young.

In contrast to Tati's story, all women do not feel that sterilization is a perquisite for success. In order to contextualize her life history a little, almost all of the women Tati knew were sterilized. Like many other women she was also misinformed about the permanency of this operation. She was 25, she had four children, two of whom were in a foster home, and she had a deep desire to go back to school and get her GED.

Tati's story demonstrates the way that women assert agency, but also the ways that agency and constraint intersect. It also illustrates that what may appear at first glance to be an exclusively "individual" or "cultural" factor also has its origins in the social and economic base. In addition to attitudes about who should control their bodies and their perceptions that they have been sterilized "voluntarily," population policy, class, and poverty play a critical role in limiting the fertility options of Puerto Rican women.

Men's role in the decision-making process

Most women in this study did not feel that they had to ask the men in their lives for permission to get sterilized. Men rarely objected to a woman's decision to become sterilized unless the couple disagreed about the number and/or gender of the children desired. Most of the couples in this study agreed that it was difficult to raise and provide for more than three children. In other words, most men were as conditioned and predisposed as the women to *la operacion*.

The perception that most women felt that sterilization was their decision and the fact that they felt they had no viable options are two separate issues. When I asked who had influenced the decision to get sterilized, only one out of ninety-six women responded that her husband directly influenced her. This does not mean that these women do not consult with their husbands/companions about the sterilization decision. In most cases they did. It means that, regardless of the man's view, most women felt they had the right ultimately to make the final decision about sterilization, because they were the ones who were going to have the baby and were the primary caregivers. They either decide independently, or with their companion/husband, that they do not desire and/or cannot afford to have any more children. These women tend to use sterilization as fertility control because of their social and historical predisposition toward this technology but also because of a lack of viable options. Given the conditions of their lives, they saw sterilization as the most reasonable decision they could make. It is possible that if some of these women had a viable alternative, they might still have opted for sterilization. However, for the majority of the women in this study, viable options did not exist and the conditions of reproductive freedom were not met.

You should have your children while you are still young and can care and play with them

The tendency either to marry or to have their children while they are still relatively young precipitates their decision to get sterilized at a younger age: 66 percent of these women were sterilized between the ages of 25 and 29. Moreover, most of the women in this study married and had their children before the age of 25. They had already achieved their desired family size by their mid-twenties but still had approximately twenty years of fecundity left. Since the most effective method available to curtail fertility is sterilization, their choice was to accept it or continue using temporary methods of birth control for the next twenty years. Women in this study had on average two or three children, the common perception of the ideal family size. More than half (56.7 percent) claimed that they were completely responsible for their fertility and child rearing. While this may appear as an issue of individual choice, it is really the construction of the nuclear family in a patriarchal society, in which the brunt of the responsibility for child rearing and birth control is relegated to women. In part this is accomplished by providing birth control mainly to women and few if any contraceptives for men. In addition to caring for their children, women are responsible for the domestic work and their husbands' needs. Once again, this is one factor, among many, that has led Puerto Rican women to opt for or accept sterilization.

Lack of access to quality health care services

On a local level, a person's resources profoundly affect both the type of health care services to which an individual has access, as well as knowledge of the options. On a microlevel, the quality of care and information that middle-class women receive in private hospitals broadens their choices by enabling them to make informed decisions within the limits of the contraceptive technology that is available. Conversely, the inadequate quality of care that poor women receive diminishes their ability to make informed reproductive decisions and in this way further restricts their already limited options. For instance, because public hospitals have fewer health care providers and facilities, and less time to spend with their patients, poor women are not always informed about all of the contraceptives that are available. This is particularly true about the diaphragm.

From informal discussions with health care providers, I found that there is a prevalent belief among them that Puerto Rican women reject the diaphragm because of women's cultural aversion to the manual manipulation involved in its use. While this may be true for some Puerto Rican women, there are other equally compelling reasons why a large number of low-income Puerto Rican women do not use the diaphragm. Some of the women in this study had never heard of the diaphragm. In order to prescribe it, the health care providers must show the women how to use it properly. This requires a minimum of ten to fifteen minutes as well as a private space. Time and space are commodities that are at a premium in municipal hospitals. Moreover, if the health care providers believe that the diaphragm is a culturally unacceptable method of birth control for the poor then they are not going to recommend it. Finally, there is also the attitude among health care providers that it is better to recommend mechanical and surgical forms of fertility control to the poor because they do not have sufficient initiative or responsibility for controlling their fertility.

Problems with birth control

The quality of health care services a woman has access to significantly influences her knowledge of contraceptives and attitudes about them. The lack of safe and effective temporary methods of birth control prompted many women in this sample to get sterilized. Although 76 percent of the women used temporary methods of birth control before getting sterilized, they expressed dissatisfaction with the contraceptives available, especially the pill and the IUD. As one woman stated: "The pill made me swell up. After three years, I had an IUD inserted. It made me bleed a lot so I had it removed. I was sterilized at the age of 25 because I couldn't use the pill or the IUD. I tried using Norforms and the withdrawal method before I was sterilized but neither method worked very well."

One woman died because of an unnecessary hysterectomy that was performed when her IUD became dislodged and her doctor could not find it. In her sister's words:

My other sister had an IUD inserted in her. It got lost. This sister planned to have another baby in the future. A doctor performed a hysterectomy on her because he said that the lost IUD had caused cancer. My sister died from this operation. I don't know why she ever used an IUD. Her husband worked and she only had two children. I never wanted to use birth control after her experience.

Cognizant of the constraints that their economic resources, domestic responsibilities, and problems with contraceptives place on their fertility options, many women feel that sterilization is the only feasible "choice," given the conditions of their lives. Hilda, for example, migrated from Puerto Rico. In Pennsylvania she worked as a migrant worker picking mushrooms with her husband. Even though Hilda loves children dearly she was sterilized at the age of 23 after her third consecutive baby refused to breast feed. Although this was the catalyst to her getting sterilized at that particular time, her fertility decision was based on her longer-standing economic and marital problems – her husband was an alcoholic and used to beat her – coupled with the hazards of living in a poor neighborhood, and her distrust of chemical/mechanical forms of birth control. Her distrust was based on the bad experiences two of her sisters had had with contraceptives.

I've gone through a lot of hard times with my family. I don't want to think about what it would have been like if I had more children. I was married at the age of 18. My first child was born at the age of 19. When my first child was a year and six months, I became pregnant again. The following year my second child was born. Then I become pregnant for the last time.

At the time my husband worked seven days a week. He picked mushrooms in a migrant camp. That was the only job available. He never had a day off, not even when he was sick. Have you ever seen mushrooms? Well, you have to cut them by the stem. By the time you get to the other side of the field, they are growing again. We used to get up at three in the morning. By four a.m. we were in the field. We worked till six in the evening. God life was hard in those days [sign].

I think a woman should have her children when she gets married. A child is the nicest thing that can happen in a marriage. Children bring happiness to a home. I don't believe in avoiding children because perhaps when you really want one you might not be able to have one like what happened to my sister.

As long as I breastfed my children, I didn't get my period. After eleven months, my third child refused to suckle. I immediately got my period. I lived in Kings Square, Pennsylvania and the hospital was in Delaware, Pennsylvania.

My husband is a good man. He's helpful around the house. He has his flaws but in the evening, he would help me with the children. Sometimes he'd even mop or wash the dishes. He helped me with the household chores a lot. But ever since we came to Brooklyn, my husband began to change. I realized that my husband was not the right man to financially care for too many children. We discussed it and he agreed that I should get operated on. I got sterilized because I did not want to increase his economic burdens. Yet financial problems still led to our divorce.

Yo practico la religion a mi manera – I practice religion in my own way

Although Puerto Rico is a Catholic country, Catholicism does not appear to have a direct effect on most women's decisions to be sterilized. Eighty-seven percent of the women in this sample were raised as Catholics. Of these women only 32 percent felt that sterilization goes against their religious beliefs. In contrast, however, women's familiarity with *la operacion* has had a profound effect on predisposing them toward sterilization.

The prolonged use of tubal ligation has transformed it into part of the cultural repertoire for a large segment of the Puerto Rican population. *La operacion* is frequently recommended by a doctor or health care provider as well as by a friend or family member. In Bobbie's words: "Women tend to talk to their mothers or someone that they know." Women's perceptions about *la operacion* are also strongly influenced by the large number of females within their own families who have been sterilized.

The effect that almost six decades of exposure to this operation has had on predisposing Puerto Rican women to sterilization cannot be underestimated. To acknowledge that sterilization has a cultural dimension to it does not, however, make the decision to become sterilized one based on free will since free will does not exist in a vacuum. Nor does such a decision suggest that it originates from women's "folk" culture, as some scholars have implied through the language that they have used to describe this phenomenon (Presser 1973). For Puerto Rican women sterilization became part of their cultural repertoire because of the political, social, and economic conditions that favored it, creating the conditions for their predisposition toward sterilization through the use of population control policies and initiatives. Through time this method of fertility control has become part of women's cultural repertoire maintained and perpetuated through need to control their fertility and their life circumstances.

Misinformation

Puerto Rican women's social and economic conditions, their familiarity with sterilization, their cultural and religious views about it, and problems with temporary methods of birth control all contribute to their decisions to get sterilized. In addition to all of this, Puerto Rican women have a very high rate of misinformation about the permanency of *la operacion*. This is important because it is one of the main factors that maintains and perpetuates the high rate of sterilization. The rate of misinformation among the women in this study is very high. Eighty-two percent of the women in this study made a distinction between the "tying" and the "cutting" of the fallopian tubes – a distinction that does not exist. According to one woman:

I feel that if a woman is not sure if she wants anymore kids, then she should have her tubes tied. Because of birth control pills, women get cancer or veins on their legs. It's a different situation when you get your tubes tied. At least then you can feel relatively safe that you will not have any more children until you want to. If a woman really has decided she absolutely does not want to have more children, then she should have her tubes cut.

The misinformation issue is complicated because of its multifaceted dimensions. In some cases women have these beliefs and do not communicate them to doctors or health providers. In other cases doctors and health care providers do not tell women about the permanent nature of this operation.

With the introduction of tuboplasty, a method used to try to reverse a tubal ligation, a new form of misinformation is developing among

Puerto Rican women. Women claimed that if they underwent a tuboplasty they could have a successful full-term pregnancy again. Almost two-thirds (63.8 percent) of the women in this study claimed that it was possible to have a child after undergoing an operation where a set of "plastic tubes" was inserted. Once again, this belief is inaccurate because only a very small number of these reversals are successful. Despite this, most women are not being properly informed about the low rate of success of this operation and the high risk of ectopic pregnancy.

Regret

Of the ninety-six sterilized women, a third (33 percent) regretted that they were sterilized. Twenty percent do not regret their decision. The others (47 percent) were somewhere in the middle. Although they felt they made the best decision they could under their given conditions, they did not regret their decision but they were not happy with it either.

To an extent, regret is a barometer of the constraints and social coercion involved in the decision-making process. Even though they felt that they had made the best or, in some cases, the only decision that they could under the given circumstances, in general terms the data show that, at some level, women are well aware that their decisions were based on their existing social conditions.

Regret is conditional upon myriad factors such as the early age at which some women are sterilized, marital status, health of their children, a change in their economic circumstances, and the conditions under which they make the decision. "If I could make that decision again today, I wouldn't do it. I was operated on when I was 18 years old. I did it because in order to work, I couldn't take pregnancy leave. Now I've met a good man, and I'd like to give him a child, but I can't."

Some women regretted they were sterilized not only because of changes in their economic and/or marital status but also because of the death of a child and/or because they felt they had made a hasty decision. As the data indicate, before the New York City sterilization guidelines were issued in New York City in 1975, many women were sterilized shortly after making this decision. In this study, 49.4 percent of the women were operated upon between one to seven days after the decision had been made. Women who waited seven days or less had a higher percentage of regret than those who waited longer. Although the issue of regret is complicated, those women who deliberated longer over this decision tended to show less regret.

Theoretical discussion: agency, resistance, accommodation, and constraint

As we have seen from the ethnographic material, Puerto Rican women experience sterilization in many different ways. Sterilization may give one woman freedom, but be oppressive to another. A woman may perceive sterilization as empowering at one point in her life because it gives her a degree of independence, but at another point in time she may perceive it as oppressive. For example, she may regret having been sterilized if her child dies, or she remarries and wants more children. A woman who opted for sterilization because she thought it was a temporary method of "birth control" may feel oppressed once she finds out that *la operacion* is for the most part irreversible. As I noted previously, a large number of Puerto Rican women in this study believed a tubal ligation could be reversed.

Different realities can, and often do, coexist within the same context. A Puerto Rican woman may decide to get sterilized because she does not want any more children. From her perspective, this is a vital decision giving her more control over her body and her life. Her decision is encouraged, however, by a state which considers her fertility a burden because of her dependence on welfare. In this sense, her interests and those of the state coincide and produce an apparent consensus between the woman and the state over the need to control her fertility. Her sterilization is a source of resistance and empowerment for the woman, but is simultaneously an expression of her oppression by a state motivated by considerations of economics and politics.

In other cases a woman may get sterilized in order to resist one oppressive situation only to subject herself to another potentially oppressive situation. For example, a woman may choose sterilization as a way of resisting forced maternity, preferring to accept a health practitioners' recommendation on sterilization (Colon *et al.* 1992).

Finally, it is also important to consider that there are Puerto Rican women who are not using sterilization as an element of resistance at all. These women may get sterilized because they have achieved their desired family size and they decide either independently or with their companion/husband that they do not want and/or cannot afford to have any more children. Most of these women may tend to use sterilization as a birth control policy that they have been conditioned or predisposed to use. It is a method of fertility control they are familiar with and, given their socioeconomic condition, the method they may be the most comfortable with, and/or they feel is the most viable. And, in these cases, sterilization may be the most reasonable decision they can make.

There is also the possibility that even if these women had viable alternatives and their conditions were different, they might choose sterilization. However, this is not the case for the majority of women.

Conclusion

In Puerto Rico, state policies such as sterilization developed within a social and historical context of colonialism. Whereas colonialism restructured Puerto Rican society as a whole, sterilization, used as a form of population control, medicalized and commodified Puerto Rican women's reproductive practices. To understand fully the insidious impact of sterilization on the Puerto Rican community, we must transcend the individual as the unit of analysis and examine women's reproductive decisions within a larger social and historical context while at the same time respecting women's reproductive decisions. My perspective enables us to transcend women as the unit of analysis, and to consider the complex and often contradictory layering of individual, social, and historical forces that shape and constrain women's reproductive behavior.

Focusing on individual and sexual rights to the exclusion of community rights obfuscates the insidious nature of sterilization as population control and keeps us locked into the individual paradigm, whether or not we consider the larger social and historical forces. There can be no individual rights, as long as the Puerto Rican community does not have basic rights such as reproductive freedom. Until community rights become an entitlement, individual rights will continue to be a moot point.

REFERENCES

Abramovitz, Mimi 1988, *Regulating the Lives of Women: Social Welfare Policy from Colonial Times to the Present*, Boston: South End Press.
Colon, Alice, Davila, Ana Luisa, Fernos, Maria Dolores, Bonilla, Ruth Silva and Vicente, Ester 1992, "Salud y derechos reproductivos," Tercer encuentro de investigadoras auspiciado por el proyecto de Intercambio CUNY-UPR.
Hartman, Betsy 1987, *Reproductive Rights and Wrongs: The Global Politics of Population Control and Contraceptive Choice*, New York: HarperCollins.
Henderson, Peta 1976, "Population policy, social structure, and the health system in Puerto Rico: the case of female sterilization," Ph.D dissertation, University of Connecticut.
Lopez, Iris 1993, "Agency and constraint: sterilization and reproductive freedom among Puerto Rican women in New York City," *Urban Anthro-*

pology and Studies of Cultural Systems and World Economic Development 22(3–4):299–323.

Mass, Bonnie 1976, "Emigration and sterilization in Puerto Rico," in Bonnie Mass (ed.), *Population Target: The Political Economy of Population in Latin America,* Toronto: Latin American Working Group, pp. 87–108.

New York City Health and Hospital Corporation 1982, Sterilizations reported in New York City, Department of Biostatistics.

Perales, Cesar and Young, Lauren 1988, *Too Little, Too Late: Dealing with the Health Needs of Women in Poverty,* New York: Harrington Park Press.

Presser, Harriet 1973, *Sterilization and Fertility Decline in Puerto,* Population Monograph no. 13, Berkeley: University of California.

Ramirez de Arellano, A. and Seipp, C. 1983, *Colonialism, Catholicism, and Contraception: A History of Birth Control in Puerto Rico,* Chapel Hill: University of North Carolina Press.

Rodriguez-Trias, Helen 1978, *Women and the Health Care System,* New York: Committee Against Sterilization Abuse.

Scrimshaw, Susan 1970, "The demand for female sterilization in Harlem," paper presented at the 69th Annual Meeting of the American Anthropological Association, San Diego, California.

Stycos, Mayone, Hill, Reuben and Back, Kurt 1959, *The Family and Population Control: A Puerto Rican Experiment in Social Change,* Chapel Hill: University of North Carolina Press.

Vasquez-Calzada, José 1982, *La Poblacion de Puerto Rico y Su Trajectoria Historica,* Puerto Rico: Universidad de Puerto Rico.

11   Situating resistance in fields of resistance: Aboriginal women and environmentalism

John D. O'Neil, Brenda D. Elias, and Annalee Yassi

The problem

In June 1985, approximately a hundred people from the largely Dene community of Wollaston Lake (Hatchet Lake Band) in northern Saskatchewan set up a blockade camp on the road leading into the Rabbit Lake and Collins Bay uranium mines. They were joined by other Aboriginal people[1] from Saskatchewan and Manitoba, and by approximately thirty-five non-Aboriginal anti-nuclear "activists" from across Canada and Europe.

In a book entitled *Wollaston: People Resisting Genocide*, Mary Anne Kkailther, wife of the Chief at the time of the Hatchet Lake Band, is quoted at length from a statement she made at a community meeting on the day before the blockade (Goldstick 1987:172–3):

The Lac La Hache Band asked these people to come here to support us in opposing the uranium mining at Wollaston Lake . . . We were against uranium mining since 1972. When mining companies and governments came to our community to talk about the mines they only told us good things about the mines. Things like giving people jobs and medicines. They never talked about uranium wastes that are dangerous to all living things. They never talked about how uranium is used in making bombs, but we know how dangerous it is . . . We cannot sit back and let them go on destroying our land and water. We live off the land, on animals, fish and berries. Some people and some newspapers say that people here are not against the mines. The majority of people here signed petitions to the government of Saskatchewan to stop all uranium mining on our land.

The blockade lasted nearly four days. Although non-violent, tensions were high as the blockade was under police observation, and mining officials threatened legal action. The blockade ended with a promise of negotiations to involve the Wollaston Lake First Nation community in the economic benefits of the mining activity. It ended as well amidst rumors and accusations that the protest was organized by "Greenpeacers" and other outside agitators who manipulated local opinion for external ends.

In the evening of November 6, 1989, Chief Edward Benomie was flying back to Wollaston Lake from Points North (the principal staging area for mining in the region), when he noticed a large pool of discolored water near the mill of one of the uranium mines. He asked the pilot to circle the area and realized he was looking at a large spill of contaminated water from the mine. He flew on to Wollaston Lake and waited all the next day for a phone call from the mine, to indicate that the spill had occurred. He called the mine in the evening and was told that no spill had occurred. He continued to press for information, calling head offices and government officials throughout the country. Finally, under pressure from the media, the federal government sent officials to investigate (who, according to local informants, arrived in Wollaston Lake drunk, wearing rubber boots, and carrying bottled water). The people of Wollaston were assured they were at no health risk, and the mining company was forced to make a public admission of the error and clean up the problem as best they could. But many people in Wollaston cite this incident as evidence that no one from the industry or government can ever be trusted to protect the interests of the people of Wollaston Lake.

The research relationship

In August 1991 Annalee Yassi was invited to serve as an expert in environmental health on a Joint Federal-Provincial Environmental Assessment Review Panel to investigate the environmental impact of expanding the uranium mining activity in northern Saskatchewan, a responsibility that required working closely with a tribal chief from the area and attendance at community meetings in the region throughout 1992 and 1993. John O'Neil was contracted by this Panel in the summer of 1992 to conduct a "health risk perception study" in the communities of northern Saskatchewan. This inquiry required a series of interviews with key informants in all communities in the region; nine interviews were done in Wollaston Lake and included some of the same people who had been involved in the 1985 blockade. In 1993, Brenda Elias was hired as a research associate on a study of environmental risk perception directed by O'Neil and Yassi. She spent three months in Wollaston Lake, interviewing residents about their perceptions of health risks associated with the uranium mining industry.

This chapter is based on the results of these various inquiries. The results are generated from the different perspectives in the context of our different relationships with the community of Wollaston Lake. Our particular interest in this chapter is in how the women of Wollaston Lake have approached the problem of uranium mining.

Theoretical perspectives

This chapter will also explore the character of "resistance" from several converging perspectives. In the environmental "risk analysis" literature, interest in the "social construction of risk" has generated interest in attempts to situate risk analysis in the central debates related to modernist and postmodernist articulations of social theory. Rappaport (1988) argues that current interest in lay discourse on risk represents a "post-modern turn" in risk analysis. Webler, Rahel and Ross (1992) suggest, alternatively, that concepts of Habermasian critical theory such as legitimation crisis and communicative action are useful to an understanding of state interest in environmental risk management. Throgmorton (1991) compares the relevance of Foucault and Habermas to a critical analysis of rhetorical discourse in risk communication, and argues that Habermas in particular provides a useful critical framework for understanding current approaches to "risk management" which he claims distort the "resistant" nature of public discourse on risk and obscure the actual structures and dynamics of power.

Similarly, debate within feminist theory continues to consider the relative "alignments" of an analysis of power and domination from socialist feminist/Marxist (modernist) vs. postmodern perspectives. Harstock, for example, argues that Foucault fails to understand his position as a colonial intellectual in the colonizer/colonized structure of power. She contends that Foucault's claim that biopower can only be resisted, not transformed, "reinforces the relations of domination in our society by insisting that those of us who have been marginalized remain at the margins" (Hartsock 1990:168).

Ecofeminists embrace the postmodernist deconstruction of universalistic discourse on materialist understandings of progress, but also reject non-transformational approaches to an analysis of power (Mies and Shiva 1993). Their version of political ecofeminism, grounded in the materialist survival experiences of colonized women in the South, further challenges the so-called "luxury spirituality" which they claim has been expropriated by Western feminists.

In this paper we pick up the editors' challenge to reconsider resistance to biopower from women's perspectives, but we will focus primarily on the nature of resistance, with reference to perceived health risks associated with the technology of uranium production. We intend to frame this paper in a "critical postmodernist" perspective, a perspective which relies primarily on Foucault, but continues to draw on the critical theory of Habermas and others, and is convergent with a political ecofeminism grounded in the analysis of colonialism and gender.

The chapter will attempt to describe the experience and perspectives of the Dene women of Wollaston Lake, as First Nations women resisting the destruction of their land, as mothers, sisters, and daughters resisting threats to their families and community, and as women resisting marginalization and asserting a central role in the affairs of their society. We recognize that this report is at best an "approximate" account of the lives of Dene women in Wollaston Lake, biased through the filter of Western, non-Aboriginal science. Our goal is not to exploit their experience for academic or political purposes, but to represent our understanding of the complexity of everyday life in Wollaston Lake as "truthfully" as possible.

Uranium mining in Saskatchewan

Northern Saskatchewan is classic Canadian shield topography. Granite outcroppings, small coniferous trees, and myriad lakes, rivers, and streams provide shelter and food for fish, ducks, geese, deer, moose, and bear among other species. Flying over the region, the first impression is that there is more water than land, that the water system is entirely interconnected, and that human habitation is minimal.

In fact, there are twenty-one Cree and Dene First Nations reserves in northern Saskatchewan (252,432 square kilometres lying north of the 54th parallel), housing approximately 8,000 people or 25 percent of the population in the region. The remainder of the population, both Aboriginal and non-Aboriginal, live in small towns and cities in the more southerly part of the region (ESAS 1992).

Uranium was first discovered in northern Saskatchewan in 1946. Between 1948 and 1960, two large underground mines (Eldorado Nuclear and Gunnar Mining Ltd.) were brought into production just north of Lake Athabasca, located approximately 40 km south of the border with the Northwest Territories (Sibbald 1981).

By 1958, the Lake Athabasca mines were producing 3,835 tonnes of uranium, nearly all of which was exported to the United States. The population of Uranium City, situated on the shores of Lake Athabasca and the processing centre for about thirty producing mines in the area, boomed to 4,500 people. In 1959, the US Atomic Energy Commission instituted a uranium self-sufficiency policy, resulting in a collapse of the world uranium market. By 1964, most Canadian mines had closed, and

Saskatchewan production was down to 460 tonnes. The population of Uranium City fell to 2,000 (Salaff 1983).

Despite a depressed world market, uranium exploration continued at a frantic pace in northern Saskatchewan. By 1969 almost all of northern Saskatchewan had been claimed by mineral permits and several large uranium deposits were discovered, stretching from Lake Athabasca south along the west side of Wollaston Lake (collectively referred to as the Rabbit Lake deposit). In 1977, the United States began to import uranium again and an expanding international nuclear power industry created new demand for Saskatchewan resources. The Eldorado operation near Uranium City attempted to expand during this period but declining ore quality and fluctuating prices led to Eldorado ceasing operations in 1982. Thousands of people in the area lost their jobs and homes; by 1987 there were 250 people, mostly Aboriginal, remaining in Uranium City (Canada Employment and Immigration Council 1987).

The Rabbit Lake deposit on the west side of Wollaston Lake came into active production in 1975. The project was a joint venture of Uranerz Canada Ltd. (jointly owned by several German energy producers: 49 percent; Gulf Minerals Canada Ltd.: 45.9 percent; and Gulf Canada Ltd.: 5.1 percent). Mining the deposit required the draining of Rabbit Lake and the creation of the third largest open-pit uranium mine in Canada, with an annual production of 2,000 tonnes of uranium.

By the early 1980s, the quality of ore in the Rabbit Lake mine had fallen below profitable levels. In 1982, Eldorado Nuclear Ltd., a federal crown corporation, merged with the Saskatchewan Mining Development Corporation to form Cameco (Canadian Mining and Energy Corporation), and purchased the Rabbit Lake operation as well as other deposits and processing facilities owned by the Uranerz/Gulf joint venture. These assets included the Collins Bay "B" deposit, situated *under* the water of an inlet on Wollaston Lake. This deposit was accessed by an underground mine and an elaborate series of dams and dikes along the shores of Wollaston Lake.

By the late 1980s, there were three major uranium mining operations active in northern Saskatchewan, including the Rabbit Lake/Collins Bay operation on the shores of Wollaston Lake. Cluff Lake in northwestern Saskatchewan and Key Lake in the south central region comprise the other operations. In 1989, Canada was producing nearly one third of the world's uranium concentrate, and the majority came from northern Saskatchewan owing to the superior ore quality (0.58 to 2.04 percent in Saskatchewan compared to an average of 0.07 percent elsewhere in Canada and globally; ESAS 1992).

The Panel to which Dr. Yassi was appointed had as its mandate to review five uranium mine proposals, which included by far the world's largest and richest ore bodies in the world. Cigar Lake, for example, has an ore body of 353 million pounds at an average grade of 9.2 percent U_3O_8 with zones as high as 25.6 percent U_3O_8; McArthur River has 416 million pounds of ore body and regions with an average grade of 15 percent U_3O_8.

The uranium industry also has a complex history of corporate ownership, the details of which are beyond the scope of this chapter. Ownership has gone through several transitions from primarily foreign in the early seventies (Uranerz Ltd.), to primarily a Canadian federal crown corporation in the early 1980s (Eldorado Nuclear), with an increase in Saskatchewan government ownership (Cameco) in the late 1980s and early 1990s, to the current situation where Cogema Resources Ltd., a subsidiary of the French government's power corporation, has purchased a controling interest in all proposed new mines (89 percent Cluff Lake DJ extension; 70 percent McLean Lake Project; 56 percent MJV; 36 percent Cigar Lake; 16 percent McArthur River).

The uranium industry in Saskatchewan has been actively promoted and subject to supportive review procedures by both New Democratic (socialist) and Conservative governments over the past several decades. In Saskatchewan, the perceived importance of the industry to one of the smallest provincial economies in Canada seems to have outweighed environmental and health concerns.

The economic realities of the uranium industry in Saskatchewan are, however, more ambiguous. In 1991, essentially urban-centered and secondary economic activities such as finance, real estate, public administration, transportation and communication, and trade contributed approximately 70 percent to the Saskatchewan economy. Of the remaining "primary" economic activities, approximately 40 percent was manufacturing and construction, 35 percent was agriculture and forestry and 25 percent was mining – or approximately 7.5 percent of the total economic activity. Within the mining sector, uranium ranked well behind petroleum and potash (fertilizer). In 1990, uranium mining contributed only 10 percent of the total mining-related revenues of the province (Saskatchewan Bureau of Statistics 1991).

In real terms, the uranium industry contributed $18,692,308.00 in royalties to provincial coffers in 1990, and approximately $330 million over fifteen years (Saskatchewan Energy and Mines 1990). Other analysts claim that when royalties are combined with indirect benefits associated with reduced unemployment and social assistance, individual taxation, etc. which result from employment at the mines (1,500 direct and indirect jobs in 1990), the industry contributed $166 million to the gross domestic product of the province in 1990 (Ernst and Young 1991). However, critics have suggested that these benefits are much less than the industry predicted ($1.5 to 3 billion) in its applications for licensing in the late 1970s (Harding 1993).

Benefits and costs to the Aboriginal people of northern Saskatchewan are difficult to calculate, not surprisingly because many provincial departments fail to keep statistics which would identify ethnicity or northern residence. It would appear that approximately 40 percent of employees working at the mines in 1991 were northern residents (both Aboriginal and non-Aboriginal); in 1991, seven people from Wollaston Lake were employed at the mines (Saskatchewan Education as reported in ESAS 1992).

Industry sources also claim that northern businesses, including an increasing number of businesses either partially or exclusively owned by Aboriginal individuals and organizations, benefited directly by "purchase north" policies. In 1989, the uranium industry claims to have spent approximately $20 million on goods and services from northern businesses (Midwest Uranium Project 1991). Both the Prince Albert Grand Council and the Meadow Lake Tribal Council (First Nations political organizations representing most Bands in the region) are partners or owners of businesses that have benefited from this economic activity.

Public costs of the uranium industry include everything from provincial development of infrastructure such as roads, occupational safety programs, and training programs, to the more difficult to measure social costs of changes to the Aboriginal subsistence economy and culture. Some of these costs will be addressed in depth in the remainder of this chapter.

In summary, the uranium industry in northern Saskatchewan has played a significant role in defining the discourse on economic development for the province over the last several decades. Despite evidence that the industry may not be as important or as stable a contributor to the provincial and national economy as the discourse might suggest, political support for the expansion of the industry has been widespread, including socialist and conservative governments, and the Aboriginal leadership.

Biomedical discourse: health risks associated with uranium mining

It has long been recognized that uranium mining can pose serious health risks to persons who are employed at the mines, as well as risks to the public. People can potentially be affected by a variety of means such as direct exposure to mine wastes, the spread of contaminants by wind or water, and the absorption of contaminants into the food chain.

Air containing a variety of contaminants, including radioactive substances, has been a long-standing problem at most mines, particularly underground mines. However, mines which produce radioactive minerals such as uranium may contain a greater hazard than other mines from air contaminated with radioactive gases which occur as part of the decay process of radionuclides such as uranium-238 and thorium-230. These gases are naturally present in the environment, though they and their decay products are more concentrated in many mineral deposits, especially uraniferous deposits. They emanate into mines from rock faces, broken rock, and mine water (Ham 1976). *Bergkrankheit*, a mysterious disease which afflicted silver miners in Joachimsthal, Czechoslovakia, was first recorded in the early sixteenth century (Kunz 1992). However, the first specific reference to the disease came only in 1913 when it was found that, of 665 Erzgebirge Mountain miners who died between 1875 and 1912, 40 percent died of lung cancer. For the next few decades, the focus remained largely on mines and miners in Europe. By the 1940s, it shifted to North America when large-scale mining and milling of uranium ore for weapons production began in the United States. By then, the relationship between uranium mining and lung cancer was recognized by the international scientific community, though it was still given little heed by government and industry (Bates 1980; Yih *et al.* 1995).

While the health effects of mining for uranium and other minerals in unventilated or poorly ventilated mines has been recognized for some time, the adoption of standards designed to limit exposure to radon and its decay products is relatively recent, and came on the heels of what was termed a lung cancer "epidemic of major proportions" among former miners. The conclusion that such an epidemic existed was based on a number of studies. For example, in 1950 the United States Public Health Service (USPHS) established a study of miners and millers in the Colorado plateau area (Wagoner *et al.* 1964). In May 1952, the USPHS released an interim report reporting the high lung cancer mortality in miners in German and Czechoslovakian mines, where concentrations of radon and its decay products were similar to those in

US mines, and warned of the dangers in the Colorado mines (Yih et al. 1995). Conditions in the mines did not improve. In 1964 the USPHS published its first research paper, reporting on cancer mortality for 5,370 miners and millers followed through the end of 1962. This study noted an excess mortality from accidents (mainly mine-related) and for cancer of the respiratory system, with up to a tenfold increase in lung cancer for underground miners with five or more years of underground experience (Wagoner et al. 1964). The first published evidence of a substantially increased risk for lung cancer in American-Indian miners was reported by Archer et al. (1976), and detailed further by Gotlieb and Husen (1982) and Samet et al. (1984). A study conducted by New Mexico miners also found that lung cancer risk increased with cumulative exposure to radon decay products (Samet et al. 1989). In addition, non-malignant respiratory disease was also found to be elevated (Waxweiler et al. 1981). It is, of course, well known that underground miners have a higher risk of silicosis (a scarring disease of the lung).

Studies conducted in Canada also confirmed an increased risk of lung cancer and silicosis. These health effects in fact became a major focus of a royal commission on health and safety in Ontario mines (Ham 1976). Even closer to home, a study was conducted of 8,487 workers employed at Beaverlodge Mine in northern Saskatchewan between 1948 and 1982 (L'Abbé et al. 1991). A total of sixty-five miners in the cohort died of lung cancer in this period, compared to thirty-four expected; this constituted a significantly elevated risk of dying of lung cancer from working in northern Saskatchewan uranium mines. In addition, some of the Saskatchewan uranium mines have high concentrations of both arsenic and nickel, as noted above, posing an greatly increased risk of lung cancer.

From these studies, it is evident that uranium mining and milling process a variety of radioactive materials which are harmful to human health. It is important to note, however, that these materials are in the environment before the mines begin operation, but usually they are far underground and dispersed in the substrate. Any radiation which may reach the surface is typically of a low level and is considered a form of background radiation. What uranium mining does is bring these materials to the surface in quantity. Milling then concentrates and contains them as a product, rubble, mine water, or tailings, and also releases small proportions of them into the environment.

Tailings can have immediate somatic or genetic health effects if people are exposed to them. The American western states, and especially the Colorado plateau states, have experienced significant health effects from old uranium mines and improperly decommissioned tailings. Evidence of health effects from living near uranium mines and mills has been difficult to conduct and interpret. Shields *et al.* (1992) studied birth data for 13,329 Navaho children born between 1964 and 1981 at the Indian Health Service Hospital in Shiprock, New Mexico. They found a statistically significant increase in adverse health outcome such as birth defects, stillbirths, and deaths from illnesses during infancy in the offspring of mothers living near mine dumps and mill tailing areas. However, this increase was not related to reported duration of exposure, and other possibilities may explain the increase, including paternal employment in the mines, which was marginally significantly associated with the elevated risk for adverse outcome. Nonetheless, clearly these sites pose a risk to the people of the area. Parts of the Navaho Reservation in Arizona are pock-marked by numerous uranium mines, the remnants of small "mom and pop" uranium mining operations encouraged by the US Government in the 1950s. Many of these abandoned mines have filled with water over the years, providing attractive, although clearly hazardous, summer swimming holes for Navaho children (Taylor 1983).

It is noteworthy that over 125 radioactive spills were reported to Saskatchewan's Spill Control Program (Dirschl *et al.* 1992) and from 1975 to 1977 almost 2 million litres of untreated waste were released into Wollaston Lake. (This is described further by Yih *et al.* 1995). In addition, worrisome levels of polonium-210 and lead-210 were found in the bones and organs of caribou north of the decommissioned and abandoned uranium mines at Uranium City, Saskatchewan (Thomas *et al.* 1993).

Concentrations of radionuclides can also take a very long time to become harmless. Though they may become diluted in the process, radionuclides can spread via the atmosphere and hydrosphere. Over a long period, barriers can break down and contaminants can leach into aquifers and eventually find their way into surface waters. This may not pose a serious threat in a region if mining is short-lived, but if mining continues for several decades, the end result could be a substantial rearrangement of harmful radionuclides and significant accumulations over an extensive region.

The discourse on indigenous environmentalism: global dimensions

Global resistance to the nuclear industry, including uranium mining and refining, nuclear power generation, weapons production and testing, and nuclear waste disposal first became visible at the beginning of the 1970s as part of the student movement, ecocultural (i.e., alternative lifestyles/ecology and ecofeminism) movement, and the peace movement (see Nelkin and Pollak 1982; Babin 1985). The nature of this resistance in large part involved the idea that technological optimism had blinded government, the uranium industry, and science to the potential problems of something so powerful and technologically sophisticated. Indigenous people were brought into this global fold because many of these activities occur in different parts of the world on lands occupied by indigenous peoples. In particular, northern Australia, Polynesia, central Brazil, southwestern United States, and northern Saskatchewan are both primary homelands for indigenous peoples world-wide, and also the primary international sites for various aspects of the nuclear industry.

To describe this resistance as discourse, however, situates this chapter squarely in the center of current debates about modernist and postmodernist approaches to the critical analysis of social movements (Fraser 1989). Anthropologists such as Baer (1990) and Nash and Kirsh (1986) have articulated clearly a structural critique of the political economy of state and corporate collusion in the exploitation of hazardous materials. This critique is situated in the context of "partisan observation," as Baer describes his role as an academic activist with a "commitment to the empowerment of people in their struggle against hegemonic institutions" (Baer 1990:237). Similarly, Nash and Kirsh develop their analysis in support of a community whose actions have resulted in profound social changes in the patterns of political power and wealth in relation to the use of polychlorinated biphenyls in the electrical machinery industry (Nash and Kirsh 1986:137).

In this chapter, we are interested in the critical analysis of risks associated with uranium mining, but we are principally interested in the ways in which this analysis is articulated as a global discourse of resistance, and we are interested in the ways in which the women of Wollaston Lake are "colonized" by this discourse. We intend to show that just as the local political economy has been colonized by the "megaproject" global industrial economy of uranium mining, so too have local expressions of resistance been colonized by global opposition to the industry.

In the 1980s, several anti-uranium/anti-nuclear texts appeared, some of which included a discussion of the situation of Aboriginal people from some of these geopolitical regions. A critical text by Falk (1982:259), for instance, discussed the conflicts over nuclear power and the case of Australian Aborigines. He reported that the 1970s:

were marked by an increasing recognition by whites of the plight of the Aborigine. In particular, there was a gradual recognition of the desperate need of the Aborigine for "land rights" – the right to unspoiled land still related to the culture of surviving Aborigines. The Labour government responded to this by enacting an Aboriginal Land Rights Act [1976]. Under that act no new uranium mining could take place until agreement had been obtained from the "traditional Aboriginal owners" of the land in which the uranium deposits lay.

Goldstick's book *Wollaston: People Resisting Genocide* followed in 1987. It reported his involvement in facilitating the blockade and involving the indigenous people of Wollaston Lake with the World Uranium Congress's anti-nuclear campaign against the Canadian uranium mining industry in northern Saskatchewan. Other acts of local indigenous resistance were reported by Mackay (1988) in his analysis of the north–south dimensions of "People's Détente." He summarily suggested that such local indigenous campaigns as the ones in Brazil and Malaysia had given people a better understanding of nuclear issues.

In 1992, the "World Uranium Hearing" published the first edition of the *World Uranium Hearing Grey Book* (Krumbholz and Kressing 1992). This 135-page volume provides a global survey of uranium-related activities throughout the world, with a particular focus on impacts on indigenous peoples. The book was produced as background documentation for the World Uranium Hearing Conference in Salzburg, Germany, September 13–19, 1992. It is the work of numerous agencies and individuals who collectively are concerned with the environmental effects of the uranium/nuclear industry. The World Uranium Hearing maintains offices in Munich, New York, New Mexico, and Montreal, with contacts in Paris, Salzburg, and Moscow. Contributing organizations include the Office of the Dalai Lama (who writes the foreword to the volume), Akwesasne Notes (Mohawk Nation), Canadian Coalition for Nuclear Responsibility, Friends of the Earth (Australia), Greenpeace International, Survival International (UK), and the Tribal Research and Training Centre (India) among more than thirty contributors. The central theme of the document is summarized well by one of the editors in the preface:

This year marks two historic commemorations: 500 years of European colonialism in the Americas, and 50 years after the beginning of the nuclear age. The World Uranium Hearing is set up to give people a voice who are suffering from the effects of the nuclear industry, and are also the victims of colonialism. Most of the world's uranium production is carried out on the lands of indigenous peoples. Nearly all atomic weapons have been tested on or under Native people's lands. Their territories are now considered to be "appropriate" to host the deadly leftovers of nuclear technology: the radioactive waste. (p. 8)

The volume then begins with a deconstructive analysis of another discourse: "nukespeak." Nukespeak is the language of the nuclear age, providing a vocabulary of terms and constructs which allow for a seemingly rational discussion of the conditions and consequences of nuclear technology which supports the thesis that human control over nuclear power is possible, e.g., "limited nuclear war." It is also considered to express the world view of dominant class interests to the exclusion of alternative modes of discourse which are rendered naive (Chilton 1985). The World Uranium Hearing Grey Book is offered as an alternative discourse to Nukespeak.

The connection between Wollaston Lake and this global alternative discourse on the nuclear industry is established early in the Grey Book. Miles Goldstick, the author of *Wollaston: People Resisting Genocide*, and one of the main participants in the organization of the 1985 blockade of the Rabbit Lake mine, is both the author of the first chapter, and acknowledged for his general contributions to the volume. Although much of the alternative discourse on the nuclear industry is oriented to end-use problems (such as weapons and reactors) which threaten urban, industrial societies, Goldstick focuses the discourse on the potential health effects of mining activities, and particularly the disposal of large volumes of waste material from the milling process. This theme is key to establishing a unified discourse which incorporates indigenous peoples. Although nuclear weapons testing has had an historical impact on indigenous peoples, end-use concerns are generally not important to indigenous communities in the contemporary context.

Discursive fractures in resistance perspectives in Wollaston Lake

In his presentation to the Environmental Impact Hearings in Wollaston Lake in 1994, Joe Tsannie, Chief of the Hatchet Lake Band, makes a thinly veiled reference to one effect of this global environmental discourse on the people of Wollaston Lake:

> It would be safe to say that other groups and other organizations have had a negative influence which has killed most of our local economy. For example, the fish industry. That publicity and the media has had an effect on our fish industry. It is said that Wollaston produces uranium and it keeps going on, so it is hard for consumers to buy our fish products. It has a lot of downfall also on the fur industry as well.

Chief Tsannie is making reference here to the impact of the environmental protest against the use of animal furs as clothing, together with the international publicity about uranium mining, generated largely by environmental groups, which has reduced consumer demand for both commercial fish and sport fishing opportunities in the region.

Chief Tsannie also articulated the perspective of the political and economic interests of Wollaston Lake. He suggests that the community is divided between the younger generation who are desperate for training opportunities and employment prospects, and the older generation who wish to protect their traditional way of life. While balancing these concerns is difficult, Chief Tsannie indicates that the community must provide economic opportunities for future generations and suggests his community is willing to support uranium mining in the region as long as several conditions are met. In general, the community wants compensation for traditional economic activities impacted by mining, a greater share of mining revenues, joint development of community infrastructure such as improved roads, housing, and recreation facilities, technical training, renewable resources development (a fish processing plant), and mining-related business opportunities for the people of Wollaston Lake.

In contrast, Sophie Denedchezhe and Sarazine Josie, two women from Wollaston Lake, made presentations to the same hearings which emphasized the health dangers associated with the uranium industry. However, both of these women had recently returned from the World Uranium Hearing in Austria. Ms. Denedchezhe's presentation specifically describes her experience in Austria:

My presentation is about my trip to . . . [T]he World Uranium Hearings . . . The indigenous people from all over the world were . . . at the conference . . . I didn't hear anything good about uranium mining, industrials or refineries or nuclear reactor. I found out there were a high rate of health problems . . . cancer, birth defects and spontaneous abortion of pregnancy of healthy women . . . There is no such thing as low radiation level after the uranium mines are done . . . It will never be safe for the environment.

Ms. Denedchezhe also read from a prepared statement which was apparently signed by all the indigenous people participating in the Salzberg Conference:

We the indigenous peoples of different communities of the earth, our mother . . . are concerned for our health and well-being and future generations. We have heard from the people of the mountain, the forest, the desert and the ocean who have suffered daily from the nuclear mining, I mean uranium mining, nuclear weapons testing and nuclear power generation and radioactive wastes.

Sarazine Josie confirmed the impact of the World Conference on the understandings of Wollaston women. She stated that at first she could not believe some of the ill effects of uranium. She reported on seeing pictures of birth deformities and hearing from other indigenous people about their health problems. Ms. Josie also challenged the idea that economic development associated with the uranium industry would produce positive benefits in the community:

And also, you said that people will benefit from the mine, but the people that are working in the mine are causing social problems here in our community and in the other community such as bringing booze and drugs. I myself have known about this and the community knows about the social problems around our communities and the Athabasca region.

In these presentations, two themes have emerged. One is the perception of some people in Wollaston Lake that "outside agitation" contributes to both misunderstandings about the real health risks of uranium mining, and the destructive effects of the global environmental discourse on the local renewable resource economy. The second theme is the apparent difference between the male leadership, who are advocating a negotiated economic benefits package as their condition for supporting the uranium mining industry, and women in the community who are concerned that "social problems" like substance abuse will increase with continuation of mining activities. The first theme supports the notion that global environmental discourse is having a colonizing effect on women's understandings of health risks. The second theme suggests that women, in turn, are resisting the colonizing effects of industrialization on the community economic system. The apparent contradiction between these themes will be explored further in the rest of this chapter.

Gender differences in health risk perception

Before proceeding with a narrative consideration of women's resistance to either of these colonizing forces, we will briefly review the findings of a risk perception survey that was administered to forty-six men and fifty women in Wollaston Lake in 1994. This questionnaire asked respondents to respond on a five-point scale to a variety of statements describing risks associated with a wide range of activities, some associated with the uranium mine and some reflecting everyday life in the town and on the land. Although the results of this survey are not entirely consistent with the narrative accounts of risk understandings collected during fieldwork, they do suggest a framework for interpreting these narrative accounts.

In general, the people of Wollaston Lake express a high level of uncertainty when asked to determine whether an activity is risky. In most risk perception surveys, uncertainty is usually reported as insignificant and treated as a methodological problem. The "Don't Know" response is considered a product of poor interview technique and is usually reported as less than 5 percent of responses. In our view, uncertainty in risk perception is also culturally constructed, as a reflection of cultural values as well as a political response to surveillance activities. However, a full exploration of these issues is the subject of another paper.

In our survey, uncertainty was generally high in response to all questions, but decreased in relation to knowledge about traditional land-based activities. For example, 45 percent of respondents indicated they were uncertain as to whether the transport of processed uranium ("yellow cake") created a health risk for their community. However, 31 percent of respondents were also uncertain as to whether there are health risks associated with smoking, and 15 percent were uncertain whether hunting alone in winter should be considered dangerous. While the first and second indicators could be explained as a lack of familiarity with the issue, the last indicator suggests that uncertainty is an appropriate cultural response to questions about risk. Although our respondents seemed more confident about defining risks related to traditional activities, people in Wollaston Lake have also been exposed to substantial amounts of information related to more modern understandings of health risks through television and public health promotion campaigns.

Despite a high general level of uncertainty, however, people in Wollaston recognize profound differences in risks associated with various activities. Whereas 89 percent of people indicated it was dangerous to consume alcohol when pregnant, only 61 percent felt that smoking was dangerous to health, and only 8 percent felt that there were risks associated with a hospital birth. Similarly, 68 percent of respondents indicated that boat travel in the late fall was dangerous but only 15 percent indicated that travelling on the land in January was dangerous.

Perceptions of risks associated with uranium mining also varied. Whereas 46 percent of respondents indicated they thought animals near the mine would get sick from radiation, only 20 percent indicated there were health risks associated with eating country food from near the mine. While 73 percent of respondents indicated they thought alcohol problems in the community would rise with continued uranium mining, only 25 percent thought birth deformities would increase.

Given both the high level of general uncertainty and broad variation in risk perception, we would expect that men and women might have different estimations of health risks associated with uranium mining, particularly in light of the foregoing discussion. The results of the

Table 1. *Variations in risk perception by gender (total = 96; women = 50; men = 46)*

Risk perception issue	Dangerous		Don't know/ no opinion		Not dangerous	
	Women	Men	Women	Men	Women	Men
Smoking*	76.0	45.7	22.0	41.3	2.0	13.0
Hospital birth*	6.0	10.9	24.0	52.1	70.0	37.0
Spring fishing*	22.0	10.8	32.0	15.2	46.0	74.0
Hunting alone in winter*	42.0	19.6	20.0	8.7	38.0	71.7
Trap near mine*	48.0	26.1	42.0	50.0	10.0	23.9
Eat fish harvested near the mine*	58.0	39.1	40.0	43.5	2.0	17.4
Work underground in mine	76.0	63.0	22.0	28.3	2.0	8.7
Transport yellow cake	50.0	63.0	50.0	32.6	0	4.4

* Significant at P < .05

Table 2. *Variations on agreement with expressed risk perceptions by gender (total = 96; women = 50; men = 46)*

Risk perception issue	Agree		Don't know/ no opinion		Disagree	
	Women	Men	Women	Men	Women	Men
No one will buy our fish	34.0	32.6	24.0	30.4	42.0	37.0
Increase in family violence	56.0	65.2	34.0	23.9	10.0	10.9
More childbirth deformities	32.0	17.3	42.0	58.7	26.0	24.0
Get cancer if work at mine	44.0	50.0	50.0	39.1	6.0	10.9

survey are somewhat surprising. In general, while there are differences in risk perception related to areas of everyday life associated with men's or women's activities or specialized knowledge, perceptions of development related risks are not significantly different. Tables 1 and 2 summarize gender differences on several key questions representing several broad domains.

Although statistical significance is weak, these results show that women in general are more concerned about health risks associated with uranium mining. However, the results also suggest that while the "activist" men and women in the community may differ markedly in their perspective on uranium mining, the "silent majority" of men and women in the community may share a more concerned perspective on the potential health risks associated with uranium mining. However, it is the "activist" women who give texture to these concerns in the public sphere, as the next section will describe.

The character of risk and women's resistance

In this section we will explore the various dimensions to women's health concerns and ground these concerns in the historical and everyday experience of the local community.

For women in Wollaston Lake, the experience of risk is an everyday occurrence. One woman described the following experience:

On a Sunday [in August] the weather was very stormy. My husband picked me up at the Barge Landing [on opposite side of lake] with our boat. We started to make our way back but the weather got worse, and the lake got rougher. We ended up staying overnight on an island where other people were stranded. No one had any camping gear. All we had was a tarp and two blankets. We stood around the fire in the rain until 3:00 am. Then we put the tarp over the two boats pulled up on the beach. We joked about the contrast between the luxurious hotel rooms in La Ronge and the sandy beach. The next day the men went in the boats to Wollaston but the women stayed behind. We were afraid of travelling in the stormy weather. The men made it to the community and arranged for a float plane to pick the women up off the island.

Travelling on the land to hunt, fish, or trap, or to travel away from the community, entails different kinds of risks at different times of year. Women do not take these risks for granted; the story described above ended well, but nearly every year someone drowns or is lost. As the results of the survey suggest, it is women who worry most about these risks, although it is usually men who experience them directly.

To some extent these concerns are related to the interdependence of the family unit and the fear of losing a husband. Most of the wage-related jobs in the community are held by women (because most are in education, social services, and administrative and clerical support to government). At the same time, given the relatively undeveloped infrastructure of the community, maintaining a household is still a full-time domestic task. One woman describes the interdependence of men and women, and the impact of losing a husband even for a short time:

Working to make a home here is hard work. Why do you think more women work than men? My husband stays home to look after the house as well as look after the kids. Water has to be hauled in by hand. Wood has to be cut for the winter. He even does the laundry. He goes out on the land and gets meat and fish. The mines are another thing. I have two boys working at the mine. When one of my boy's wife was pregnant, he was told by Cameco [uranium mining company], that he had to go down south to take his three month apprenticeship training. It was winter. His wife was due. Who was going to haul water in for her? Cut wood? Help with the laundry? There was no one. Other family members are busy with their own problems. So he didn't go. So how can our people get ahead. I think the companies do that on purpose, so they have an excuse not to hire us.

This interdependence is also evident in political affairs in the community. Although the Chief and Band Council are usually men, the Band functions according to custom, rather than the regulations of the federal government. Elections can be called at any time if community members are unhappy with the current Band government. In several cases related to us, the election of a new Chief and Council was strongly influenced by the perspectives of women in the community. One such election occurred during our fieldwork and the following observation was made:

At the meeting to decide whether to get rid of Chief and Council, the women of the community overall did most of the talking. Only two male elders spoke. The rest of the men just watched and made comments to each other. I asked people standing by me if this was always the case. They said it was and like tonight there was always much arguing. They explained the two women elders involved in the debates represented different families in the community. When they spoke, they spoke against the other families and what they represented in the community in terms of their behavior. Other women spoke and they too represented different families.

Despite this interdependence, however, the primary political division in the community seems to be in regards to the risks and benefits associated with uranium mining. As previously indicated, the current Wollaston Lake leadership has generally taken the position that uranium mining will be beneficial to the community as long as the companies involved enter into agreements with the community which produce real economic benefits. Resistance to this position is situated in the activities of the Wollaston Lake Environmental Committee, comprised mostly of women working in the health, social service, and education fields in the community. Several of these women have participated in the international World Uranium Hearings and see themselves as providing a moral alternative to the pro-development forces in the community. One woman explained her relationship with the political leadership as follows:

Its hard to say. He [the new Chief] will probably be supportive of mines because he worked there. He was one of the people who was against me when I spoke out at the time of the blockade. A lot of people believed him because he was working out at the mine. It's funny to say but the ex-chief [current chairperson of the Environmental Committee] was against me too. He was working out at the mine. But he now knows what's happening and he will never work in the mine again.

In our interviews with women in Wollaston Lake, fears of health problems associated with uranium mining were not restricted to the direct biological effects of radiation. Women articulated a broad socially constructed view of health that integrated various domains of everyday life as possibly impacted by uranium mining. While fears of direct poisoning of the primary food source – fish and wildlife – were foremost in their minds, concerns were also expressed about the sensitivity of animals to any industrial activity in their territories:

There are a lot of animals that are getting scarce. Like before the mining started you could go anywhere and there were a lot of animals around but not now. There used to be a lot of porcupines on the road in the old days. And now you don't hardly see any.

Relations with the surrounding society are also a fundamental component of women's concerns. Fears of contacts with dangerous "white men" were seen as a pervasive threat from the expansion of southern industrial activity in the north. Women described a general fear of contact with white prospectors or construction workers who might be encountered accidentally during hunting, fishing, or camping trips in the bush. These fears often assumed almost mythical status with stories exchanged from one community to another across the north:

One story she heard while she was visiting Uranium City. It was about a group of seven or eight men, who people thought might be escaped convicts, who were in a bar getting drunk and bragging about how they were "killing Indians" when they went out on the land. The story went that they were bragging how they terrorized and killed Dene women, children and men who were out living on the lakes throughout Black Lake, Fond du Lac and Wollaston Lake.

Women also challenged the view that an increase in wage-related economic opportunities necessarily contributes to an improvement in social well-being. Drug and alcohol abuse is of particular concern to women, since they and their children are most often the victims of the domestic violence that frequently occurs. Some women identified the rotational employment system, where mine workers are employed on a one week in, one week out arrangement as a particular problem in this regard:

The social problems are not getting better, they are getting worse because of the mining and the road across the lake. I mean that when they go back to the mine they come back with drugs and we raised that question a lot of times but it still happens.

Perceptions of health threats associated with exposure to uranium and other by-products of mining were characterized by some women as the direct cause of many diseases. While cancer was identified as the primary disease linked to exposure to uranium, disease causality was considered in more general terms. Virtually all disease is understood as infectious, an understanding that is in part a legacy of public health education over the past few decades, and one woman explained that the health effects of exposure to uranium can be passed from one person to another:

Everything around the mine that comes out of D-Zone causes disease. If one person gets it, the next person who they come in contact with would get it. It's contagious. Everything around D-Zone will be diseased.

Attribution of blame to the uranium mines for all health problems is extensive. In one case, a mother explained the death of her son as a direct result of exposure to tailings from the processing of uranium ore, when the official cause of death was listed as excessive consumption of alcohol.

These general concerns about the possible health risks associated with uranium mining have emerged in a context of distrust and misinformation. Most of the women to whom we talked were sceptical of information they had received from any official source. Most felt that the provincial government and the mining companies had systematically withheld information from them about the potential risks associated with uranium mining. They cited occasions where officials had presented information which emphasized the beneficial uses of uranium in medical technology, and the potential economic benefits of mine employment, as particularly devious attempts to convince the community to support the industry:

The first time we had a meeting here about the mining was when [an Aboriginal public relations officer working for a mining company] was translating. They talked about all the benefits . . . jobs. They gave reasons why they wanted to mine. They wanted it for electricity and medicine. But they never ever mentioned about the contamination. They never told the people anything.

In contrast, environmentalists have introduced a different understanding of the risks and benefits of uranium mining. Environmentalists have portrayed the consequences of uranium mining as catastrophic. The discourse conflates the experience of indigenous peoples living downwind from open-air atomic weapons testing with the experience of people travelling on roads used by trucks transporting yellow cake, and equates the effects:

Like what we heard from those people is that nothing good comes from uranium mining industry. Some people say that its good for your health. But I don't believe them. From what the people told us their lands had been destroyed because a nuclear reactor had blew up. It *infected* the land. All the lands are radioactive, and they have radioactive waste problems downstream . . . We have *proof* that the people they [mining companies] hire are not telling the truth so [yellow cake] is blowing everywhere like salt. It's scattered all over the place and people and kids are playing in it.

Particularly for women who have been participants in various environmental forums, the stark contrast in these messages has eroded trust in all outside agencies:

I don't know. I don't know anymore. I'm so confused all the time. I don't know what to believe anymore . . . People tell us what had happened to them by the mining industry. But the mining industry tells us that didn't happen. Only good things came out of it. People are working. I don't see people working from Wollaston. There is just a handful of people, and they said they are going to hire more workers and northern people. I don't see it . . . I see it as an empty promise. They say that they are going to do it and then they say that they did it because they had done just a little bit . . . I guess that is the reason why people are hesitating to get interviewed. I guess they talk and talk but nothing is done. So they are fed up with everything . . . A lot of times people have really good information. And they talk to people and they are just tired of answering all those questions. What's the use of saying it. I said it before and nothing was done about it. I guess that's why people don't want to talk.

This acute perception that neither the government, industry, nor environmentalist agendas could be trusted was also extended to our research. Several members of the community felt abused by the characterization of the community as portrayed in the 1987 book by Miles Goldstick, *Wollaston: People Resisting Genocide*:

His wife emerged from the bedroom and spoke quite adamantly (in Dene) to the community researcher. He explained later that she had forcefully told him that she was very apprehensive to talk to a white person because of what was published in the Goldstick book. Her husband and she agreed that they would speak to us providing that the Chief said it was okay.

Some members of the community felt that the publication of this book had done more harm to the community than the uranium mine. Some men in particular felt that the mining companies punished Wollaston Lake for the negative publicity associated with the publication of the book by hiring few people from Wollaston to work at the mines. Others felt the local commercial and sport fishing economy had been negatively affected by southern fears of contaminated fish raised by the book's publication. Some women who were deeply associated with the blockade and the book's publication found themselves under attack by other members of the community:

When we had the blockade a man from the federal government came up. But before the blockade we never got support from anyone. They [community] didn't even know what was happening. Only a few of us know what was happening. But we had to blockade the road to be heard. A lot of people [community] were really against it. They were against me. They were against what I was doing. There is a lot of support from down south. There is the Inter-Church Uranium Committee. People there are concerned about the environment. But here they never realized it and spoke out against it. But the people here never knew what was happening even though the mine was close by.

Hegemony, discourse, and resistance: an anthropological solution

In this chapter, we have described the character of Dene women's concerns about the health risks associated with uranium mining in northern Saskatchewan. We have argued that these concerns reflect significant dissonance in the discursive frameworks that structure the issue for First Nations people in northern Saskatchewan. We suggest that women in Wollaston Lake struggle to articulate a perspective on this issue that is in resistance to the hegemonic influences of both an industrial and an environmental discourse, neither of which is grounded in the everyday realities of life in a remote reserve community in the 1990s.

The chapter also engages the conceptual problem of synthesizing a postmodernist analysis of cultural discourse with a critical reflection on the transformative potential of discursive resistance. Dene women in Wollaston Lake do not accept the capitalist rhetoric of industrial development that their fathers, husbands, brothers, and sons sometimes seek to control. Neither do they see themselves as the passive victims of an international conspiracy to destroy the environment. They struggle to articulate an understanding of community well-being that is both grounded in their traditional cultural experience as well as resistant to the hegemonic and colonizing effects of global discourse.

We are not suggesting that this resistance should be characterized as conflict between men and women in the community. As the survey data suggest, men and women generally express shared health concerns. Where disagreement exists it is more in relation to the identification of points of resistance to the hegemonic character of global discourses on either industrial development or environmentalism. While some Wollaston men are attempting to resist the exploitation inherent in a global capitalist system, perhaps somewhat naively, by negotiating for greater local control over the "means of production," women are attempting to broaden the local discourse on health risks to challenge the simple notion that increased economic opportunity equals better health. Local women's health discourse is also both produced by, as well as resistant to, global discourse on environmental health.

We also suggest that this analysis is situated in the context of an anthropological project to examine the interactive and constructive aspects of global and local influences on cultural formation. In many applications of Foucault's ideas, resistance is characterized as seamless, and as non-transformational. That is, local discursive resistance to global discursive hegemony is usually cast as oppositional, relatively homogeneous, and rarely successful in transforming relations of power. Alternatively, local discourse is constituted as the local expression of a resistant global discourse, but nonetheless with limited transformative capacity.

We argued in the introduction to this chapter that we wished to embrace the theoretical tension explicit in merging modernist, e.g., critical theory, with postmodernist perspectives in order to understand not only the constituent features of discursive practices surrounding the uranium industry in northern Saskatchewan, but also the global and local conditions which produce, and are produced by, these practices. We see similar attempts to synthesize these perspectives at work in socialist and ecofeminist thought, where global feminist discourse is critiqued in similar terms. From this perspective, local communities of colonized women resist the totalizing tendencies of a global feminist discourse which has been produced in the context of global capitalism, and, while resistant, is nonetheless limited in its transformational potential by these delimitations. Alternatively, local feminist discourse, while perhaps less consistent in relation to global capitalist hegemony, is also potentially more transformative in affecting the conditions of life at the local level.

NOTES

1 In Canada, "Aboriginal" is the current acceptable term when referring collectively to the indigenous peoples of the country who are referred to specifically as First Nations, Métis, and Inuit. "Native" and "Indian" are considered derogatory by many Aboriginal groups. However, Canadian Aboriginals are distinct both biologically and culturally from Australian Aborigines, although both populations have experienced similar colonial histories.

REFERENCES

Archer, V. E., Gillan, J. D. and Wagner, J. K. 1976, "Respiratory disease mortality among uranium miners," *Annals New York Academy of Sciences* (271):280–93.
Babin, Ronald 1985, *The Nuclear Power Game*, Montreal: Black Rose Books.

Baer, Hans 1990, "Kerr-McGee and the NRC: from Indian Country to Silkwood to Gore," *Social Science and Medicine* 30(2):237–48.

Bates, D. V. (Chairman) 1980, *Royal Commission of Inquiry: Health and Environment Protection – Uranium Mining,* Commissioners' Report, Vol. 1, 1980.

Canada Employment and Immigration Council 1987, *Canada's Single Industry Communities: A Proud Determination to Survive,* Ottawa.

Chilton, Paul (ed.) 1985, *Language and the Nuclear Arms Debate: Nukespeak Today,* London and Dover: Frances Pinte.

Dirschl, H. J., Novakowski, N. S. and Burgess, L. C. N. 1992, "An overview of the biophysical environmental impact of existing uranium mining operations in Northern Saskatchewan," ESAS, Inc., Ottawa, Canada.

Ernst and Young 1991, *Economic Impact Study,* Uranium Saskatchewan, Saskatoon, Saskatchewan.

ESAS 1992, *Health in the Context of Uranium Mining in Northern Saskatchewan,* Ottawa.

Falk, Jim 1982, *Global Fission: The Battle over Nuclear Power,* Melbourne: Oxford University Press.

Fraser, Nancy 1989, *Unruly Practices: Power, Discourse, and Gender in Contemporary Social Theory,* Minneapolis: University of Minnesota Press.

Goldstick, Miles 1987, *Wollaston: People Resisting Genocide,* Montreal: Black Rose Books.

Gotlieb, L. S. and Husen, L. A. 1982, "Lung cancer among Navajo uranium miners," *Chest* 81:449–52.

Ham, James M. (Commissioner) 1976, *Report of the Royal Commission on the Health and Safety of Workers in Mines,* Toronto: Government of Ontario.

Harding, J. 1993, *Presentation to Joint Federal-Provincial Panel on Uranium Mining in Northern Saskatchewan,* Regina, Saskatchewan.

Hartsock, Nancy 1990, "Foucault on power: a theory for women?," in Linda J. Nicholson (ed.), *Feminism/Postmodernism,* New York: Routledge.

Krumbholz, Esther and Kressing, Frank (eds.) 1992, *The World Uranium Hearing: Uranium Mining, Atomic Bomb Testing, Nuclear Waste Storage – a Global Survey,* Munich: The World Uranium Hearing.

Kunz, Emil (1992), *Czechoslovak Epidemiological Studies of Miners Exposed to Radon,* International Conference on Radiation Safety in Uranium Mining, Saskatoon, Saskatchewan. May 25–8.

L'Abbé, Kristan, Howe, G. R., Burch, J. D., Miller, A. B., Abbott, J., Band, P., Choi, W., Du, J., Feather, J. and Gallagher, R. 1991, "Radon exposure, cigarette smoking, and other mining experience in the Beaverlodge Uranium Miner's Cohort," *Health Physics* 60(4):489–95.

Mackay, Louis 1988, "Lines of longitude: people's detente, north and south," in Louis Mackay and Mark Thompson (eds.), *Something in the Wind: Politics after Chernobyl,* London: Pluto Publishing Ltd.

Midwest Uranium Project 1991, *Environmental Impact Statement,* Vol. 2, *Project Description,* Midwest Joint Venture, Denison Mines Limited (operator).

Mies, Maria and Shiva, Vandana 1993, *Ecofeminism,* Halifax: Fernwood Publications.

Nash, J. and Kirsh, M. 1986, "Polychlorinated biphenyls in the electrical machinery industry: an ethnological study of community action and corporate responsibility," *Social Science and Medicine* 23(2):131–9.

Nelkin, Dorothy and Pollak, Michael 1982, *The Atom Besieged: Antinuclear Movements in France and Germany*, Cambridge: The MIT Press.

Rappaport, R. A. 1988, "Toward postmodern risk analysis," *Risk Analysis* 8(2):189–91.

Salaff, Stephen 1983, "The prospects for Canadian uranium," Working Paper no. 27. Kingston, Ontario: Centre for Resource Studies, Queens University.

Samet, J. M., Kutwirt, D. M., Waxweiler, R. J. and Key, C. R. 1984, "Uranium mining and lung cancer in Navajo men," *New England Journal of Medicine* 310:1481–4.

Samet, J. M., Pathak, D. R., Morgan, M. V., Marbury, M. C., Key, C. R. and Valdivia, A. A. 1989, "Radon progeny exposure and lung cancer risk in New Mexico U miners: a case control study," *Health Physics* (56):415–21.

Saskatchewan Bureau of Statistics 1991, *Economic Review*.

Saskatchewan Energy and Mines 1990, *Mineral Statistics Yearbook*, Miscellaneous Report 90–3.

Shields, L. M., Wiese, W. H., Skipper, B. J., Charley, B. and Benally, L. 1992, "Navajo birth outcomes in the Shiprock uranium mining area," *Health Physics* (63):542–51.

Sibbald, T. I. I. 1981, *Saskatchewan Uranium Field Trip Guide*, Calgary: Geological Association of Canada.

Taylor, Lynda 1983, "Resources for self-reliance, uranium legacy," *The Workbook*, 8(6), Southwest Research and Information Centre, Albuquerque, New Mexico.

Thomas, P., Sheard, J. W. and Swanson, S. 1993, "Uranium series radionuclides, polonium-210 and lead-210 in the lichen–caribou–wolf food chain of the Northwest Territories." Prepared for Environment Canada, Atomic Energy Control Board, Department of Indian Affairs and Northern Development, and Department of Renewable Resources (NWT). Ottawa: Environment Canada, March 1993.

Throgmorton, J. A. 1991, "The rhetorics of policy analysis," *Policy Sciences* 24:153–79.

Wagoner, J. K., Archer, V. E., Carroll, B. E., Holaday, D. A. and Lawrence, P. A. 1964, "Cancer mortality patterns among US uranium miners and millers, 1950 through 1962," *Journal of the National Cancer Institute* 17:373–80.

Waxweiler, R. J., Roscoe, R. J., Archer, V. E., Thun, M. J., Wagoner, W. K. and Lundin, F. E. 1981, "Mortality follow-up through 1877 of the white underground uranium miners cohort examined by the United States Public Health Service," in M. Gomez (ed.), *Radiation Hazards in Mining: Control, Measurement, and Medical Aspects*, New York: Society of Mining Engineers, American Institute of Mining, Metallurgical, and Petroleum Engineers, pp. 823–30.

Webler, Thomas, Rahel, Horst and Ross, Robert J. S. 1992, "A critical theoretic look at technical risk analysis," *Industrial Crisis Quarterly* 6:23–38.

Yih, Katherine, Donnay, Albert, Yassi, Annalee, Ruttenber, A. James and Saleska, Scott 1995, "Uranium mining and milling for military purposes," in Arun Makhijani, Howard Hu and Katherine Yih (eds.), *Nuclear Wastelands: A Global Guide to Nuclear Weapons Production and Its Health and Environmental Effects*, Cambridge: The MIT Press, pp. 105–68.

12 Women, resistance, and the breast cancer movement

Patricia A. Kaufert

Yet once I face death as a life process, what is there possibly left for me
to fear? Who can ever really have power over me again.
(Audre Lorde 1980:61)

Analyses of the impact of medical knowledge on women's health and
well-being typically focus on issues of reproduction, such as the control
of fertility, childbirth and pregnancy, menopause, or the new reproductive technologies. In this literature, feminist researchers have denounced
the contraceptive pill and hormone replacement therapy as iatrogenic.
They have rejected the new technologies as a form of cooptation by
science of women's reproductive powers. They have decried the
application of medical knowledge in the management of birth as an
intrusion upon the natural processes of the female body. The histories
of the Dalkon Shield and Diethylstilbestrol (DES) have been used to
give dramatic expression to a world view in which women are betrayed
and injured by medical science.

In describing the malevolent impact of science on women's bodies,
many feminists have framed resistance in terms of the rejection of
medicalization, the validation of experiential knowledge, and the
reassertion of women's traditional wisdoms. They propose to women an
alternative vision in which they birth naturally, become fertile with ease,
traverse menopause without problem, and age with grace. Their well-
being as women is constant, preserved through good nutrition, the
maintenance of spiritual balance, the use of herbs and other forms of
alternative medicine. Home birth, in which a woman removes her body
totally outside the sphere of medical control, becomes the ideal model
of resistance.

This vision of health as the natural state of woman is both beautiful
and powerful; unfortunately, it is as much imagery as actuality. The
reality of most women's experience – whether of the self or others – also
includes the knowledge that birth can be dangerous, fertility is not
always assured, breasts and uteri are vulnerable to the growth of tumors

and fibroids, the body is difficult to proof against the aches and pains of aging. A philosophical commitment to resist medicalization is easy to make, but difficult to maintain in the face of unanticipated trauma. A sense of well-being and spiritual balance may become elusive with the onset of chronic disease.

If all women have some consciousness of the body as potentially vulnerable, a woman with breast cancer has proof of it. Once diagnosed, she finds herself trapped in an intimate, emotionally draining, and often painful relationship with medicine, science, and technology. Whatever her commitment to a feminist perspective, she cannot exit cancer care in quite the same way as a woman might exit obstetric care by choosing home birth. To the extent that withdrawal is virtually – if not absolutely – impossible, she must either abandon resistance or conduct it from within the system, guerrilla-style.

This essay is an exploration of the various forms of resistance developed by women with breast cancer.[1] For over the past ten to fifteen years, women with breast cancer have gradually put together an oppositional discourse in which they have reinterpreted the meaning of being a woman with cancer, challenged existing stereotypes of how they should behave, and demanded recognition of a new paradigm. Initially focused at the microlevel of the individual encounter with the cancer care system, resistance subsequently turned into a demand for the reformulation of the relationship between women and the medical and scientific research establishment.

My interest in the emergence of the breast cancer movement developed during work on a longer-term project in which I am examining the public health discourse on risk and its assumption that all bodies, male and female, are actually or potentially diseased. While searching for information on the North American debate over mammography screening for breast cancer, I reviewed the writings of women with cancer, looking for their descriptions of the screening and diagnostic experience. I also gathered more general material on the politics of breast cancer, including the emergence of the breast cancer movement. In tracking the history of this movement, I collected newsletters produced by breast cancer consumer groups, articles written by leaders in the breast cancer movement, transcripts of their speeches and interviews with media, the briefs presented to a sub-committee of the Canadian Parliament on the subject of breast cancer.

All this material is in the public domain, but none of it was produced for an academic audience. Speeches by leaders in the breast cancer movement, for example, were aimed at "outsider" audiences of politicians and policy makers, health professionals, research scientists, and journalists. Part of a larger lobbying effort, one of their aims was to challenge the medical research community, but their other purpose was to gain political and public support. By contrast, the newsletters were written for an "insider" audience of members in breast cancer organizations, primarily women with breast cancer and their supporters. The autobiographies written by women with breast cancer had their own objectives. While sometimes discussing the political and public context of breast cancer, the primary purpose of these books is to provide an account of a personal odyssey, retold for other women with cancer. Far too often, they exist also as an elegy for those who wrote them.

In treating this collection as research material, I am breaking away from the preference given in feminist methodology to the in-depth interview, that personal and private conversation between researcher and researched. But women with breast cancer have their own voice and tell their own stories; they do not need another academic researcher seeking to reframe their experience through her questions.

Yet, the breast cancer movement has importance within the wider discussion of women and biopower, providing a different perspective on medicalization and women's struggle for control over their own bodies. Rather than withdrawing from medical control, these women confronted the power of medicine by seeking to impose their own objectives on the research community. Seen from this perspective, the history of the breast cancer movement offers a rare example of the emergence of a formal, structured, highly self-conscious resistance movement, put together by women and in defense of their lives. I want to use this chapter to explore the social and political context of this movement, the sources of its power, its vulnerabilities, its emergence out of acts of individual protest into a mass movement.

Social identities and social movements

The breast cancer movement began with individual women meeting, forming small groups, committing themselves to sharing knowledge and listening to each other talk. Groups expanded, joined, formed regional and national coalitions. Looking for a way of construing this process, I used Nancy Fraser's (1992) discussion of the formation of social identities and the emergence of social movements. Writing about the relationship between French discourse theories and feminist politics, she describes social identities as "discursively constructed in historically specific social contexts; they are complex and plural; and they shift over time" (1992:178). Group formation occurs as people come together, assume collective identities, and "constitute themselves as collective social agents . . . Preexisting strands of identities acquire a new sort of salience and centrality. These strands, previously submerged among many others, are reinscribed as the nub of new self-definition and identity" (1992:179). A reading of Nancy Fraser suggested the following questions: "Why did the identity of being a woman with breast cancer change from passivity to action?" "What were the strands in a woman's previous identities which went into the creation of a breast cancer activist?" "What impelled women with breast cancer to break out of their isolation and assemble under the banner of a new social movement?" "What was the historically specific social context in which this movement emerged?" Looking for answers, I started from the initiation of a woman into her new identity as a woman with breast cancer.

From passivity to action: becoming a woman with breast cancer

As women with breast cancer have abandoned silence to speak or write about their experience, they usually start their narratives at the moment when first told they had cancer. Rosalind MacPhee wrote: "I was in a bubble. I saw his mouth moving and I was aware of a flow of words, but I was unable to process most of the information. He might as well have been speaking a different language. The diagnosis of breast cancer had taken over" (1994:41). Barbara Rosenblum recalls: "I shut my eyes and saw absolute black, no line of red or purple. My agitation lifted me off the table and I started walking around the examining room in small steps, working off the tension, I thought I might put my fist through the wall" (Butler and Rosenblum 1991:10).

Reading through the autobiographies of women with breast cancer provides some sense of the intensification of fear that accompanied diagnosis, turning the thing dreaded into reality. As women lived through the experience of their disease and treatment, they learned at first-hand what science and medical care had to offer by way of treatment and cure. Yet, this form of experiential knowledge was a source of fear rather than power. The body became untrustworthy, concealing truth. "When the body, like my body, is no longer consistent over time, when it gives different signals every month, when something that meant one thing in April and may have different meaning in May, then it's hard to rely on stability – and therefore the truth – of the body" (Butler and Rosenblum 1991:136). Rosalind MacPhee (1994) wrote about how hard she found it to reconcile knowing that a cancer had been growing silently within her body for months with her memory of a sense of total wellness during that same time.

The treatment process is described as all-consuming of time and energy. A deeply disorienting experience, treatment transforms not only the inner sense of self, but also the outer image. The person in the mirror is no longer recognizable: "I didn't know I would be sick, nauseated, frightened, unable to sleep, irritable, have strange mood swings which have alienated my family, get terrible hot flashes, lose my hair on my head and other places, and feel exhausted." A woman describes her body after mastectomy as half still her own and half the body of a boy, a strange and alien presence.

As they write about living through attempts to cut, poison, and burn out their cancer, women use their autobiographies to explore what it was like to enter a strange, medically dominated, world with its own language and culture, and its own definitions of appropriate behavior. Implicit in these descriptions of diagnosis and treatment is the construction of a new identity, crafted out of the number of lymph nodes involved, the type of surgery done, the type of chemotherapy given, the number of radiation treatments. The woman under treatment exists as an extreme exemplar of Foucault's "docile body," whose "forces and energies are habituated to external regulation, subjection, transformation" (Bordo 1989:14).

Marianne Paget (1993) had leimyosarcoma rather than breast cancer, but has written brilliantly on the experience of going through treatment for cancer. A social scientist, she used her training to observe and comment on what was happening to and around her. Writing about the chemotherapy room, for example, she describes the loss of social identity and basic rights: "Patients, whatever their sex, race or class are treated there without distinction and without recognition of normal rights to privacy provided in this culture" (1993:56). In another passage, she refers to herself during treatment as in a "liminal" state, using a term taken from anthropology to suggest an analogy between the cancer treatment process and the rituals of initiation, as described in the following passage from Victor Turner: "The passivity of neophytes to their instructors, their malleability, which is increased by submission to ordeal, their reduction to uniform condition, are signs of the process whereby they are ground down to be fashioned anew" (Turner quoted in Davis-Floyd 1992). For Paget, the pressures to conform and behave as prescribed by the cancer care system have a similar power and purpose. Sharon Batt is another woman who has described how isolated, frightened, dependent on their physicians women become during treatment. She suggests that most women "shrink from any action that could be interpreted as a lack of gratitude," while others fear being labeled as a troublemaker (1994:366). She continues: "Even women who identify with an activist philosophy may feel too vulnerable in the months after their diagnosis to speak out and run the risk of antagonizing their treatment team" (1994:366). As described in these autobiographies, each stage in the treatment process is another rite in the passage from being the "well" woman to being this other woman, the cancer patient, passive and compliant.

Yet, Batt herself made the transition from passivity to action, speaking out and becoming a leader in the Canadian breast cancer movement. Her existence, and that of other women like her, suggest a change either in the cancer clinic or in the women who came to it for treatment. As there is no evidence of a change in the clinic, the difference must presumably lie in women. This next section explores how some women started to weave their new identities as patients with breast cancer into the warp of their previous selves, and created a new phenomenon – the breast cancer activist.

Weaving a new identity

The breast cancer movement started with a few individual women who not only refused to behave as expected, but developed their own oppositionary and public discourse around breast cancer. Audre Lorde wrote: "Off and on I kept thinking. I have cancer. I'm a black lesbian feminist poet, how am I going to do this now? Where are the models for what I'm supposed to be in this situation? But there are none" (1980:28). Finding no model, but refusing to allow her previous identities to be erased, Audre Lorde chose to reinscribe them "as the nub of a new self-definition and identity" (Fraser 1992:179). In essence, Audre Lorde reconstructed herself as still a black, lesbian, feminist poet, but now also as a black, lesbian, feminist poet with breast cancer.

Although years and countries apart, Eva Bereti was like Audre Lorde in having already forged a strong identity as a member of one of Canada's First Nations communities. Angered by her racist treatment in a Canadian hospital, she decided to go home. "For weeks, burning sweet grass every day, I tried to cleanse my mind and regain my strength. I was caught between two worlds. Staking my life on the old ways, I returned to my people, to the sweat lodge." (Amesbury 1995:41–2). Her previous identity as a healer in touch with traditional ways is rewoven with her identity as a woman with breast cancer. Rather than accepting a role as victim, she set about healing herself, using the smell of the burning sweet grass and the sweat lodge.

Another Canadian woman, Mary Drover, simply refused to discard her identity as a competent adult. She recalled: "Cancer made me an activist. I was given my diagnosis in a crowded emergency room – then left in the dark. With surgery scheduled for the following week and absolutely no idea what my options were, I was expected to make what seemed to be life-and-death decisions. Look, I'm a smart person. Maybe not brilliant, but I can read a medical journal. I needed information, not condescension. I deserved better" (Amesbury 1995:21–2). These three individuals – Audre Lorde, Eva Bereti, and Mary Drover – refused to allow their sense of self to be eclipsed by becoming a woman with breast cancer. Rather their prior identities, as poet, healer, competent woman, became the foundation of a new self.

Audre Lorde was among the first to recognize the importance of becoming visible as a woman with breast cancer. Despising the convention that she should hide her identity as a woman without a breast, she wrote: "I refuse to have my scars hidden or trivialized behind lambswool or silicone gel. I refuse to be reduced in my own eyes from warrior to mere victim, simply because it might render me a fraction more acceptable or less dangerous to the still complacent, those who believe if you cover up a problem it ceases to exist" (Lorde 1980:60). Some years later, Louise Lander described her refusal to wear a prosthesis as an act of resistance to the "subtle coercion to pass as having two breasts" (Lander 1993:21). The famous cover of the *New York Times Magazine*, showing a picture of Matuschka with the long scar of her mastectomy uncovered, accompanies a story with the title, "You can't look away anymore." The Matuschka picture and the almost equally well-known photograph of the tree of life tattooed over Dena Metzger's mastectomy scar, have acquired the status of icons, possessing great power and beauty, but existing also as statements of loss and pain. Above all else, they make visible what breast cancer does to a woman's body.

Audre Lorde wanted voice as a woman with breast cancer as well as visibility; she describes writing the *Breast Cancer Journals* because "I do not wish my anger and pain and fear about cancer to fossilize into yet another silence, nor rob me of whatever strength can lie at the core of this experience, openly acknowledged and examined" (Lorde 1980:9). She was probably not the first woman with breast cancer to keep a journal of her experiences, but her journals were unusual in being published. Her example has been followed by others and several autobiographies have appeared over the last few years. Easily available in bookstores and public libraries, they are unlike the academic and medical literature on breast cancer, partly in being relatively inexpensive, easy to find, and written in accessible language. The informational literature handed by cancer societies has some of these characteristics but is designed to soothe and placate. The autobiographies are often angry, and their purpose is to uncover, rather than conceal. The women who wrote them name their pain, loneliness, and fear. Wittingly or unwittingly, these are books of resistance, in the sense of making women privy to secrets previously hidden within the cancer treatment centre. As a result, women facing treatment for breast cancer may now learn – should they so choose – what others have gone through before them, step by step.

No one knows how many women read the *Cancer Journals* and turned from victim into warrior, willing to speak out their fear and anger. What is clear, however, based on the history of breast cancer support groups, is that increasing numbers of women started breaking out of the isolation of the cancer patient and assembling together, first in small, but then in larger groups, gradually transforming into the breast cancer movement.

From individual protest to networks of resistance

According to Nancy Fraser, the explanation of a social movement lies in the "historically specific social context in which this movement emerged" (Fraser 1992;178). In the case of the breast cancer movement, this context includes the political and ideological history of the 1950s and 1960s. An increasing number of the women diagnosed with breast cancer in the late 1970s and early 1980s had grown up during the period of women's liberation and some will have participated in the self-help and consciousness raising groups characteristic of that time. They believed in the value of bringing women together, breaking down their isolation, promoting a sense of sisterhood based on shared experience. Formed by this experience, some women turned naturally to the idea of mutual support groups when they developed breast cancer.

The occasional account of the beginnings of a breast cancer support group suggests a pattern in which two or three women would meet, then decide to form a group to which they would recruit other women. Formations at the grassroots, these were community groups, sometimes in the sense of a geographical entity and sometimes in the sense of a community of shared identity; for example, the roster of support groups includes the African-American Breast Cancer Alliance and the Mautner Project for Lesbians with Cancer, as well as groups based on a common treatment centre or living in the same town.

The next step in these histories is the development of group identity, fund raising, and sometimes the publication of a newsletter. The latter were used partly as a means of raising money, but also to distribute information and keep members in touch. Typical examples of material in the newsletters sent out by Y-ME, a Chicago-based support group, include an article on breast cancer and pregnancy, a discussion of mind-body connection in breast cancer, a note on new legislation in Illinois to provide better drug coverage, a calendar of forthcoming fund-raising activities, a request from the Y-ME wig and prosthesis bank for medium-sized prostheses, and a valedictory essay for a woman who had died. The overall tone is akin to a church parish broadsheet, except the parishioners are all women with breast cancer.

All these different activities – the education sessions, the support groups, the fund-raising activities and newsletters – are typical of voluntary organizations. They would have been familiar to many of the women in these support groups, part of the social and community fabric of their lives. The difference was that their sense of collective identity came not from having children in the same school or going to the same church, but from shared experience and knowledge of the treatment process. Women were bound also as witnesses to the deaths of other women and through fear of their own mortality.

Groups formed, disappeared, or flourished. Survival was always fragile, as members became too sick to continue or, recovering, quit participation, but those who left were often replaced by other women, the newly diagnosed. Rather than disappear, some groups expanded, taking on a regional or national identity. Y-ME, one of the oldest of these support groups, was started by two women, Ann Marcou and Mimi Kaplan, in Chicago in 1979. By 1992, it had become "the largest consumer-based support program for breast cancer in the United States" with chapters in eleven other states. As described by its director:

We have a lot of administrative structure and I think that's what made us work. Making it a "mom and pop" organization won't work if you want it to continue. It works fine for a group of women who want to support each other for several months. It's a wonderful thing, but once they heal, many of them just want to get on with their lives. It's not a sign of rejection that it fell apart, it's just that it met its need and it's time. (Green 1992:109)

Although Y-ME organized support groups, ran education sessions, and published a newsletter, it became best known for running a national telephone information hot-line. Women telephoned when they wanted a list of specialists in their community, needed information on what forms of treatments were available, or wanted to talk to someone who had been through the treatments they had been offered. Some sought clarification of what they had been told by their oncologist, but in terms they could understand.

The leader of the first wave in the formation of the breast cancer movement, Y-ME was a relatively conservative organization compared with the more activist, feminist groups which came later. Y-ME prided itself, for example, on working closely with its local medical community; it had an advisory board of medical specialists and claimed cordial relationships with the American Cancer Society. Its executive director, Sharon Green, described the boundaries the organization set for itself in a testimony before a Canadian Parliamentary Sub-Committee: "I think they [doctors] trust us not to step beyond our bounds; we don't give medical advice, we help explain in lay terms what the medical issues are, and we give someone an opportunity to talk to women who've made the same type of choices they're going to have to make" (1992:7). This is not the talk of revolution, yet for all this tone of caution, Y-ME's hot-line was an attempt to change, even if slightly, the asymmetry of the accepted power relationship between women and physicians. To appreciate why simply providing women with information qualifies as an act of resistance requires thinking back to the period when Y-ME first started its hot-line.

Breast cancer, knowledge, and resistance

The ability of an oncologist to control access to information, coupled with her isolation, promoted dependency and passivity in the woman with breast cancer. Kathryn Taylor (1988), who studied the communication styles of oncologists during the 1980s, described two approaches. One of these was practiced by research oriented clinicians, who said they favored full disclosure, but were observed talking to women using medical terms they could not understand and a mass of statistics. The majority of the oncologists in her study, however, favored a paternalistic style, relying on the use of euphemisms and avoiding answering direct questions. Taylor quotes one of her informants: "I always try to tell just enough so they realize this is no joke, but not enough to scare them out of their wits" (Taylor 1988:129). The control of oncologists over the information available to women was broken by groups like Y-ME. They could now learn about the debates over the relative merits of lumpectomy versus mastectomy, or radiation plus chemotherapy or radiation alone. Sylvia Morrison, a Canadian activist and member in a group modeled on Y-ME, speaking before the same Parliamentary Sub-Committee, asserted the rights of women to information:

To know and understand to the greatest possible extent what the situation is and what the options are, and to be intimately involved in the decision process. Unfortunately, there often seems to be a paternalistic attitude on the part of the physician that implies the patient is not capable of understanding the explanations and options or of making rational decisions on her own behalf . . . Surely, it is a fundamental right to have information appropriate to the control and management of one's own body. (1992:44)

Women learned how to prepare a list of questions for their oncologists and to take a partner as a witness and recorder. They consulted with other women, phoned Y-ME, did their own literature search. Women became not only better informed but more skeptic, particularly if they discovered that their treatment options depended less on the clinical evidence, and more on their insurance coverage, or the age and personal preferences of their oncologist. Asking questions, querying treatment, changing physicians counts as resistance, but confined at the micropolitical level of the physician–patient encounter. Resistance might have remained there, but for the emergence of a small, highly vocal network of support groups, which took as their model, not Y-ME, but the AIDS movement. These groups moved protest out of the clinic and into the public domain.

Going radical: feminism, AIDS, and the breast cancer movement

The historical context of the breast cancer movement includes not only women's liberation, but the civil rights movement, Vietnam war protests, the women's health movement, gay rights, and the AIDS movement. Many of the women who emerged as leaders in these other, more political groups, such as Jackie Winnow, who created the Women's Cancer Resources Center, and Elenore Pred, a founder of the San Francisco Breast Cancer Action, were former peace activists and committed feminists. A diagnosis of breast cancer may have forced them to accept a new identity, but they brought to it their past experience as political radicals. Susan Shapiro wrote that "cancer is clearly a feminist issue. We need an organization – of women, for women – that will encompass political action, direct service and education" (quoted by Steingraber 1993). Jackie Winnow embodied the combination of feminism and AIDS activism: "And I took some of what I learned doing AIDS work and a lot of what I learned from feminist organizing and women's liberation, and with other women, created the Women's Cancer Resources Center" (Winnow 1991:27).

The AIDS movement provided women with breast cancer not only another model of a single-disease, consumer-based group, but also with a blueprint for action, which included a target (the medical and research establishment) and objectives (better-quality care and more money for research). The linkages with the AIDS movement were based sometimes on personal ties and were in the form of practical help. A member of ACT-UP, for example, gave workshops on successful advocacy tactics for Breast Cancer Action in San Francisco. Another AIDS activist showed Eleanore Pred how to do computer-based research (Batt 1994:313).

More often the ties were indirect and based on example. The very public presence of the AIDS activists in the media or in the community demonstrated to women that there were other ways of dealing with disease and treatment than becoming the compliant patient. Sharon Batt, for example, has described the effect on her, while undergoing treatment for breast cancer, of watching protesters from ACT-UP at an AIDS conference in Montreal. The images served as a catalyst for her own anger and frustration, setting her on the road to activism.

Two years later, Sharon Batt joined with two other women to found Breast Cancer Action, Montreal, modeled on similar groups in California and Vermont (Batt 1994). These groups attracted women whose ideological and political perspectives encompassed environmentalism, support for alternative health care, and various forms of new age feminism. Compared with Y-ME, the newsletters of these groups read less like parish journals and more like radical tracts. Typical examples from Breast Cancer Action, San Francisco include articles discussing herbal therapies, meditation, the higher than average rates of breast cancer in San Francisco, and the relationship between chemical pollution and breast cancer.

Already politically aware, conscious of the effectiveness of the AIDS movement, it was natural for the women who formed Breast Cancer Action and similar groups to think in terms of political protest. They moved the breast cancer discourse beyond the microlevel of the clinic and refocused it at the interface between practice and research. The main targets for their anger were the traditional cancer agencies, the American Cancer Society and the National Cancer Institute. These institutions were condemned partly for their reluctance to support studies on less toxic methods of treatment or to do research on the occupational or environmental causes of breast cancer. The activists focused their main attack, however, on the overall neglect of research on breast cancer. Faced with the refusal of the cancer research agencies to change funding practices, the breast cancer activists looked to the example of the AIDS movement and began to talk in terms of national political action. It was at this point, that the two streams – the one represented by Y-ME and this other one represented by the Breast Cancer Action groups – came together.

Going national

The National Breast Cancer Coalition was formed in 1991 by Susan Love, an oncologist, Susan Hester and Amy Langer. The mission statement of the new organization was: "to work to eradicate breast cancer through focusing national attention on breast cancer and by involving patients and caring others as advocates for action, advances and change" (Langer 1992:207).

The timing of the Coalition's entry onto the Washington scene was well chosen. Women's health was becoming a key political issue, partly because of the lobbying efforts of the Society for the Advancement of Women's Health Research. Created in 1990 in response to a recommendation from the Public Health Service Task Force on Women's Health Issues, the new society had promptly hired a Washington lobby firm to present the case for increased investment in women's health research. In the same year, National Institutes of Health had announced an Office of Research on Women's Health with a mandate to increase "research on diseases, disorders and conditions that affect women."

Working effectively and rapidly, the Coalition was successful in recruiting over 150 different organizations as members, including such diverse groups as Y-ME, Breast Cancer Action in San Francisco and the American Cancer Society. The Coalition provided an organizational framework for these different groups and a centre through which to coordinate their activities. The potential power of the Coalition lay in the ability of its member organizations to tap into a diverse network of women, extending through grassroots America and linked through support groups, newsletters, fundraising, and other volunteer activities. The first task was mobilization.

The more extreme forms of protest associated with the AIDS movement were deliberately avoided. Sharon Batt has suggested that the main reason lay in women's traditional discomfort with the open display of anger, coupled with a reluctance to engage in activities which might offend other women and dissuade them from joining (Batt 1994). Instead, the Coalition and its member groups adopted a more traditional, but highly effective program based on public demonstrations, marches, candle-lit vigils on the steps of State Capitols. Rallies were held at which many of the speeches were given by women with breast cancer, standing together with their husbands and their children, speaking of their desperate hope for a cure. This was Audre Lorde's demand for visibility transferred from the individual to the public forum.

In addition to the planned program, other factors also played into the hands of the Coalition and contributed to the rapid politicization of the emerging national movement. One was the continued refusal by leaders in the major cancer research institutions to agree to requests from women that funding be targeted specifically for breast cancer research. Seen from the perspective of an activist, such as Sharon Batt, it seemed that: "All cancer funding agencies have the same general views about public involvement in their affairs: they don't like it. Scientists know best they argue, and imposed guidelines impede excellence in research. They do not like to allocate basic research funds to anyone type of cancer" (Batt 1992:24). In retaliation, the Coalition attacked the way in which research priorities were set and money allocated, borrowing some of their criticisms from ones used earlier by the AIDS movement. In addition, it used the argument that the largely male research establishment had neglected breast cancer simply because it was a disease of women. Susan Love, one of the leaders of the Coalition, threatened the American Cancer Society with the withdrawal of the women's labour on which they depended for their fund raising activities: "No more politeness. We [women] are not going to be cheerleaders and fundraisers for the same old system. Our intention is to become experts about the breast cancer establishment. We need to demand a place in the design of trials and hold researchers accountable for women's lives" (quoted by McGregor 1993:5). In resistance terms, this might count as a guerilla tactic aimed at the workings of the system.

The actions of government provided an unintended lesson to women on sexism, power, and politics. Deciding to organize a letter writing campaign directed to the President and members of Congress, the Coalition planned for 175,000 letters – a number based on the number of cases of breast cancer diagnosed in the previous year – but received 600,000. To maximize the impact of the campaign, it was agreed that letters would be hand-delivered by volunteers, many of whom had breast cancer. One batch was directed to the White House. Sharon Green recalled that "we were disappointed that the Bush administration barely responded. We had over 100,000 letters for George Bush. With great difficulty, we finally got an aide from the White House to accept letters on his behalf. So this was an eye-opener for a lot of women" (Green 1992:12).

The second lesson was serendipitous. The volunteers arrived on Capitol Hill while the Anita Hill–Clarence Thomas hearings were in process. This chance juxtaposition – women from the breast cancer movement and Anita Hill – made for powerful political theatre. For the volunteers, as for women across the United States, these hearings were the equivalent of watching a morality play on the forces of patriarchy played out on their television screens. Sharon Green describes the impact of this experience on her own politics: "If you were any type of a woman activist and had been dormant, that came through loud and clear. I became a flaming liberal that day, and all those latent things came to the front" (Green 1992:12). The combination of Hill–Thomas hearings, plus not being acknowledged by their President, offended many women. Over the following few months, the Coalition became an effective Washington lobby group. Working with women members of Congress and some male members, it was successful in obtaining an agreement from the National Cancer Institute that money be targeted for breast cancer research; the quid pro quo was an increase in funding for NCI. The impression was that the research establishment appeared to have surrendered to women's demands in exchange for a mess of money.

The Coalition's greatest triumph, however, was the Harkin Amendment by which $210 million for breast cancer research was attached to the Defense Appropriation Act. The amendment passed with sufficient votes to ensure its survival past presidential disapproval. Describing the situation, a commentator from the Coalition wrote:

Thanks in part to Anita Hill, this is the Year of the Woman on Capitol Hill. With many female candidates mounting aggressive campaigns, the Harkin transfer amendment passed because many senators did not want to appear to be insensitive to women's needs and concerns, especially to a highly visible health issue such as breast cancer research. (McGregor 1992:3)

Possibly the symbolism of the amendment was almost more important than the money. The defense budget, the ultimate expression in economic and political terms of male power, had been coopted by and for women.

The Coalition continued in existence, but this $210 million marked its apotheosis, the high point of its mission. For this reason, the Harkin Amendment serves as a convenient point at which to end this history. In the remainder of the chapter, I want to return to questions raised at the beginning and discuss what the breast cancer movement can tell us of women and resistance, the darker as well as the lighter aspects. Recognizing the success of the breast cancer movement entails also recognizing some of its weaknesses and failures, the darker side of resistance.

The breast cancer movement as an exemplar of resistance

As quoted earlier, Nancy Fraser described social movements as constructed within "historically specific social contexts" (1992:178), but they are also constructed out of the particular histories of specific individuals. The emergence, continuation, and growth of the breast cancer movement depended on choices and decisions to resist and challenge, or remain quiet and compliant, made by hundreds of women with breast cancer. The manner of these decisions was certainly a product of the times – as Nancy Fraser would argue – but also of each woman's personal autobiography, her demographic characteristics, and her emotions. The courage and will of women helped form the movement, but it was also affected by the occasional narrowness of their vision and the compromises they made among themselves to maintain consensus.

Many of the women who joined the movement had a very different perspective on medical care than their mothers' generation. Some had followed political creeds in their youth based on notions of civil disobedience and resistance. Others had been influenced by the women's health movement and were accustomed to being critical of health professionals, hostile to the medicalization of women's bodies, and mistrustful of technology. The tendency of women like Audre Lorde or Jackie Winnow was to fight against loss of control over what happened to their bodies and to reject compliance. Both were too influential to be dismissed as members in some radical fringe, but many women who supported the breast cancer movement will have been politicized at a different depth and level of consciousness. To be effective, women had to work together and inevitably this led to compromise. The nature of this compromise is evident in another passage from Sharon Green's statement before the Canadian Parliamentary Sub-Committee, speaking about the early days of the Coalition: "We were naive. We also had some disagreement among ourselves, whether we were going to act up and be radicals, or try to work the system. The consensus was to first go through the system and see how it worked so we wouldn't look dumb and do something really wrong" (1992:11).

One of the consequences of building a coalition across diverse groups was a subtle shift in the previously close relationship with activists in the AIDS movement. It is doubtful that the Breast Cancer Action groups and others of similar ilk would have emerged and taken the form they did, but for the model provided by the AIDS movement. Yet, when the

Coalition eschewed the more radical tactics of ACT-UP, it is likely that the decision owed something to a shrewd sense that it was important to draw a distinction between themselves and the AIDS activists. The Coalition's influence lay in emphasizing the very "ordinariness" of their members, a microcosm of American womanhood, angry but neither threatening nor contentious. Although denying that more money for breast cancer should reduce the amount spent on AIDS, the Coalition gained from contrasts drawn in the media between the monies invested in research on AIDS and breast cancer relative to the far higher number of women dying from breast cancer. The moral worthiness of the breast cancer victim became part of a sub-text: the young mother dying with breast cancer contrasted against the public stereotype of the AIDS patient, gay, male, and radical.

The other field of ambiguity lies in the relationship between "race", "class," and the breast cancer movement. Breast cancer was presented as a disease to which all women were vulnerable regardless of race, income, or education. Yet, the movement itself was largely a construct of educated, middle-class women. As such it benefited enormously from being able to draw on the support and talents of individuals powerful in many different areas of American life, including politics, science, and the arts. These women helped raise funds, lobby, organize. In terms of the class representation of its members, the Coalition was typical of other new social movements (including the AIDS movement) in which middle-class professionals played a key role. As a group, they bring many skills to the movements they join; they are "highly articulate, very capable of manipulating ideas and concepts, well suited to the task of innovating new types of political and social outlook" (Day and Robins 1987:245).

Yet while the middle classes bring skills and good intentions and commitment, their vision of problems and solutions is relatively narrow because of the limited range of their experience and culture. To borrow old terms from old political dialogues, the middle-class women of the breast cancer movement tended toward reform rather than revolution. These women wanted access to information, a more supportive care system, acknowledgment of their psychosocial needs. Above all else, they wanted a cure and they expected this would come through medical research. These are very middle-class goals, displaying a middle-class faith in the power of scientific knowledge, an assumption that should a cure be found it would be available to them, and the luxury of taking access for granted and focusing on a more "user-friendly" model of care. These attitudes contrast with the following passage from an interview with a Mexican American woman talking about the relationship between money and care seeking: "I don't have insurance. In my opinion, if one does have insurance, it's bad because, well, here cures are expensive and, well you know, sometimes for many people, what we earn is not enough even to eat and live. So when we have these types of illnesses, we don't go to the doctor because of lack of money" (Chavez *et al.* 1995:57). A cure for breast cancer, should it be found, would be no use to her, if not affordable. More empathic health professionals will not help her, if she cannot access the health care system. More money for cancer research will not solve either problem.

Reading through the newsletters, the autobiographies, the media interviews with leaders in the breast cancer movement, the overwhelming image is of all women joining together in common cause. It is easy to miss the relative invisibility of Hispanic, Asian, or African American women. The reasons why the breast cancer movement attracted primarily middle-class women are presumably much the same as any other movement. The effect, however, is that despite Audre Lorde and the African-American Breast Cancer Alliance, despite its commitment to inclusivity, the breast cancer movement was not really in touch with the problems and issues faced by women who were not middle-class, not insured, not white and whose survival time after a diagnosis of breast cancer was, according to the epidemiological data, significantly shorter. (The most likely explanation of this particular statistic is late diagnosis and poorer quality care once diagnosed.)

The relatively narrow class base of the breast cancer movement is not unusual. Accusations that someone, whether scholar or activist, has ignored or neglected the "other" woman are endemic within women's studies. The "other" may be defined by her poverty, or her disability, or her label as an immigrant or refugee, but she is the shadow presence whose needs and interests have been ignored. These criticisms are often justified. Even some of feminists' most cherished causes, such as the home birth movement, are largely middle-class phenomena. Their model of home birth, for example, ignores the reality of the lives led in conditions outside their own expectations of safe, warm houses and incomes adequate to paying a midwife.

Saying the breast cancer movement is class-bound in no way negates the commitment of women within the breast cancer movement (or within the home birth movement). They genuinely believe that they are fighting for the rights or needs or life of "everywoman." They are blinkered, however, by their education and their security and, therefore, restricted in their ability to see and acknowledge the needs of the "other."

Finally, there is the question of women's emotions and the role played by the breast cancer movement in the construction of fear. Many of the autobiographies trace a trajectory from the initial diagnosis, mapping the complex path from fear to anger to defiance. Yet, the fear of breast cancer exists long before diagnosed or even present in the body.

Breast cancer is an old rather than a new disease, but women's fear of breast cancer has escalated rapidly in the last fifteen to twenty years, far out of proportion to the epidemiological evidence. For although the incidence of breast cancer has risen, there has not been an equally marked change in mortality rates. The main difference is in the visibility of breast cancer.

At an individual level, a new openness in speaking about breast cancer meant that women no longer heard simply that someone went in hospital or died; they were now told that a woman went into hospital for a mastectomy or died of breast cancer. Each announcement made a woman aware of the presence of cancer within her own circle of "known" women, made up of relatives, friends, acquaintances, colleagues, but also women seen on television or known by reputation. All these different acts of naming gave breast cancer a frightening reality for women.

The media have played their own role in intensifying women's sense of risk. Stories about women with breast cancer, or women's risks of breast cancer, became commonplace during the 1980s and early 1990s. Billboards, television, and women's magazines carried advertisements telling women of the dangers of breast cancer and warning that their only protection lay in early detection. Paid for by the American Cancer Society, as part of its commitment to persuading women to have mammograms, these advertisements were deliberately designed to increase women's sense of vulnerability. Health activists and environmentalists have also had a part in creating fear, publicizing associations between breast cancer and the contraceptive pill or breast cancer and chemical pollution. The basics of living – food, water, air – became sources of risk. Finally, the breast cancer movement wanted to make women angry enough to demand more money for research, but inevitably helped exaggerate women's sense of being at risk.

Conclusion

A recent summary of the history of the Coalition since the Harkin Amendment noted that the membership had increased to 300 organizations and boasted that:

The NBCC [National Breast Cancer Coalition] has built a grassroots network of advocates across the country, with members in every state; successfully fought for a five-fold increase in federal funds for breast cancer research; targeted President Clinton with 2.6 million signatures which resulted in his commitment to create a national action plan to end breast cancer; established working relationships with the nation's lawmakers and prestigious medical and research institutions. (*Nabco News* 9, October1995)

Yet, some of the excitement of the original years of the Coalition was over. A new political climate in Washington discredited lobbying by special interest groups. Media attention switched to the discovery of breast cancer genes. There are rumors suggesting a split in the Coalition, dissension within the leadership, complaints that the movement had been coopted and made safe.

Possibly because of the primacy they have given to capturing the individual voice, feminist anthropologists have made little attempt to analyze large-scale interest organizations, such as the breast cancer movement. But rather than having to search for evidence of women's resistance in hidden acts of defiance, this movement is an opportunity to look at resistance played out on a very public stage.

Resistance would not have taken the form it did, if women had not believed in the possibility of a cure. This was the generation which heard Nixon's proclamation of the "War on Cancer"; it was the generation which had been told repeatedly that the best hope for cure lay in more money for research. If a cure had not been found, logic suggested inadequate funding. Faced with their own death or the death of friends, women did not see the problem of breast cancer as insoluble, but as neglected. They had been betrayed, left to die, simply because this was a disease of women. Anger turned into resistance, expressed not through withdrawal, but through a concerted effort to make the scientific system work for women. Challenging the scientific establishment yet maintaining faith in the scientific enterprise is a singularly American, yet also middle-class, stance.

Like the AIDS activists, who wanted "more science rather than less science, and that science to be about them and their disease" (Emke 1992:72), breast cancer activists sought ways of intensifying the search for a cure and prevention. Emke's statement on the AIDS movement can be applied also to the breast cancer activists. He wrote:

What is special about AIDS is that PWAs possess, for a complex of reasons . . . the political power needed to confront the therapeutic system with a case for the rights of all catastrophically ill patients . . . [T]hey have added their powerful voice to what has traditionally been a silent or politically disorganized constituency. (Dixon 1990, in Emke 1992: 72)

In seeking to curb the power of the research foundations and check the independence of the scientific community, women were challenging the tacit contract between the scientist and the state, between women and the medical establishment. In this sense, this history can be read as an account of a popular movement of resistance by women and for women, focused at the interface between "body-politic and body self, the dynamics of knowledge and power" (Kirmayer 1992).

Women like Audre Lorde challenged existing cultural meanings, replacing the image of the tragic victim – passive, hidden, suffering – with a woman visible, angry, demanding attention. Individual resistance became group resistance, became a mass movement, intent on challenging power at the level at which scientific knowledge is produced and policy is set. No one knows whether the money won and the influence gained will translate into a cure for breast cancer, or a safe method of its prevention – the real objectives of the women who brought this movement into existence. But success must also be counted in Sharon Batt's defiant words: "The research organizations have basically owned the disease. We're saying that we're the ones who should be at the centre, it's our disease, we're the ones living with it and we're not going to be marginalized" (Nemeth 1994:43).

NOTE

1 I have used the phrase "women with breast cancer" throughout this chapter. Some prefer the term "survivor," but Barbara Brenner (the President of Breast Cancer Action, San Francisco) rejects this term because it implies that breast cancer is curable (Brenner 1995:2). She describes herself as a "woman living with breast cancer." I have shortened this by leaving out "living" but see it as still implicit.

REFERENCES

Amesbury, Barbara (ed.) 1995, *Survivors - In Search of a Voice - The Art of Courage*, Toronto: Woodlawn Arts Foundation.
Batt, Sharon 1992, "Women act up over breast cancer," *This Magazine* 26(1):22–6.
1994, *Patient No More: The Politics of Breast Cancer*, Charlottetown: Gynergy Books.
Bordo, Susan R. 1989, "The body and the reproduction of femininity: a feminist appropriation of Foucault," in Alison M. Jaggar and Susan R. Bordo (eds.), *Gender/Body/Knowledge*, New Brunswick, New Jersey: Rutgers University Press, pp. 13–33.
Brenner, Barbara 1995, "Hope, politics, and living with breast cancer," *Breast Cancer Action Newsletter* 31, August, p. 2.

Butler, Sandra and Rosenblum, Barbara 1991, *Cancer in Two Voices*, San Francisco: Spinsters Book Company.

Chavez, Leo R., Hubbell, F. Allan, McMullin, Juliet M., Martinez, Rebecca G. and Mishra, Shiraz I. 1995, "Structure and meaning in models of breast and cervical cancer risk factors: a comparison of perceptions among Latinas, Anglo women, and physicians," *Medical Anthropology Quarterly* 9(1):40–74.

Davis-Floyd, Robbie E. 1992, *Birth as an American Rite of Passage*, Berkeley: University of California Press.

Day, G. and Robins, D. 1987, "Activists for peace: the social basis of a local peace movement," in C. Creighton and M. Shaw (eds.), *The Sociology of War and Peace*, London: Macmillan.

Dixon, John 1990, *Catastrophe Rights: Experimental Drugs and AIDS*, Vancouver: New Star Books.

Emke, Ivan 1992, "Medical Authority and its discontents: a case of organized non-compliance," *Critical Sociology* 19(3): 55–80.

Fraser, Nancy 1992, "The uses and abuses of French discourse theories for feminist politics," in Nancy Fraser and Sandra Lee Bartky (eds.), *Revaluing French Feminism*, Bloomington: Indiana University Press, pp. 177–94.

Green, Sharon 1992, Testimony presented to the Standing Committee on Health and Welfare, Social Affairs, Seniors and the Status of Women, no. 10, House of Commons, Ottawa, Ontario.

Kirmayer, Laurence J. 1992, "The body's insistence on meaning: metaphor as presentation and representation in illness experience," *Medical Anthropology Quarterly* 6(4):323–46.

Lander, Louise 1993, "Coming out as a one-breasted woman," in Midge Stocker (ed.), *Confronting Cancer, Constructing Change: New Perspectives on Women and Cancer*, Chicago: Third Side Press.

Langer, Amy S. 1992, "The politics of breast cancer," *Journal of the American Medical Women's Association* 47(5):207–9.

Lorde, Audre 1980, *The Cancer Journals*, San Francisco: Spinsters Book Company.

McGregor, Marilyn 1992, "From Anita Hill to Capitol Hill," *Breast Cancer Action* Newsletter 15, pp. 2–3.

1993, "Funding for breast cancer research," *Breast Cancer Action Newsletter* 19, p. 5.

MacPhee, Rosalind 1994, *Picasso's Woman: A Breast Cancer Story*, Vancouver: Douglas and McIntyre.

Morrison, Sylvia 1992, Testimony presented to the Standing Committee on Health and Welfare, Social Affairs, Seniors and the Status of Women, House of Commons, Ottawa, Ontario.

Nemeth, Mary 1994, "The new war on breast cancer," *Maclean's Magazine* July 11, 42–4.

Paget, Marianne A. 1993, "Life mirrors work mirrors text mirrors life," in Marjorie L. DeVault (ed.), *A Complex Sorrow - Reflections on Cancer and an Abbreviated Life*, Philadelphia: Temple University Press.

Steingraber, Sandra 1993, "Life styles don't kill: carcinogens in air, food, and water, do: imaging political responses to cancer," in Midge Stocker (ed.),

Cancer as a Women's Issue: Scratching the Surface, Chicago: Third Side Press, pp. 91–102.

Taylor, Kathryn M. 1988, " 'Telling bad news': physicians and the disclosure of undesirable information," *Sociology of Health and Illness* 10(2):109–32.

Winnow, Jackie 1991, "Lesbians evolving health care: our lives depend on it," in Midge Stocker (ed.), *Cancer as a Women's Issue: Scratching the Surface*, Chicago: Third Side Press, pp. 23–35.

13 Selective compliance with biomedical authority and the uses of experiential knowledge

Emily K. Abel and C. H. Browner

The connection between concepts of knowledge and women's oppression is an increasingly central focus of feminist inquiry. Growing numbers of scholars examine what kinds of knowledge count as legitimate and which social groups are entitled to produce, control, and circulate it. Lorraine Code argues that stereotypic representations of women as incapable of abstract thought have helped to exclude women from those processes. In addition, the kinds of knowledge considered "authoritative" tend to be abstract and universalistic and transcend the particularities of individual experience, but most knowledge accessible to women is experiential and particularistic (Code 1991:223).

A common assumption is that women inevitably accept authoritative knowledge even when it contradicts their own experiences. Yet some evidence points to a different conclusion. Historians examining the processes by which biomedicine expanded to establish authority over childbirth and mothering in the first part of the twentieth century in the United States show that African American, American Indian, and European immigrant women often resisted the messages of biomedical advice givers; many expressed contempt for knowledge derived from formal education rather than personal experience (Sicherman, 1984:119; Muncy 1991:114–15). Even many women who welcomed the new advice produced by medicalization viewed it as a resource to be used selectively (Abel and Reifel 1996).

Understanding women's relation to such advice is particularly important because medicalization frequently is considered a major form of social control (Conrad 1992). Parsons's conceptualization of the sick role as an institutionalized form of deviance and Szasz's analysis of the sharply widening realm of psychiatry (Parsons 1951) laid the theoretical groundwork for a number of case studies elucidating the processes by which a wide variety of phenomena began to be regarded as medical problems (Conrad 1975; Scull 1975; Pfohl 1977; Schneider 1978). Such studies view medicalization as imposed, rather than as a set of dynamic processes involving the interaction of lay people and professionals.

This paper, by contrast, examines how women either facilitate or block biomedicine's expansion in two areas – prenatal care and family care of frail elderly people. Although ancient and historical records contain abundant instructions for the care of pregnant women and make a multitude of suggestions, organized prenatal care became common only during the expansion of biomedicine in the early twentieth century (Oakley 1986). This care remained largely in nurses' and health educators' hands in Europe and the United States until the latter part of the twentieth century (Browne and Browne 1960; Thompson *et al.* 1990). Several factors help to explain physicians' success in gaining authority over the prenatal period. Rapid technological advances during the past twenty years have given physicians new tools for diagnosing, monitoring, and intervening in pregnancy (Oakley 1982; cf. Wright 1988). In addition, as Arney shows, a new metaphor of the body transformed the conceptual basis of medicine near the end of World War II:

> The body was no longer looked upon as a machine which was made up of other machines; instead it became a system composed of systems articulated at many points and levels. Furthermore, the body existed as a single component in other, higher-level, systems. An ecological metaphor replaced the mechanical one. (Arney 1982:8)

The understanding that social, economic, political, and cultural dynamics affect birth outcomes meant that birth was no longer defined primarily by the site in which it took place. These transformations were accompanied by a transition from childbirth technologies based on domineering control to technologies of monitoring and surveillance (Arney 1982:8).

State interests also influenced the development of prenatal care. Industrialized nations with government-funded health care systems typically support expanding such services as a way to reduce postnatal costs and contribute to the production of a healthier population. The continued ambivalence about governmental responsibilities in the United States, however, frequently results in a reluctance to finance the costs of poor women's prenatal care.

All US women nevertheless are encouraged to see physicians as soon as they suspect they are pregnant. In this era of widely available home pregnancy testing, those with private medical insurance frequently visit physicians within days after missing their first menstrual periods. Most women either covered only by Medicaid or lacking any health insurance experience lengthy delays obtaining care. The vast majority of US women, however, eventually enroll, although poor women of color remain less likely than others to receive first-trimester prenatal care (Braverman *et al.* 1989).

The standard recommendation is for monthly prenatal visits during the first six months, biweekly visits during months seven and eight, and then weekly visits until the onset of labor. The initial consultation is the lengthiest. Providers obtain medical, family, and pregnancy histories, perform physical exams, and either administer or schedule tests for a wide variety of conditions including cervical cancer, sexually transmitted diseases, diabetes, and anemia. In addition, a prenatal diagnostic screening test to help detect birth defects may be offered.

Most women also receive informational materials at their first prenatal visits. One large California health maintenance organization (HMO), for example, distributes the 96-page booklet "Preparing for a Healthy Baby," that they themselves publish, as well as advertising circulars, coupons, and samples of a wide range of products including ointment to prevent diaper rash, a bottled-water delivery service, and toys.

During subsequent prenatal visits, providers weigh women, take their blood pressure, retest their urine, and evaluate the fetus's growth and heartbeat. An ultrasound exam increasingly is routinely administered between the sixteenth and twentieth weeks of pregnancy to confirm the expected due date, detect fetal heart motion, and check for gross fetal malformations.

Women who receive prenatal care at clinics or HMOs may be offered or required to attend one or more group prenatal education classes, the costs of which are borne by the HMO. Taught by nurses, health educators, and/or dieticians, these classes describe the physiological and psychological changes associated with pregnancy, the nature of prenatal care, and the providers' recommendations for diet, exercise, weight gain, and rest. The classes typically last three or more hours and combine lectures and video presentations.

In addition to their formal prenatal care, US women have at their disposal a wide range of books. The average chain bookstore carries between thirty and fifty titles, including *Mayo Clinic: Complete Book of Pregnancy and Baby's First Year* (Johnson 1994), *What to Eat When You're Expecting* (Eisenberg *et al.* 1986), *Making Love During Pregnancy* (Bing and Colman 1989), *Trust Your Body! Trust Your Baby! Childbirth Wisdom and Cesarean Prevention* (Henkart 1995), and *Unassisted Childbirth* (Shanley 1994). There also are subscription magazines, free "throw away" magazines that are little more than advertising supplements, and ubiquitous T.V. and radio shows on such topics as drug use during pregnancy and cesarean delivery. These various sources are multivocal. Although some, like Henkart and Shanley, challenge prevailing biomedical understandings, most buttress its claims.

Daughters caring for frail elderly parents also can receive a wide array of advice and information. We have noted that, in the late nineteenth century, physicians sought to establish authority over mothering. Since then, the contours of women's caregiving responsibilities have changed dramatically. The elderly were just 4 percent of the population in 1900, but they increased to 8 percent in 1950 and 12 percent in 1984 (Feldblum 1985; Siegel and Taeuber 1986). Although most people aged 65 and over can care for themselves and their households without assistance, approximately one-quarter require at least occasional help (Liu et al. 1985). Like other forms of domestic labor, care for the elderly continues to be allocated on the basis of gender. Women represent 72 percent of all caregivers and 77 percent of the children providing care. Almost one third (29 percent) of all caregivers to frail elderly parents are adult daughters (Stone et al. 1987).

It would, of course, be impossible to subject caregivers to the same regimentation as pregnant women. Nevertheless, as care for the aging gains a central place in women's lives, a new industry is emerging, devoted to counseling and educating relatives of the frail elderly, especially of those suffering from some form of dementia. Financial concerns can help explain the proliferation of such services. Caregivers who are asked what programs would be most helpful to them express a preference for supportive services, including transportation, home maintenance and chore services, personal care services, and adult daycare (Horowitz and Shindelman 1983). A critical demand of many caregivers is respite services, which can provide temporary relief from the burdens of care (Montgomery 1988; Wallace 1990). But it is far cheaper to establish a ten-week course of lectures for caregivers than to provide them with the services of homemakers and home health aides over a period of months or even years. Moreover, many educational programs promote personal adjustment. A major governmental concern is that women will attempt to unload responsibilities on the state, astronomically increasing its financial burden. Policy makers are aware that caregiving is not without cost to women; it frequently reignites family conflicts, imposes financial strains, and encroaches on both paid employment and leisure activities (Abel 1991). One purpose of many educational programs is to help women cope better with the stresses caregiving creates.

What distinguishes both areas we are examining is that, although doctors can make diagnoses, they can offer little in the way of treatment.

Although dramatic new technologies have markedly increased physicians' ability to diagnose fetal defects, they have little power to ameliorate most problems they may find unless women opt for abortions. Physicians today seeking control over pregnancy have nothing comparable to the anesthesia and forceps physicians used in the nineteenth century to establish dominance over childbirth (see Leavitt 1986).

Similarly, a diagnosis of dementia typically follows an evaluation by a physician. Once the diagnosis has been made, however, medical science can offer little aside from prescribing medication to control agitation. Physicians can neither cure the disease nor slow its progress. Unable to offer therapeutic intervention, doctors focus on providing information and advice. They encourage caregivers to disregard their own knowledge of their relatives, view the relatives' behavior as manifestations of a disease, and learn standardized techniques for dealing with them.

In offering information and advice in areas where treatment is unavailable, doctors simultaneously expand their turf and leave themselves open to challenge.[1] Andrew Abbott argues that professions are especially vulnerable to encroachment from other professions at the boundaries of their jurisdictions (1988). Professions gain authority by claiming, in Magali Sarfatti Larson's words, a "monopoly of competence" (1977). In areas peripheral to their jurisdictions, however, professions rarely enjoy exclusive rights to expertise. In fact, social workers, nurses, and health educators have taken the lead in producing a burgeoning advice literature for both pregnant women and caregivers. For example, the authors of the most popular book for pregnant women, *What To Expect When You're Expecting* (Eisenberg et al. 1991), include three laywomen, one of whom has a bachelor's degree in nursing science. Although nurses, social workers, and health educators frequently invoke doctors' authority to legitimize their works, they rely heavily on their own professional training and experiences. Many of the women we interviewed received advice from this literature as well as from a variety of lay sources.

Because Abbott focuses on struggles among professions for dominance over cognitive areas, he slights client production and acquisition of knowledge. We suggest that women are especially likely to draw on experiential knowledge to maintain critical distance from biomedical authority at the margins of physicians' jurisdictions.

The first study on which we rely involved a group of pregnant women, who used "embodied" knowledge as the basis for either incorporating or refusing to incorporate clinical recommendations regarding their prenatal care. By "embodied knowledge" we mean knowledge derived from women's experiences with and perceptions of their bodies as they change throughout the course of pregnancy or knowledge derived from their previous pregnancies. Embodied knowledge can also be drawn from other women's reports of their own pregnancy experiences. The second study focused on women caring for frail elderly relatives; these women rely partly on what we call "empathetic knowledge." Evelyn Fox Keller has described empathy as "a form of knowledge of other persons that draws explicitly on the commonality of feelings and experiences in order to enrich one's understanding of another in his or her own right" (Keller 1985:117). Family caregivers give credence to their own understandings of relatives, produced by a lifetime of close association. This permits caregivers to challenge physicians' recommendations regarding their relatives' care.

These two kinds of experiential knowledge thus differ in important ways. One derives from direct sensory experience, the other from close emotional ties between individuals. In addition, each type can take various forms. Women obtain embodied knowledge not just from current pregnancies but also from memories of past physical changes. Both pregnant women and caregivers derive knowledge from the personal experiences of people with whom they identify as well as from their own experiences. One element that unites these different types of knowledge is their particularity. Although most accounts of medicalization processes assume that people accept biomedicine because it is more effective than any other paradigm, we suggest that pregnant women and caregivers use diverse forms of experiential knowledge to retain critical distance from biomedical authority.

Our two studies were conducted in the late 1980s and early 1990s in southern California. Data were collected through lengthy, open-ended interviews in women's own homes or in other places of their choosing. For the prenatal study, we interviewed 158 women. The sample consisted of European American, Mexican American, and immigrant Mexican women from middle- and lower-class backgrounds (see Browner and Press 1996 for more information on sample selection). These groups historically have had very different relationships to the health care system; according to Emily Martin (1987), poor women and women of color are more resistant to biomedical frameworks. Nevertheless, our study found no significant differences by ethnicity or social class in women's use of different types of knowledge in connection with prenatal care. Ellen Lazarus reports similar results from her research on Puerto Rican and European American obstetrical patients at a US inner-city hospital (Lazarus 1988:36).

For the study of elderly caregiving, fifty-one primarily middle-class women were interviewed (see Abel 1991 for a description of the study population). There is an urgent need for research examining how factors of class and race affect the caregiving experience. Until that research is completed, we will be unable to determine to what extent the findings from this study are generalizable.

It is important to note the impossibility of completely disentangling the two types of knowledge – professional and experiential – we have described. In the first place, both pregnant women and caregivers indicated that physicians helped them trust their own perceptions. As one woman in the prenatal study explained:

I told the nurse, "You know, I'm always tired . . ." [And] she goes, "Well, you do have three kids and they're kind of small." And I said, "Yeah, well, yeah, and then I cook, clean, wash. I do all that. Nobody helps me do all that." She goes, "Well, that has a lot to do with it." I was thinking, maybe something's wrong with me. I'm always tired. . .

Biomedical authority helped to validate this woman's feelings of fatigue. Similarly, a caregiver noted that a medical evaluation confirmed her sense that her mother had changed:

We suspected, and we didn't think we had a right to suspect without a professional opinion . . . We used to swap stories of "guess what mother did now" and it wasn't cruel. [The doctors] reconfirm that it's not you, because sometimes when you're in with someone who's not dealing with things properly, you begin to feel: "Was it me? Did I hear that? I don't believe she said that."

Moreover, women seek biomedical information partly to help explain their own experiences. Both pregnant women and caregivers asserted that one reason they sought the advice of doctors was to gain a sense of control by learning what to expect. A woman caring for a mother with dementia remarked, "At the hospital, there was a wonderful doctor, and he said: 'Watch for these signs. When you come to pick her up and she has to brush her hair or brush her teeth, she's beginning to deteriorate. And then watch for her doing this and wandering off and not being able to get home.' So we watched for all the signs to come." Similarly, a pregnant woman said, "It comforts me to [learn] this is how you're going to be feeling."

Caregivers are especially anxious to find a new way to make sense of their parents' behavior. Although the women we spoke to drew on their intimate relationship to their parents in order to care for them, some felt overwhelmed by the emotions the caregiving experience provoked. Judith Kegan Gardiner notes that, according to some psychologists, "empathy is not the same as but opposite to projective identification in which one person insists that the other is an extension of the first. This . . . view of empathy entails no merging, blurring, or loss of self for adults" (Gardiner 1987). But many caregivers acknowledge that they continue to experience themselves the way they did as children in relation to their parents and project inappropriate emotions onto the parents. Medical information enables such caregivers to disengage. Susan Jackson[2] reported:

We always viewed my mother as somewhat crazy and tried to get her to see a psychiatrist, but to have it be a clear dementia in some ways makes it easier to relate to her . . . My coping mechanism had always been to distance myself, but there was always some doubt that maybe that was invalid, it always got to me eventually. This way, it's objective, so there is no way it could get to me.

When some caregivers learned from clinicians that their parents' actions were unintentional, their own emotions changed. Evelyn Baker recalled how her anger at her mother's behavior faded:

I took my mother to the doctor . . . He's the one who told me about the book, *The 36–Hour Day* . . . Because . . . it was so difficult not to be mad . . . And then when I read the book, I realized that she was just like a model case . . . all these things that were in this book were happening to her . . . I was seeing that she can't help it . . . and then our whole relationship and my attitude to her really changed.

By offering a framework for understanding experience, biomedical information shapes that experience. The following quotation demonstrates that some information pregnant women receive changes their interpretation of sensory experiences. In explaining why she thought it important for pregnant women to receive prenatal care, Ana Martínez said, "If I'm feeling real weird, like I get a kick and it feels really warm after the kick but only in one spot . . . to me it's like, is that normal?" To the extent that experience includes not just "raw" sensory data but also the meanings attached to them, we can say that medical information transformed this woman's experiential knowledge (Weedon 1987:85; Gunew 1990; Canning 1994).

As we have seen, medical information also alters the way caregivers understand elderly parents suffering from dementia. As caregivers' medical knowledge grew, some increasingly spoke of their parents not as unique individuals but rather as part of the large group of victims of dementia. In answer to questions about their own parents, they discussed adults with dementia in general, occasionally referring to "them" or "these people." One woman lamented her inability to spend more time talking with her mother "because this is what an Alzheimer's disease patient needs." Another woman explained why she had found the right aide for her father: "She is aware of how to take care of Alzheimer's people. It would be a real problem for some if they didn't understand Alzheimer's disease and the nature of it and how people are when they have that disease."

But the power of biomedicine should not be exaggerated. If biomedicine transforms experiential knowledge, it does not substitute for that knowledge entirely (cf. Duden 1993). "Substitution" implies the existence of a finite amount of knowledge in a particular domain. Our interviews reveal not only that biomedicine is the dominant medium through which pregnant women articulate their experiences but also that women seek to negotiate a variety of different knowledges, and many achieve uniquely syncretic accommodations (Root *et al.* n.d.).

Jaber F. Gubrium and Robert L. Lynott (1987) argue that once medical assessments of demented adults have been conducted, caregivers tend to "see impairment everywhere," implying that they cease relying on their own experiential knowledge. A study by Betty Risteen Hasselkus (1988), however, suggests that family members are less easily swayed by medical labels. The caregivers she interviewed occasionally used their special knowledge of elderly relatives to cast doubt on the diagnoses.

A few women we spoke to pointed to faculties their parents retained in order to question the medical diagnosis. Some who accepted the diagnosis nevertheless faulted biomedical expert judgments that attributed to disease behaviors that were exaggerations of lifelong personality traits. Others insisted that their parents' unique personalities effectively transcended the disease. Alice Holt explained why she enjoyed the time she spent with her father: "He's real sweet, he's not like sometimes Alzheimer's people get, kind of angry . . . I mean, to me, he's fun, and even with his Alzheimer's, he'll say really funny things." Marsha Jordan similarly continued to respond to her mother as an individual, despite her mother's failing mental capacities. She commented, "I've just realized that there are things my mother can't grasp. My dad set up a trust in his will when he was ill, and I explained it to her so many times over so many months, and she still doesn't understand it . . . [But] I think in matters of the heart she probably could still advise me. She just can't balance her checkbook very well." As Marsha struggled to accept that her mother's mental capacities had diminished, she continued to know that her mother possessed wisdom in other important areas.

One reason neither pregnant women nor caregivers simply surrender to biomedical authority is that some advice rendered to both groups of women is too vague to provide a useful guide for action. Also, doctors often disagree about the details of specific recommendations (Chalmers *et al.* 1989) and women who change physicians may receive conflicting advice from each. Women obtain information from a wide variety of other sources as well. Thus, when Kristin Robinson had to decide whether or not to consume artificial sweeteners during her pregnancy, she considered the vast array of information she obtained from her own reading and the advice pregnant relatives reported having been given by their own physicians. Given an increasingly medicalized society with its ubiquitous sources of health information, it is impossible for women to accept all the information and advice they receive.

Women in both groups used experiential knowledge as a basis for accepting or rejecting clinicians' recommendations, even as the biomedical paradigm shaped that knowledge. Kitty Carson, for example, explained why she refused to stop smoking during pregnancy, despite being repeatedly urged by her physician to do so: "I smoked during my first pregnancy and I had a nine pound baby . . . [And the baby] had a nine on the APGAR which the highest is ten. So for *me* it was like okay." Similarly, Rachel White explained, "After my first child what came out was I was born to have babies . . . so I'm not as rigid [about following prenatal recommendations] as I was before."

Embodied knowledge was also the basis on which some pregnant informants rejected biomedical advice that proved not to bring about promised changes. In her first pregnancy, Karen Brooks enthusiastically had followed a prenatal exercise program recommended by her provider. Interviewed during her second pregnancy, she stated, "I was told that if I exercise a lot that my labor would be easy. So I was still in labor for 17 hours. This time I'm not doing anything. Who knows, maybe this baby will just pop out." Although Karen initially was willing to accept biomedical authority unquestioningly in this area, its failure to bring about the hoped-for results led Karen to reject this specific advice.

Caregivers used empathetic knowledge of their parents to override physicians' advice. Thus, Marge Ellison scoffed at a physician who recommended that she give her mother a sense of security by imposing routines on her mother's life. "My mother never has lived by routines," Marge explained. The medical recommendation most commonly rejected was that relatives be placed in nursing homes. Despite the widespread belief that family members are overeager to exile the elderly to institutions, many women complain about and resist pressure from physicians to do so. One who did accept a physician's counsel to put her mother in a home later bitterly regretted her decision. Thinking back over her experience, she asserted she would have made a better decision had she trusted her own understanding of her mother's needs:

The worst thing I ever did was to put her in a nursing home and not let her stay with me anymore. I was given advice by professional people that I respected . . . The doctors convinced us that this was the only thing that we could do . . . So it wasn't a question of listening to ourselves, it was a question of listening to professionals tell us that this was the way it had to be or should be.

So far we have examined two types of knowledge women gain from direct experience. Both pregnant women and caregivers also rely on experiential knowledge obtained indirectly. Pregnant women often place special trust in the embodied knowledge of female kin with whom they believe they share physiological traits. One pregnant woman explained: "Exercising is very important . . . I've noticed like, my sisters and my aunts, when they were pregnant, they talk about body-aching. Even myself, my body aches. It's just because your body needs exercise." Another remarked, "I take a lot of my mother's advice because she had ten kids and went through ten pregnancies so I believe her a lot of the times more than I do some of the nurses and some of the doctors . . . With ten pregnancies she should know." It is noteworthy that both these women came from Mexican American working-class backgrounds, where a family culture of pregnancy as counterpoint to the biomedical may remain intact.

Caregiving tends to be a much lonelier endeavor than pregnancy, providing fewer "natural" opportunities to draw on the experiential knowledge of others. Nevertheless, some daughters rely on siblings to make sense of parental behavior because they have the same family history. In addition, some caregivers seek assistance from support group members who share a common experience and can empathize with them. Several caregivers we interviewed stated that, as they heard others narrate personal experiences, they drew comparisons with their own situations and began to reinterpret them. A woman whose mother suffered from recurrent bouts of depression described how she gained critical distance by listening to members of her group and relating their accounts to her own life:

This caregiver group is the one place that I feel I could go and I could tell whatever was happening and people would really understand. I don't think, unless you're going through it yourself, that you can understand it. So I would say that's my biggest resource, to be able to go every week to that meeting, and even if I don't talk very much about what's going on with me, I'll listen to the other people and I can identify so much with what they're going through, and that helps me.

Another woman explained how she was able to contemplate institutionalizing her mother. Support group members "really opened my eyes to realize that I wasn't a bad person, I wasn't evil because I wasn't dumping my mother." She managed "just by listening to them, and the way they felt and what they were going through, and what they were doing, and I thought, 'Well, I've done that,' and it just really opened up everything for me to realize that I'd done all I could do. I couldn't do anymore." When she announced to the group that she finally had resolved to find a nursing home for her mother, the other members bolstered her decision. Because all the members shared her experiences, she invested them with authority and attached enormous significance to their judgment.

Support groups do not undermine biomedical authority in any simple or straightforward way. Some physicians encourage caregivers to enroll; some support groups are run by health professionals and invite doctors to address them. Nevertheless, the power of these groups derives from the exchange of experiential knowledge, not from whatever information leaders or guest speakers dispense.

Conclusion

Despite the denigration of knowledge derived from individual perceptions and feelings, an ongoing and dynamic tension exists between the two types of experiential knowledge we have examined and biomedical knowledge. Pregnant women experience sensory data partly through the interpretive frame provided by biomedicine. At the same time, however, attention to their own physical sensations, and those of other women who have experienced pregnancy, makes pregnant women reluctant to surrender all authority to biomedical experts. Caregivers employ a type of thinking that incorporates emotion and intuition as well as reason. Although a diagnosis of dementia changes some caregivers' feelings about the care recipient and alters the way caregivers interpret his or her actions, caregivers refuse to view frail elderly relatives simply as a set of symptoms. To the extent that caregivers rely on their own empathetic understandings of care recipients, they retain distance from biomedical experts' pronouncements.

These studies lend support to Jana Sawicki's assertion that the expansion of power can create "new possibilities for disruption and resistance" (Sawicki 1991:88). Sawicki adopts Foucault's view of power as an unstable and shifting set of relations rather than a primarily repressive force; people may simultaneously be victims and agents within systems of domination. We have seen that biomedicine transforms women's experiential knowledge and that women help to extend biomedicine's power even as they appropriate it for their own purposes. Biomedicine also expands as doctors offer information and advice in areas where they cannot provide therapeutic interventions. Spurred by a variety of motives, women seek this information and advice not only from their own doctors but also from the popular literature that buttresses doctors' claims to authority. The more information women acquire, however, the more they realize the lack of unanimity among professional thinking (see also Lock 1994). The fissures in medical expertise provide opportunities for women to rely on their own experiential knowledge. Our analysis points to a need for feminists to examine the extent to which women in other arenas use various forms of particularistic knowledge to resist authority.

It is important not to romanticize women's resistance to biomedical authority. Much of the recent emphasis on resistance stems from a desire to describe patterns of domination without casting subordinate groups solely as victims. But our desire to restore agency to such groups may encourage us to find instances of resistance where none exists (Abu-Lughod 1990; Lewin 1996). Moreover not all forms of resistance advance women's interests. Some of the advice about behavioral change pregnant women spurn may have the potential to promote better outcomes. Caregivers who continue to tend extremely disabled parents at home may jeopardize their own well-being. Even the use of empathetic skills can disadvantage women. Some evidence suggests that such skills are unequally divided between genders; as a result, women often provide more care to others than they can expect in return (Miller 1976; Belle 1982; Miller 1990). Nevertheless, these studies caution us against assuming that the expansion of biomedicine inevitably results in women's loss of control. At least in the two areas we have examined at the margins of physicians' jurisdictions, the relationship between women and medical expertise is fluid and complex.

But we also should note that some women do cling tenaciously to biomedical authority. Particularly in the case of life-threatening illnesses such as breast cancer, patients want there to be someone or some body of knowledge they can unambiguously trust. In US society, knowledge derived from scientific experimentation and its technological applications, such as biomedical knowledge, fits this description. Moreover, the diagnosis of serious illness highlights what we try to deny at other times, namely the fragility of human life. This creates a fundamental contradiction. Although US society celebrates mastery, control, and predictability, life, particularly for the seriously ill, is inherently uncertain. Unwilling to acknowledge that life is ultimately unmanageable, we instead look to science to eliminate, or at least better control, this uncertainty and ambiguity. In order to understand women's relationship to biomedicine fully we must examine not just how women maintain distance from biomedicine authority but the circumstances under which they are most likely to place inflated trust in it.

ACKNOWLEDGMENTS

The prenatal study was supported in part by NICHD grant No. HD11944 and grants from the Academic Senate and Chicano Studies Research Center at UCLA. The caregiving study was funded by the Alzheimer's Disease and Related Disorders Association and the UCLA Center for the Study of Women. Browner thanks Nancy Press for her outstanding collaboration in all aspects of the prenatal research from inception to conclusion. She also thanks the administration and staff of the HMO for graciously facilitating the project and the women we interviewed for their generosity and patience. We also wish to thank Francesca Bray, Sondra Hale, Sandra Harding, Linda M. Hunt, Margaret Nelson, Arthur J. Rubel, Mariko Tamanoi, and Sharon Traweek for thoughtful and constructive comments on earlier drafts. Earlier versions of this chapter were presented at the 1994 Annual Meeting of the American Ethnological Association in Santa Monica, California and at the Feminist Research Seminar at UCLA.

NOTES

1 Of course, as managed care expands in the United States, doctors will have less opportunity to dispense information and advice. One of the major criticisms of managed care as it exists in the US today is that it sharply curtails the amount of time doctors can spend with each patient.
2 All proper names are pseudonyms.

REFERENCES

Abbott, Andrew 1988, *The System of Professions: An Essay on the Division of Expert Labor*, Chicago: University of Chicago Press.
Abel, Emily 1991, *Who Cares for the Elderly? Public Policy and the Experiences of Adult Daughters*, Philadelphia: Temple University Press.
Abel, Emily and Reifel, Nancy 1996, "Interactions between public health nurses and clients on American Indian reservations during the 1930s," *Social History of Medicine* 9:89–108.
Abu-Lughod, Lila 1990, "The romance of resistance: tracing transformations of power through Bedouin women," *American Ethnologist* 17:41–55.
Arney, William Ray 1982, *Obstetrics and the Power of the Professions*, Chicago: University of Chicago Press.
Belle, D. 1982, "Social ties and social support," in D. Belle (ed.), *Lives in Stress*, Newbury Park, California: Sage, pp. 133–43.
Bing, Elizabeth and Colman, Libby 1989, *Making Love During Pregnancy*, New York: Ferrar, Straus, and Giroux.
Braverman, Paula, Olive, Geraldine, Miller, Marie Grisham, Reiter, Randy and Egerton, Susan 1989, "Adverse outcomes and lack of health insurance

among newborns in an eight-county area of California, 1982–1986," *New England Journal of Medicine* 321:508–13.

Browne, F. J. and Browne, J. C. McClure 1960, *Antenatal and Postnatal Care*, 9th edn, London: J. and A. Churchill Ltd.

Browner, C. H. and Press, Nancy A. 1996, "The production of authoritative knowledge in American prenatal care," *Medical Anthropology Quarterly* 10:141–56.

Canning, Kathleen 1994, "Feminist history after the linguistic turn: historicizing discourse and experience," *Signs* 19:368–404.

Chalmers, Iain, Enkin, Murray and Keirse, Marc J. N. C. (eds.) 1989, *Pregnancy*, Vol. 1, *Effective Care in Pregnancy and Childbirth*, Oxford: Oxford University Press.

Code, Lorraine 1991, *What Can She Know? Feminist Theory and the Construction of Knowledge*, Ithaca: Cornell University Press.

Conrad, Peter 1975, "The discovery of hyperkinesis: notes on the medicalization of deviant behavior," *Social Problems* 23:12–21.

1992, "Medicalization and social control," *Annual Review of Sociology* 18:209–32.

Duden, Barbara 1993, *Disembodying Women: Perspectives on Pregnancy and the Unborn*, Cambridge: Harvard University Press.

Eisenberg, Arlene, Murkoff, Heidi E. and Hathaway, Sandee E. 1986, *What to Eat When You're Expecting*, New York: Workman.

1991, *What to Expect When You're Expecting*, New York: Workman.

Feldblum, C. R. 1985, "Home health care for the elderly: programs, problems, and potentials," *Harvard Journal on Legislation* 22:193–254.

Gardiner, Judith Kegan 1987, "Self psychology as feminist theory," *Signs* 12:761–80.

Gubrium, Jaber F. and Lynott, R. J. 1987, "Family responsibility and caregiving in the qualitative analysis of the Alzheimer's disease experience," *Journal of Marriage and the Family* 50:197–207.

Gunew, Sneja 1990, "Feminist knowledge: critique and construct," in Sneja Gunew (ed.), *Feminist Knowledge: Critique and Construct*, London: Routledge.

Hasselkus, Betty R. 1988, "Meaning in family caregiving: perspectives on caregiver/professional relationships," *The Gerontologist* 28:686–91.

Henkart, Andrea Frank 1995, *Trust Your Body! Trust Your Baby!Childbirth Wisdom and Cesarean Prevention*, Westport, Connecticut: Bergin and Garvey.

Horowitz, A. and Shindelman, L. W. 1983, "Social and economic incentives for family caregivers," *Health Care Financing Review* 5:25–33.

Johnson, Robert V. 1994, *Mayo Clinic: Complete Book of Pregnancy and Baby's First Year*, New York: William Morrow and Co.

Keller, Evelyn Fox 1985, *Reflections on Gender and Science*, New Haven: Yale University Press.

Larson, Magali Sarfatti 1977, *The Rise of Professionalism: A Sociological Analysis*, Berkeley: University of California Press.

Lazarus, Ellen 1988, "Theoretical considerations for the study of the doctor-patient relationship: implications of a perinatal study," *Medical Anthropology Quarterly* (n.s.) 2:34–58.

Leavitt, Judith Walzer 1986, *Brought to Bed: Child-Bearing in America, 1750–1950*, New York: Oxford University Press.

Lewin, Ellen 1996, "'Why in the world would you want to do that?' Claiming community in lesbian commitment ceremonies," in Ellen Lewin (ed.), *Imagining Lesbian Cultures in America*, Boston: Beacon Press, pp. 105–30.

Liu, K., Manton, K. G. and Liu, B. M. 1985, "Home care expenses for the disabled elderly," *Health Care Financing Review* 7:51–8.

Lock, Margaret 1994, *Encounters with Aging: Mythologies of Menopause in Japan and North America*, Berkeley: University of California Press.

Martin, Emily 1987, *The Woman in the Body*, Boston: Beacon Press.

Miller, Baila 1990, "Gender differences in spouse management of the caregiver role," in Emily K. Abel and Margaret K. Nelson (eds.), *Circles of Care: Work and Identity in Women's Lives*, Albany: State University of New York Press, pp. 92–104.

Miller, Jean Baker 1976, *Toward a New Psychology of Women*, Boston: Beacon Press.

Montgomery, Rhonda J. V. 1988, "Respite care: lessons from a controlled design study," *Health Care Financing Review*, Annual Supplement:133–8.

Muncy, Robyn 1991, *Creating a Female Dominion in American Reform, 1909–1935*, New York: Oxford University Press.

Oakley, Ann 1982, "The relevance of the history of medicine to an understanding of current change: some comments from the domain of prenatal care," *Social Science and Medicine* 16:667–74.

1986, *The Captured Womb: A History of the Medical Care of Pregnant Women*, Oxford: Basil Blackwell.

Parsons, Talcot 1951, *The Social System*, New York: Free Press.

Pfohl, S. J. 1977, "The 'discovery' of child abuse," *Social Problems* 24:310–23.

Root, Robin, Press, Nancy A. and Browner, C. H. n.d. "Foucault, Feminism, and the Pregnant Body." Unpublished ms. in authors' files.

Sawicki, Jana 1991, *Disciplining Foucault: Feminism, Power, and the Body*, London: Routledge.

Schneider, J. W. 1978, "Deviant drinking as a disease; deviant drinking as a social accomplishment," *Social Problems* 25:361–72.

Scull, A. T. 1975, "From madness to mental illness: medical men as moral entrepreneurs," *European Journal of Sociology* 16:218–61.

Shanley, Laura Kaplan 1994, *Unassisted Childbirth*, Westport, Connecticut: Bergin and Garvey.

Sicherman, Barbara 1984, *Alice Hamilton: A Life in Letters*, Cambridge: Harvard University Press.

Siegel, J. S. and Taeuber, C. M. 1986, "Demographic perspectives on the long-lived society," *Daedalus* 115:77–118.

Stone, R. I., Cafferata, L. and Sangl, J. 1987, "Caregivers of the frail elderly: a national profile," *The Gerontologist* 27:616–26.

Thompson, Joyce E., Walsh, Linda V. and Merkatz, Irwin R. 1990, "The history of prenatal care: cultural, social, and medical contexts," in Irwin R. Merkatz and Joyce E. Thompson (eds.), *New Perspectives on Prenatal Care*, New York: Elsevier, pp. 9–30.

Wallace, Steven P. 1990, "The no-care zone: availability, accessibility, and acceptability in community-based long-term care," *The Gerontologist* 30:254–61.

Weedon, Chris 1987, *Feminist Practice and Poststructuralist Theory*, Cambridge, Massachusetts: Blackwell.

Wright, Peter W. G. 1988, "Babyhood: the social construction of infant care as a medical problem in England in the years around 1900," in Margaret Lock and Deborah Gordon (eds.), *Biomedicine Examined*, Dordrecht: Kluwer Academic Publishers, pp. 299–329.

14 The mission within the madness: self-initiated medicalization as expression of agency

Mark Nichter

Medicalization is often thought of in terms of the appropriation of social problems by the "medical profession" which establishes standards of normality as well as acceptable parameters of deviance (Conrad and Schneider 1980; 1992; Ingleby 1982; 1988; Nelkin and Tancredi 1989).[1] Through medicalization, social disorder is domesticated and social control exerted. This is accomplished in myriad of ways from the diagnosis and treatment of individual pathology to the manner in which a population is socialized to assume appropriate sick role behavior, from medical surveillance to self-monitoring, from discourse about risk to prevention programs which index personal responsibility.[2] The dominant medical system, the reasoning goes, is engaged in micropolitics at the site of the body and is complicit in supporting the hegemonic project of the state. Science is motivated despite claims of neutrality; through the production of knowledge about health, risk, and disease, the politics of "biopower" (Foucault 1980a; 1980b) is exercised.

In this chapter, medicalization will be considered from a different vantage point. Medicalization is not just the prerogative of the medical (psychological and medico-legal) professions and it is engaged for reasons other than social control. It is embraced by people for a variety of reasons. The medicalization of disorder may be self-initiated, engaged prior to medical confirmation or contrary to the opinion of doctors. Health-care seeking may be undertaken to legitimize and validate a sick role already assumed and enacted.

When unsanctioned by the dominant medical system, self-initiated medicalization tends to be evaluated by clinicians in terms of primary and secondary gain, that is, rewards patients derive from mobilizing resources (intrapsychic, emotional, economic) as they "work the system" (both social and medical systems) for their own benefit. While these constructs have some utility, they conceal as much as they reveal.[3] Glossed over by the use of these rubrics is the social context in which medicalization is adopted. Underappreciated are instances in which

327

self-initiated medicalization is adopted as a somatic idiom of distress deployed when other avenues of communication prove ineffective in a person's lifeworld (Nichter 1981).[4] Medicalization may also constitute a means of coping with suffering through the construction of a narrative to make sense out of chaotic life events which threaten one's sense of self integrity (Cassel 1982).[5] The medicalization of disorder may diminish as well as facilitate reflexivity. It may afford one the time and space in which to experience what Dilthy has referred to as an "impression point" (Stromberg 1985), a newly inspired reading of one's life reflecting a fundamental shift in personal meaning.

Medicalizing one's own state of dis-ease through the appropriation of medical diagnosis and the production of knowledge supporting one's claims of illness present a serious dilemma for the "democratic state" as well as the medical system. Assuming a chronic sick role for reasons unsubstantiated by medical truths constitutes an act of deviance which Parsons (1976) has highlighted in his writings on the sick role. Such deviance, he argued, poses a dire threat to American values of productivity, progress, and individual responsibility. To prevent the system from being undermined, the afflicted needed to work on becoming well with the help of doctors as paternalistic agents of the state, whose job was to guide them back to a productive goal and role oriented life.[6]

Patients who suffer from sickness and have little or no inclination to recover are "borderline" in multiple senses.[7] They challenge both the centrality of mainstream values and the limits of acceptable deviance. They "split" health care providers by raising contradictions implicit in their dual allegiance to the afflicted who require care, and the hospital as a state institution regulated by fiscal bodies. The refusal of the "afflicted" to engage in the work of becoming well (or becoming as functional as possible) triggers countertransference among professionals accustomed to "fighting the good fight." Challenged is their "good object" status as healers as well as the work ethic. Such patients present double binds for which there is no happy resolution, only endless struggles.

Control battles are commonly waged over self-initiated medicalization in American hospitals. Emergent during such battles is resistance to biomedical applications of body/mind dualism and the reduction of psychosocial and sociogenic problems to psychological states and predispositions. Also brought to light during such battles is the ambiguity of entitlements available to citizen-consumers who have come to expect care, not just cure from a medical system. Perceptions of the health care system as the compassionate arm of the state are placed in relief.[8] Exposed is the soft underbelly of a society which valorizes the heroic efforts of doctors to control disease in a world replete with suffering and in short supply of resources earmarked for "social services."

Doctors in the US (if not elsewhere) are placed in a paradoxical situation by the ethics of the Hippocratic oath and their role as gatekeepers for a medical system subject to economic constraints and profit motives.[9] As physicians, they are sworn to administer to the sick. As gatekeepers, they are told to remain vigilant and to guard the system against unauthorized intruders who may mask their state of dis-ease ("illth") such that it is made to appear as disease.[10]

Only bona fide (properly diagnosed), card carrying (insured) patients are welcomed into the medical system.[11] Others, those suffering but not "diseased" or adequately insured, are treated like second-class citizens, if not immigrants suspected of being illegal aliens. In both cases there is fear that if those at the margins are treated with too much compassion (care as well as cure) the system will become overwhelmed. However, just as determined illegal immigrants find entry into the US through porous state borders, those determined to enter the medical system find points of access.[12] Knowledge of the system is required, knowledge of how to key symptoms to differential diagnosis and report complaints in appropriate language. While gaining initial entry into the medical system is relatively easy, maintaining a legitimate basis for accessing the system is more problematic. This requires some finesse.

Many lessons are to be learned from those who are "borderline," those living at the margin of society who at once engage the medical system in resistance and calculated conformity. Like the possessed who speak through spirits enabling them to challenge the status quo while appealing to higher sources of power and authority, the dispossessed who self-medicalize appeal to higher sources of authority and ethics through their distress.[13] Both call attention to social injustice and contradictions in values, remind us of social obligations, and raise fundamental moral issues. Both express themselves through cultural performances in which the agency of the subject is manifest, yet consciousness is denied. In both cases an inchoate expression of unspoken negative feelings (alienation, frustration, dissatisfaction, anger, etc.) stands the chance of becoming domesticated, transformed by the medico-religious system through diagnosis/divination.[14] In both cases, attempts at domesticating disorder and dis-ease sometimes fail. Not all cases of sickness or spirit possession abate despite the best attempts of physicians or exorcists, hospitalizations or healing rituals. The afflicted are not always rendered docile, allowing their suffering to be defined out of existence or masked by therapeutic modalities as a manageable entity. This is an issue which I wish to address in the remainder of this chapter.

Considered will be the "case" of Joan, a "problem patient" actively engaged in the work of maintaining an illness identity against the best efforts of her doctors.[15] Joan's long history of persistent somatization is a legend in one of the hospitals I have worked at as a medical anthropologist.[16] I was initially "exposed to Joan" as part of my clinical education about "borderline personality disorder, hypochondriasis, and chronic pain of psychogenic origin." While several fascinating papers could be written on Joan's "pathology" from the vantage point of various therapeutic persuasions, I want to move beyond a consideration of differential diagnosis to an examination of what Joan was trying to accomplish in her own anguished way through self-initiated medicalization.[17] Attention will be drawn not to the pathology Joan "has," but to Joan's investment in being sick; how being ill was central to her sense of agency and means of coping with suffering. Joan once spoke to me of having a mission. It is to her mission that I ultimately want to direct attention in this chapter.

By way of background, let me present two descriptions of Joan as a patient before introducing Joan as she represented herself to me in the course of telling her story. Joan's clinical profile was gleaned from (a) the notes of an attending physician conducting a chart review for a publication he was preparing on care management and a grand rounds presentation, and (b) a psychiatrist following a consult-liaison patient evaluation requiring him to review and interpret Joan's record.[18] Juxtaposed to these profiles is the personal history Joan related to me over several hospitalizations which spanned a two-year period.

Joan's narrative was motivated and populated by several different voices (the voice of helplessness, the victim, the loving mother, the vigilant patient; the autobiographer, narrator, and evaluator).[19] Her history was selective. She emphasized and downplayed various details of her life in an effort to present herself to me in specific ways at different times. Her history was revisionist; it indexed her present feelings (and no doubt agenda) as well as her past. Joan knew that I had access to details of her life which were documented in hospital records that dated back several years. The telling and retelling of her story was an expression of Joan's agency.[20] I made no attempt to challenge her about the details of her life and treated discrepancies, omissions, and silences as a subtext in their own right. The unstated was often raised later, with Joan assuming that I was familiar with details of her life "captured" in hospital records. Following a side-long glance, she might say in passing "oh you know about my anorexia or drinking several years ago" and then pass over this subject as if it were a footnote bearing mention, but not a subject she wished to dwell upon.

Following a presentation of "patient profiles" and Joan's personal history, situational stressors which triggered Joan's episodes of acute illness over the two years in which I interacted with her are reviewed. I next consider her persistent somatization as at once a mode of intrapsychic defense, an idiom of distress, and a means of resistance to modes of control and psychiatric labeling by doctors. Attention will be drawn to the power dynamics set in motion by doctors' efforts to control Joan's somatization and demands for pain killers, and her efforts to resist such control and establish a sense of moral identity and personal agency.

Joan's medical profile: a summary by her attending physician

The patient, a 60-year-old Caucasian woman, was referred to the primary care clinic with abdominal complaints and a history of extensive use of various sedative-hypnotic drugs. The patient has a lengthy history of repeated hospitalizations for diagnostic studies, weight loss, intractable vomiting, abdominal pain, and vertigo. She has undergone three abdominal surgeries: a C-section with appendectomy, a negative exploratory laparotomy (except for adhesions), and a second negative laparotomy. In addition, the patient underwent a reduction mammoplasty and a negative breast biopsy. Medical records for the eighteen months prior to her presentation at the clinic revealed eight hospitalizations, the first seven of which will be listed and the seventh reviewed:

> removal of a chronic indwelling foley catheter: 9-day admission
> two medical admissions for colon problems: a 3-day and a 5-day admission
> chronic abdominal pain and exploratory laparotomy: 48-day admission
> Ménières disease: 10 days admission
> acute anxiety and hyperventilation: 7-day admittance for psychiatric observation (Christmas holidays).

During the seventh admission, the patient's physician refused to comply with her requests for pain medications and she was discharged. The following day she was readmitted to the hospital under the care of another physician with the same complaints. Psychiatric consultation was obtained, but the patient refused follow-up with either the physician or psychiatrist, leading to her referral to the primary care clinic. The patient arrived from the medical ward via wheelchair.

A review of the patient's record has revealed a lengthy list of diagnoses, most of which have little or no objective findings. Diverticulitis had been diagnosed in spite of repeated negative barium enemas. Additional problems included spastic bladder, atonic bladder, left atrial tumor, calcific pancreatitis, irritable colon, seizure disorder, and post-surgical incisional pain. The patient has been seen by at least twenty physicians in the past eighteen months, and in one twenty-four-day period had fourteen emergency room visits.

The patient has reported being allergic to ten medications, mostly phenothiazenes or antidepressants. However, the multiple somatic complaints she has drawn attention to are not indicative of true allergic reactions. The patient was using eight medications when admitted, including dalmane, valium (40 mg/day), and acetaminophen codeine (8 tablets/day). Some doubt exists among members of her care management team as to how many of these medications she has actually been taking. The patient has a history of stockpiling medicines.

The patient has cost the state health care system in excess of a quarter million dollars for physical ailments which are medically suspect. Although listed (blacklisted) in several of the city's hospitals, she has been remarkably successful in gaining access to health care facilities.

Psychiatric note: based upon a chart review and patient evaluation

The patient is preoccupied with self-deterioration and persistent physical symptoms dominate her life. She has a long history of unstable interpersonal relationships. The patient is a barometer of situational anxiety. Anxiety attacks are provoked by the slightest situational stress, resulting in episodic decompensation. Lack of social contact and loneliness also trigger somatic distress. The patient displaces intolerable affect onto the body and this is discharged somatically. During these times, the patient regresses and makes increasing demands on clinic staff and her doctor. This inevitably results in limit setting which the patient interprets as rejection. This pattern sets in motion a cycle of depression, rage, and increased somatization. Increased somatization provides her with a defense against acute depression. Being ill removes her from situations of interpersonal stress and mobilizes attention toward her. The patient is highly analytical and obsessively aware of detail. When interacting with doctors, she takes copious notes on what is said. The patient exhibits the major characteristics of borderline personality disorder with obsessive features.[21] She has been the cause of several incidents of staff splitting.[22]

Joan's personal history

Joan described herself to me as an only child of an unwanted pregnancy. She characterized her mother as selfish, man-crazy, and constantly needing to be the center of attention. Joan's father died shortly after her birth and her mother remarried a well-to-do banker. Joan spent the first eight years of her life in the Midwest living with her grandmother, a Germanic woman remembered for her frugal living and cleanliness. Joan also spent considerable time with her favorite uncle, a "real" physician whom she greatly admired for his gentleness and sensitivity.

At age 8, Joan joined her step-family in Seattle. She described herself as a "fifth wheel" perceived by her step-family as weak and sickly. With some anger, Joan described her mother as always stealing attention from her, upstaging her even when she was ill. Her mother was subject to swooning, an act Joan despised and described as being just a "ploy" and "just psychological."

As a youth, Joan was quiet, and a good student. After completing three years of college she married a public relations man working for a large firm. She described him as a *bon vivant*, a person charming in public, but personally distant. Joan stated that he spent much of his life trying to impress the wealthy family of a woman he had once wanted to marry, but who would have no part of him owing to his lower social standing. Asked what he saw in Joan, she replied without hesitation: "He married me for my quick mind and ability to talk to important people." He relied on Joan to orchestrate a harried life of dinner parties, a role she stated was unfulfilling, but pleasurable, because it put her in contact with interesting people: "judges, lawyers and doctors." What her husband had not told Joan was that they were living well beyond their means on credit, "living in a house of cards which came tumbling down."

Joan bore one son following a traumatic pregnancy. Delivery was overdue and by cesarean "instead of being normal." The baby was allergic to Joan's breastmilk, causing him to develop colitis. Joan's husband took little interest in his son and Joan described herself as showering love and attention on the child as a means of compensating for both the love her mother had not given her and the love her husband did not give the child.

At the age of three, the child was brought to a physician for complaints of recurring constipation and impacted bowels. A consulting psychiatrist found the child reluctant to defecate because he viewed the act as dirty. The psychiatrist suggested that this was linked to Joan's compulsiveness with cleanliness and order. A question the psychiatrist posed about incest had shocked Joan and cast psychiatrists in a negative light. Taking on the voice of "evaluator" Joan noted that:

Psychiatrists are not decent god-fearing doctors, in fact they are not real doctors at all. They look for the unspeakable, dredging the shadows of life instead of dealing with real problems, problems which require immediate attention not endless questions.

The untimely death of her husband when her son was an adolescent plunged Joan into deep financial crisis and forced her to move to an ethnically mixed, poor neighborhood. Joan described the neighborhood as "unfit for her maids," "not the type of place where decent people would want to visit let alone live." Her grief for her husband was intense but short-lived, but her loss of social position was a source of immense anger and pain, emotions which caused her pain to cascade when she related her narrative to me. Joan's anger was also directed to others in her social environment who abandoned her after her husband's death. Referring to them as "fair weather friends" who had enjoyed her company when she was well placed, she spoke of her condition as more than they could handle – a reminder of their own vulnerability.

Joan related three further losses to me. First, her son exhibited little tolerance or empathy for his mother's continuing ill health. Over the past ten years, he had become increasingly distant "after taking me to the cleaners." Following her son's discharge from the army for medical reasons (a peptic ulcer), he had returned to school, shifting his studies from art to psychology to law to computer science. During two years that I interacted with Joan, he completely dissociated himself from her. A second loss revealed by Joan was her mother's death. Prior to her death, Joan had tended to her mother's needs, but was chastised and subjected to considerable guilt for not being able to give enough. The third loss, "the straw which broke the camel's back," was the death of her dog. Joan described her dog as the "only one who had ever given her real and unconditional love." She suffered considerable guilt about the dog's death. During a moment of reflection, she blamed her own self-centeredness and multiple somatic complaints as preventing her from living up to her responsibilities to both her dog and son. Interestingly, the dog suffered from a series of somatic complaints which mirrored her own.

Situational stressors triggering episodes of acute illness

During the two years that I interacted with Joan she experienced episodes of acute pain associated with two sets of situational stressors, one related to her social environment and the other to her relations with her son. Joan's social isolation was periodically interrupted by a series of short-lived relationships with live-in boarders who exchanged companionship and personal assistance for use of the spare room in her apartment. A series of such relationships with people who were themselves socially marginal (an alcoholic, a schizophrenic, a homeless teenager) lasted on average from two to four weeks. The typical scenario was that Joan ended up feeling pressured to reject a boarder, which in turn raised her anxiety level and her somatic pain, resulting in a hospital admission. During her hospitalization she would have a social worker ask the boarder to leave. Joan would bemoan the fact that these were the type of people she was doomed to interact with as a result of her poverty. After a boarder left, she would reexperience feelings of abandonment, a feeling exasperated by clinicians' attempts to get her stabilized and out of the hospital.

A second stressor was memories of her son and dog. Lack of communication with her son, who entirely dissociated himself from his mother, was incredibly painful to Joan, especially around the Christmas holidays. Joan felt her identity as a mother was negated by his avoidance of her. Motherhood, be it expressed in terms of her son or dog, was one of the only positive identities Joan had ever been able to assume. Memories of either dog or son caused her considerable pain.

Psychosocial evaluation

It fell within my scope of work as a "therapy facilitator" (Nichter et al. 1985) to evaluate social interactional and symbolic dimensions of Joan's somatization at home and on the ward. What follows is a synopsis of my notes on Joan's social interaction with doctors and her use of somatization as an idiom of distress and means of establishing moral identity as well as a mode of resistance.

Doctor–patient interactions

Over the course of two years, I identified seven themes which typified Joan's interactions with doctors through an assessment of a cycle of performances (Brodwin 1992) in the hospital:[23]

1 Entering the hospital placed Joan in the company of doctors whom

she viewed as intellectually stimulating: "people with vocabulary and grammar."[24] She felt comfortable meeting doctors on their own ground and employed a number of leveling devices as a means of establishing a more egalitarian relationship with them. For example, upon meeting a consulting psychiatrist whom she perceived as arrogant, Joan replied that she called Jesus by his first name and would be damned if she was going to refer to him as "doctor X" instead of John.[25]

2 Joan took offense at being treated like "just another patient, a statistic, a type X." It was important for her to be recognized as special, a challenging case. She went out of her way to demonstrate that she was "not your average run of the mill patient." Joan responded positively to doctors' requests for more diagnostic tests as exploratory activities, but resisted all efforts to "pigeon hole" her problems. She reminded doctors that there is individual variation in the way illness manifests and is experienced.

3 Joan took offense at being "talked down to." She demanded to be informed of even the smallest medical decision, wrote down medical terminology for future reference, and checked all medications prescribed to her in a personal copy of the physician's desk reference of medications (PDR). Catching a doctor's misrepresentation of a medicine was a source of one-upmanship for Joan. On the ward, residents were warned to pay heed to her knowledge of medicine. In the words of one resident:

You have to be careful with her, I mean this is the only game in town for her . . . She is obsessed with the details of her illness and she studies up on everything you are supposed to consider when you encounter certain sets of symptoms. She is there in your face if you don't look into everything . . . of course you can't because it would cost a fortune . . . it has cost a fortune . . . so you have to humor her . . . you know, do some of it to give her attention . . . but then you get this feeling she is setting some kind of trap and you are going to fall in sometime when you are not on your toes. You get this feeling that she is laying there waiting for you.

4 Joan's relationship with medications was paradoxical. She expressed disdain for physicians prescribing excessive medication and reported intolerance to a long list of medications. On the other hand, alterations in her medications evoked anxiety. Alterations in medicine implied changes in her relationship with a doctor and her sick role identity.[26] Medicine exchange insured the continuity of a familiar doctor–patient relationship and was a measure of her success in impressing upon her doctor the seriousness of her condition. Joan stockpiled medicines and used them at her own discretion as a form of self-regulation. More often than taking quantities of medicine above those recommended, she

hoarded medicine as "symbolic capital," tokens of her successful interactions with doctors. When necessary, she self-regulated medicines to produce symptoms warranting medical investigation.

5 Joan had little respect for "psyche types" and was irritated by any suggestion that she see a psychiatrist. Such a suggestion was interpreted by her as shifting attention from her body to her mind. Joan referred to the psyche team as "storm troopers who came to do battle in your mind when you lie there wounded in your body." She once remarked that "these people don't so much take your history as take your history from you and do with it as they please." Joan considered such "history taking" as an act of violence as doctors "got to (re)write your history any way they wanted."[27] She felt that psyche types were less interested in understanding your problems than "dissecting your past," "uprooting old problems," "opening up scars which had taken a long time to close, however imperfectly." Joan had no desire to "play their game." And yet she had become a master at doing so.

6 Joan was demanding and when her demands were not fulfilled she acted out in a manner staff interpreted as a display of passive aggression. She commonly reproached clinical staff during rounds for her lack of care only to engage them at the close of a scheduled interview. Joan was very sensitive to time politics in the hospital.[28] Doctor and staff time was as important to her as securing medicine as a measure of positive interaction. Capturing staff time was an expression of her agency. I was forewarned by one resident to wear my watch on the inside of my wrist and not to glance at it when seeing Joan. In her words, "with patients like Joan, look at your watch and it's the kiss of death, they feel totally rejected, and for her that means that her symptoms are going to escalate – and you'll be back in there before you know it."

7 Doctors who tried to reassure Joan that her pain would diminish and who cut her description of pain short, established poor relationships with her and set in motion a cycle of increased pain. Doctors who played up her pain by saying such things as "that's as much pain as I've ever seen a patient bear" or "I frankly don't know how you bear this pain alone" established closer relationships with Joan resulting in decreased reports of pain. The most successful care management plan devised for Joan involved a shift of focus from a search for "real pathology" to Joan's physical sensitivity as a constitutional proclivity easily aggravated by environmental stresses. This was framed not as a shift from the physically valid to the mentally suspect, but from simple pathology to complex interrelationships between a set of biopsychosocial concomitants. Emphasis was placed on efforts to keep Joan in "relative health" given her "condition." This management plan required

Joan to check into an outpatient facility frequently to see a doctor familiar with the specifics of her condition, rather than being subject to changing hospital staff who would not be able to understand Joan's case.[29] In other words, this plan increased doctor's surveillance of her condition and asked Joan to play a more active role in self-monitoring of her condition.

Idioms of distress

When I first met Joan, I asked her how she handled distressful feelings. Talking in terms of generalities, Joan spoke to me about her tendency to internalize bad emotions. She "swallowed anger and sadness causing it to fester inside and make her sick."[30] I observed Joan's emotional response to several stressful life events. Her chief means of processing and communicating distress to others was through the pain of bodily symptoms. Specific symptoms often served as evocative symbols for emotional states.[31] For example, on several occasions while pressing her lower abdomen, Joan referred to her personal losses as "painful emotional scars she did not want to irritate by thinking about them." Her greatest physical pains were located in regions of her body associated with traumatic memories: scars from a cesarean section and a breast which could not nurture, gastrointestinal problems and adhesions which flared up at times of social isolation and loneliness, such as times when Joan was acutely aware of having to eat alone.[32] When pain in these bodily regions occurred, Joan applied ice packs to them, ice packs which she openly displayed and frequently demanded during hospitalizations. Her desire for a foley catheter and wheelchair were symbolic expressions of helplessness and her ongoing request for laxatives was associated with her desire to "push out the poison" associated with "rotten feelings," "feelings that were festering, eating her up."

Some of the doctors whom Joan encountered attempted to decode these bodily symbols as a means of increasing Joan's insight. This only served to exacerbate her physical pain. Joan felt these doctors were attempting to discredit and preempt her experience. Joan expressed to me on several occasions her exasperation with doctors who "wouldn't listen to her body even when it was screaming with pain."[33] On one occasion she complained:

Instead of paying attention to your pain they go about their own business, their own agenda. You are a case to be poked and probed. They talk and you suffer and finally things get so bad that they just have to give you medicine. Then they act as if that is what you wanted all the time . . . Can you imagine that . . . and after they have rubbed salt in your wounds! Sometimes they apologize as they are leaving . . . as they have one foot out the door . . . and then you do want to talk to them because they recognize how much you are in pain. You have gotten through, but its too late. They are already thinking about their next damned chart!

Joan was easily angered by doctors who attempted to discredit the voices of her body and render them mute. Her primary idiom of distress was a series of chronic gastrointestinal ailments which she described in no uncertain terms as "constitutional." She defended the legitimacy of her "condition" against all forms of biomedical reductionism, speaking of her condition as a "can of worms no doctor could understand."[34] While doctors could not understand her "condition" she did feel that attentive doctors – "real doctors" – could come to appreciate her vulnerability and know how to manage her pain.

Joan resisted being labeled a "psychiatric patient." A point of particular sensitivity was any attempt to link her behavior to that of her mother. When one resident suggested to Joan that she might be predisposed to somatization because her mother had a long history of "swooning" Joan became livid and then doubled over in pain clutching her stomach. Joan's somatic idiom of distress took on meaning in opposition to that of her mother. Joan devalued her mother's actions, describing them as "only psychological." The legitimacy of her own experience was closely tied to her physical body, a body in pain which did not lie. Doctors, in their desire to search for psychological causes of her pain, challenged her identity and placed her in the same camp as her mother.

Resistance

During one hospitalization, Joan became quite agitated when it was suggested that she see a psychiatrist. She questioned a resident about whether she thought Joan was a hypochondriac. The resident replied that yes, she did think that Joan suffered from hypochondriasis. Following this interaction Joan suffered from intense pain which she associated with adhesions from a past surgery. The possibility of being referred to a psychiatrist was a direct challenge to the legitimacy of her condition and the bodily experience of pain she felt. Called in to find out why Joan was so agitated, I found that her interpretation of hypochondriasis was equivalent to malingering. The situation was defused when I had the resident clarify for Joan her definition of hypochondriasis. For the resident, hypochondriasis was a state wherein physical pain was amplified by emotional distress. Following this explanation, Joan calmed down and volunteered a description of her pain as having the characteristics of an echo:

You feel something . . . some pain deep inside . . . and you are hollow, alone. And the pain keeps repeating like an echo and you can hear your heart beating like a drum . . . sometimes a siren. Sometimes it repeats over and over and eventually it quiets down. Other times it gets louder and louder and I need a pill to make it stop. But that doesn't mean it's all in my mind. The pain, it's in my body . . . it just echoes in my mind. I'm not making it up! And I can't stop it. How do you control an echo? Don't give me that mind control crap – like fill your mind with positive thoughts. You try and have positive thoughts with my condition! It's just too hard to keep it up, too much . . . all of the time. There is just too much emptiness and hurt. It's too much to ask . . . with all the problems I have . . . and no one who really cares. You know my story, what do I have to feel positive about? The doctors have a life to feel positive about! What do they know about suffering? They should know if they are going to treat people like humans!

Some doctors spoke to Joan about developing a more positive attitude about life and told her to look around in the hospital at people who were far worse off than she was. Joan complained to me that being told to maintain a positive attitude made her feel worse because "when you can't do it you fail again." What Joan could not understand was why she was being blamed for her poor health when she was a victim of circumstances.[35] She remarked:

Look these damn doctors keep on looking for my strengths instead of seeing my weakness . . . They want me to fight my pain, but how can I, given my present state? They tell me that taking medicines makes me weaker and that they are reducing the dosage for my own good. They want to fight other people's battles at a safe distance . . . but it's me that has to pay the price. It's me that feels the pain not them . . . and then I have to suffer their disappointment . . . you can see it in their eyes . . . It's all backward you know . . . they are failing you . . . but if you tell them, you are transferred to someone else and the whole thing starts all over again. They tell me I have to learn how to cope . . . it's on their terms or else . . . but my condition is not like that.

One humanistic resident talked to Joan about alternative healing. In a discussion with me he stated: "it sure couldn't hurt and it might help, I mean it's less invasive and more interactive . . . and she'd get lots of attention." Joan was not impressed with the suggestion. While she chastised doctors for not caring and being "cocky," she viewed alternative healing as a form of medical deviance and not something with which she wanted to get involved. Joan recalled observing Judy, a patient she had met during a brief stay on the psychiatric ward. Judy championed new age healing, speaking of it as an alternative to biomedicine, a system of medicine she was convinced was engaged in mind control. Judy was hospitalized for bipolar disease after experimenting with herbal drugs instead of "taking her lithium." Judy had told Joan that "through knowing your body you could find your own cure." According to Judy, doctors prevented you from knowing your body because they numbed your senses and made you incapable of taking control of your own life.

Joan had little interest in learning to take control in the sense described by Judy. She commented: "If doctors can't find out what is wrong with you when it's their job, how are you supposed to figure it out? As for going to one of those alternative type practitioners, well I'm a good Christian." Joan also had no interest in partaking in Judy's demonization of biomedicine. Joan had a stake in the biomedical system. She sought medicalization of her condition, but on her own terms, terms which provided her a sense of dignity. What she resisted was being rendered docile, an object of psychiatric analysis and a target of interventions ordered by doctors to make her more manageable.

Joan's mission

Joan's Christianity was closely tied to her moral identity. Joan spoke of reading her Bible as a primary source of solace in the hospital. It was her "trump card in a deck stacked against her." Pointing to her Bible, which I only saw her read occasionally, Joan once remarked to me that it had greater authority and wisdom than "all the books about medicine in the world." During one memorable hospitalization, she kept a copy of the Bible and a copy of the PDR side by side next to her bed. Members of "her medical team" were in the process of trying to convince Joan of the potential benefits of a new medication. Joan looked up the medication in her personal copy of the PDR. Finding that it was an antidepressive medication, she became quite annoyed. Joan felt that through their medications, doctors were trying to redefine her illness experience as depression instead of dealing with her real pain experienced within her body.[36]

A resident had told Joan that the new medicine was very promising because it would "help her get feelings out which were locked up inside while at the same time increasing her appetite." In the resident's presence, Joan opened up the PDR to the appropriate page and proceeded to ask him why he had neglected to tell her it was an antidepressant? She then opened the Bible and remarked that it was a shame that doctors did not have the time to read the "Good Book" because it would remind them about such things as truth, honesty, and respect for fellow human beings.

One of Joan's doctors was very interested in her religious affiliation, hoping that it might prove a potential avenue for social support outside the health care system. I was sent to investigate. Joan told me that she had not participated in organized religious activities for a long time owing to her sickness. She often thought about God, however. She then confided in me that the only reason she did not commit suicide was because of her religious principles and belief in God's plan. She wished she was dead, but God had other plans for her. Suffering was her lot in life and she just had to bear it the best she could and believe that it served some purpose. It was at this point that Joan described this purpose to me as her "mission." Joan's mission was not elaborated in great detail and was thought of as emergent, just as her pain was emergent. Notably, it entailed lessons for Joan as well as lessons she was meant to deliver to doctors.

On one occasion, Joan was asked by a senior physician if she would be so kind as to participate in behavioral rounds, a learning exercise for medical students which I also attended. During behavioral rounds a patient is asked to give a short history and describe how their illness experience has affected their lives. Joan dwelled upon the pain her scar tissue caused her and spoke of how doctors did the best they could. She made it a point to state that it was not possible for doctors to "desensitize" the pain caused by old scars. All they could do was numb the pain for a time through medicines. As the students were about to leave, she added:

Well I suppose I'm a can of worms, not a neat case like the cases you find in your books . . . I'm not the patient that gets well, thanks the doctor for all he has done, and makes him feel proud to be a doctor. God did not create pain to give you doctors job security or something to conquer. God has his reasons for pain and why people must bear it, reasons we can never know. I've seen my share of doctors. Some play God and others know they are his servants. That tall doctor, the shrink who came and saw me yesterday, asked me the meaning of some proverb as a test to see if I had all my marbles. I have something for you to think about: The first degree of folly is to hold oneself wise, the second to profess it, and the third to despise counsel.

Joan was quite pleased with herself following the interview and had a good appetite. While eating her lunch she commented to me:

The least I can do is share my experience, after all I've probably seen the worst and best of this place and have learned a thing or two in the process. Perhaps the young ones haven't lost their humanity yet or its not too late for them to find it . . . It's probably good for them to meet someone like me . . . Someone their teachers can not diagnose as a classic case of this or that . . . Someone they will have to listen to in order to know how to take care of them.

Out of curiosity I asked Joan about the adage (noted above) she had presented to the team during behavioral rounds and what meaning it had for her. Joan smiled and said:

Oh I've been waiting to use that one, it's really good isn't it. It really disarms those cocky doctors carrying the big guns. I found it in some magazine . . . I can't remember who said it, but what does it matter? It makes them think. It gives them a good dose of their own medicine.

From what I could gather, Joan's mission was to foster reflexivity among doctors; to render them more humble and respectful of patients at the margin. In wanting to give doctors "a dose of their own medicine," Joan redefined her own marginality as serving a higher purpose, a purpose which provided her a moral identity.[37] At the same time, Joan was a deeply troubled, alienated, and lonely woman whose pain was agonizing, not simply strategic. Her somatization was a call for help, not just a performance. Joan's mission, to the extent it was successful and for whatever reasons it was undertaken, was her saving grace.

Discussion

In order to appreciate fully the many dimensions of Joan's self-initiated medicalization, it is important to consider how she perceived her illness. Lipowski (1970) has identified several themes commonly underlying interpretations of illness: illness as challenge, punishment, enemy, weakness, irreparable loss/damage, lesson, relief. In the present case, doctor and patient interpretations of Joan's illness were largely incongruent. Clinicians encouraged Joan to view her symptoms and pain as a challenge, something to be fought and not succumbed to. They warned Joan about losing her tolerance for pain when she requested pain medications. They also encouraged Joan to work through psychological issues and personal losses. Joan, on the other hand, complained of being "tired of coping." She viewed her bouts of illness as evidence of irreparable damage compounded by a "condition" which predisposed her to feel her losses and other negative emotions somatically. Her weak and sensitive gastrointestinal tract, "her Achilles heel," was her basic fault (Balint 1957), something she could do nothing about.[38] She had no interest in working through psychological issues related to losses, as doing so increased, rather than decreased, her pain. Joan's condition was also a source of "lessons" linked to God's plan for her.

Joan found comfort and a sense of satisfaction in the problematic nature of her illness. Her use of a somatic idiom of distress was challenged by doctors anxious to "stabilize her" and keep her out of the emergency room. Over the course of two years, I observed different doctors try to manage Joan with a variety of interactional styles and care management plans reflecting a range of different approaches to dealing with "this type of problem patient." These plans called for changes in medications, batteries of tests, the negotiation of contracts, referrals to psychiatrists, and threats of abandonment if she "didn't play ball." Joan was passed from resident to resident until a primary care doctor with an interest in chronic pain patients "took her on."

During all of this, Joan struck me as being strategically compliant when necessary as she engaged in the work of self-medicalization. She vigorously resisted subjugation through shifts in diagnosis and medication which would serve to redefine her illness experience in ways she considered untenable. Through studying medical texts and the PDR, Joan subverted the exercise of power by doctors. She appropriated medical knowledge and used her knowledge of signs and symptoms, medicines and tests, to work the system in a manner she perceived to be in her favor.

Joan once described to me how taxing it was to remain vigilant while being in the hospital. While others might see a hospital stay as rest and refuge, clean sheets, TV and meal service, Joan described her interactions with hospital staff as exhausting, "like paddling a canoe against the current while watching out for submerged rocks." I repeatedly asked myself: what did Joan get out of engaging the medical system the way she did? Beyond psychiatric considerations which no doubt run deep, one motivation strikes me as worthy of further reflection.

Perhaps it was those in power, those doctors and hospital administrators who challenged Joan, who provided her with the very means by which to express her agency.[39] Joan's sense of agency could not be experienced in the social vacuum she occupied outside the hospital. It required the participation of "those who mattered" and the challenging of relations of power embedded in routine medical practices and procedures.[40] This possibility invites us to reconsider the presence of agency in what Foucault (1980b) has described as the interplay between power and resistance.[41] Joan's sense of agency was experienced within this interplay, within the emergent space opened up by a liminal medical condition over which doctors could not exercise control, a condition described in terms of God's plan and Joan's role in the hospital.

Joan's condition gave her a mission and a sense of efficacy. Her mission involved reminding doctors of how medicine was supposed to be practiced, an idealized perception I believe she formed as a child when cared for by her good uncle. It entailed resisting being processed and reified as a "case" (object) and not a person, an issue she contended with all her life, i.e., a key issue for transference. "Doctor heal thyself"

Joan once muttered as a doctor departed from her room leaving her visibly upset. Joan recognized that it was the vocation of doctors to try and cure patients. Her mission was not conceptualized in terms of resisting biomedicine as was the case with Judy, the patient who took herbs instead of lithium. Joan embraced biomedicine. What she resisted was the way medicine was being practiced, its cure instead of care orientation. Her mission became to teach doctors to respect the uniqueness of their patients' illness experiences. It entailed altering relations of power which stripped patients of their sense of agency and dignity.

Disenfranchised by the social system she once knew, but unwilling to be "tossed aside and forgotten like some kind of derelict," "written off" or rendered invisible, Joan used medicine as a means of retaining her dignity and establishing a sense of moral identity. Her moral identity was derived from a work of illness quite different from that described by Parsons in his characterization of the sick role. Quite the opposite of being compliant and following doctors' orders to the letter, this "work" entailed monitoring the medical system for subtle and not-so-subtle applications of biopower which would render her powerless. It entailed resisting attempts to psychologize her distress (analyze her past for the presence of psychopathology) and delegitimate her somatic experience of distress.

A central reason why Joan resisted psychological evaluation of her condition was that she felt this placed the burden of responsibility for her sickness (and its management) on her "weary self." Physical illness was attended to by physicians whose job it was to "search for answers and make patients as comfortable as possible." Joan viewed a psychological interpretation of her sickness as a "cop out by doctors who really didn't care," "a way doctors wrote you off when they don't want to care for you anymore." If Joan had a crusade, it was to remind doctors that whether or not they could cure a patient's condition, it was their responsibility to care for patients like her with respect.

It is only possible to discover those meanings in one's life that one's defenses permit. While Joan was unable to be reflexive about her own life, she was quite reflexive about medicine. Being hypersensitive to contradictions in the way medicine was "practiced and preached," Joan became a problem patient in several senses of the term. She was difficult to manage and therefore costly to the system, something hospital administrators pointed out every time she gained entry to the hospital. Joan was a problem for hospital staff because she was so demanding, treating staff the way she once treated her servants. She was a problem for doctors who grew increasingly frustrated with treating her. This

resulted in referrals and problems of countertransference which influenced care management. Labeled a "tar baby," a sticky case one got
more and more entangled with the closer one got, Joan was assigned to
young clinicians (and a medical anthropologist) as part of their rite of
passage, an experience somehow meant to "build character."

Among more experienced staff in the house of medicine, Joan's
sickness became another one of those "tragic dramas you get used to
and learn not to react to over time." While Joan's admittance to the
hospital angered many staff ("My God is that woman back in here,
what idiot admitted her!"), her presence was appreciated by a few
veteran clinicians. An attending physician and a senior nurse joked
with me over lunch one day that Joan was worth keeping around for
the lessons she taught idealistic young clinicians and "doctor-knows-it-
all types."

Toward the end of my work on the ward, I was asked by a few
clinicians in training to share with them my impressions of Joan.
Mention of Joan's mission was met by nervous laughter. One resident
joked about Joan, calling her "mission impossible" to the delight of his
colleagues. The senior nurse (noted above) overheard the conversation
and made what I thought was a most insightful comment: "Dealing
with the impossible brings out the best and the worst in people."

NOTES

1 As Conrad and other social scientists have pointed out, medicalization is far
more complex than simply doctors appropriating social problems as a means
of expanding their domain of expertise and control. It needs to be
appreciated that (1) the medical profession is often pushed into medicalizing
social problems by organizational pressures and bureaucratic systems
(Daniels 1969; Ingleby 1982), the interests of moral entrepreneurs, public
sentiment and those forces which shape it, and (2) vested interest groups
within the medical system champion particular diagnoses challenged by
other factions. Biomedicine is too often reified and presented as monolithic.
Consensus on what constitutes legitimate disease (e.g. hypoglycemia, PMS,
chronic fatigue syndrome) does not exist among doctors within, let alone
across, different subspecialties. Medicalization has been studied by other
researchers in relation to lowering thresholds of discomfort (e.g., Barsky
1988a; 1988b; Nichter and Vuckovic 1994; Sonberg and Kema 1986;
Vuckovic and Nichter 1997) and shifts in medical surveillance from doctors'
tests to the self-monitoring of bodily process (Illich 1976; 1986).

2 My use of the term index connotes communication intent as distinct from
what is being overtly referred to during a communication act. For example,
calling attention to a health problem associated with lifestyle-related risk
indexes responsibility. Calling attention to a symptom may index an affective
state, e.g., loss, abandonment, anger, beyond a person's capacity to discuss

in a given context. Further, as Bakhtin has reminded us, discourse is often double voiced in that utterances come with a social history, a residue of past interactions which affect current language use.

3 Primary gain refers to the intrapsychic, psychological mechanism which defends one from unacceptable affect or conflict. Secondary gain is the interpersonal or environmental advantage which symptom(s) offer one who is recognized to be suffering (Bokin et al. 1981:331). This encompasses what Linda Alexander (1982) has described as the "new American sick role" wherein those who are ill and compensated for their illness have little motivation to give up a self-serving sick role sanctioned by public policy. As Brodwin (1992) notes, the rubric "secondary gain" more commonly refers to "the practical benefit accruing to the person in pain, than the actual rhetorical process through which pain complaints can alter the balance of power or redefine the complex dynamics of a social environment."

4 Somatization is often spoken of by doctors as providing patients with primary and secondary gain defined in terms of defense mechanisms and the manipulation of others for personal advantage. While primary and secondary gain are fairly elastic terms, they do not capture the full range of meanings associated with somatization. Somatization is often employed as an idiom of distress, a means of communicating vulnerability and/or sensitivity to unspoken issues. The way in which distress is articulated entails both the type of pain the sufferer has experienced and the manner in which this pain has been embodied. Also entailed is the response of others to expressions of pain based upon their own experiences as they are influenced by such factors as culture and family style of articulating distress. Somatization may also constitute a form of resistance to specific figures who wield power and/or representations of others (people, institutions) hailed by way of transference relations.

5 I follow Cassel in my use of the term suffering as a state of severe distress associated with events that threaten the intactness of a person's self-concept. Suffering continues until a person's self-integrity can be restored in some manner through a coherent set of meanings.

6 For Parsons (1976), health is the capacity to undertake successful goal- and role-oriented courses of action. When illness is employed as a motivated escape from the pressures and routine of normative role-driven life, it constitutes deviance society must regulate. See Scheper-Hughes and Lock (1991) for a critical rereading of Parsons which describes the need to defuse the revolutionary potential of the sick role as an act of refusal and dissent. Parsons's theory of sick role has been critiqued as (a) being medicocentric, (b) not applying to chronic illness (the sick role is not always temporary, role exemptions are not always viewed positively, stigma and perceptions of responsibility often adhere to disease and disability), (c) assuming the neutral, unbiased, and ethical role of doctors, and (d) taking as given consensus in the normative basis of the sick role which assumes a single stable value system (that of middle-class America) that overlooks gender, class, and cultural variations. Parsons's ideas about the sick role support conservative thinking in America.

7 My use of the term borderline is distinct from conceptualizations of

borderline personality disorder advanced by such psychoanalysts as Kohut and Kernberg.

8 Patients such as the one described in this chapter commonly relate to the hospital as a "mother object" in the sense of being a space of caring. Rejection by the hospital rekindles previous rejection by mother figures (including institutions) through relations of transference. Performances within the hospital are commonly multidimensional, merging the past with the present.

9 The increased surveillance of health providers, e.g., utilization review, prompted by managed care guidelines and cutbacks in personal services has intensified the double bind of accountability giving providers less latitude to negotiate care management with patients.

10 For a discussion of dis-ease as a state of "illth" see Frankenberg (1986).

11 Being welcomed into the medical system has as much to do with payment as with having a viable diagnosis. Greater research is needed in diagnosis by capacity to pay.

12 In both cases, more attention is directed to erecting fences and boundaries than rectifying conditions which lead people to cross borders as acts of desperation. Others might argue that discourse on the threat of illegal aliens is a smokescreen serving political agenda. Token gestures displace attention from the fact that aliens contribute far more to the American economy than they take out. A similar case could be made for hospitals which reject non-paying patients having "questionable diagnosis" while catering to others from whom payment may be secured.

13 I draw here on my long-term research on spirit possession in south India.

14 Scheper-Hughes and Lock (1991) speak to the problematic nature of using illness as an idiom of distress. Once dissent is expressed at the site of the body, signs of dis-ease may be translated into medical language, treated as the signs of disease, and explained in ways which distance them from the social problems with which they are associated.

15 In this case the "work(s) of illness" entails the work of instantiating an illness identity as well as the emotional work of sickness, "working" the medical system as well as working with and against doctors.

16 Somatization is a rubric which encompasses a continuum of illness states ranging from unconsciously induced or magnified symptom states to symptom states consciously produced or misrepresented. As Mayou (1976) has aptly reminded us, somatization is not a separate entity, but a psychological reaction to distress which, like anxiety or depression, ranges from a passing state to totally disabling severity. I have used the term persistent somatization as a descriptive rather than a diagnostic term following Abey and Lipowsky (1987) and Lipowsky (1986).

17 Joan's "case" would invite several different types of clinical assessment. For example, Joan could be seen as having a personality disorder along the lines of the ICD-10 (World Health Organization 1992). The ICD-10 links personality disorders to developmental conditions which emerge from strategies adopted at an early age to deal with social-environmental challenges. Adoption of a sick role as a coping strategy might be seen as a learned adaptive response engaged by those who have no other viable avenues of coping available to them. Bass and Murphy (1995) argue for

assessing the manner in which adoption of a somatic idiom of distress affects a person's cognitive style, self-image, and personality development. Joan's "case" might also be examined in light of similarities observed between hypochondriasis and obsessive-compulsive disorders.

18 Some details of Joan's record have been altered to protect her confidentiality. Clinical profiles were shared with me as a member of the team that was responsible for Joan's care management. Joan was well aware that I was an anthropologist collecting the life histories of patients and not a clinician. She often related to me as an empathetic witness (Kleinman 1988).

19 My use of the term "voice" draws both upon Goffman's (1974) concept of "figures" as personages manifest during dramaturgical presentations of self and Bakhtin's (1973) writings on the dialogic self in which a plurality (polyphony) of voices accompany and oppose one another. Lamentations of self (inner voices) are found within Joan's narrative. As Bakhtin has noted, the privileging of voice entails a conscious choice enabling the speaker to orient the listener as to her emotional state and moral identity at a given point in time. The conceptualization of a plurality of consciousness broadens an assessment of "personality" as an individual may live in multiple worlds and author multiple narratives.

20 Following Giddens (1979), I conceive of human agency as involving reflexive monitoring and rationalization of a continuous flow of conduct rather than a sequence of discrete acts of choice and planning.

21 Joan's clinical profile was characterized by various doctors (between 1972 and 1981) as falling between the diagnostic categories of Briquet's syndrome, psychalgia, and Munchausen syndrome on a somatization continuum (Nadelson 1979). Her somatization, obsessiveness, and intellectualization were characterized as maladaptive *primary* defense "mechanisms" used to cope with untenable emotion-laden psychological pain.

22 Splitting in this context refers to pitting clinical staff against each other through subtle manipulation often associated with the treating of various staff as good and bad objects-identities which was often short lived.

23 My thinking about cycles of performances has benefited from Brodwin's (1992) writing on chronic pain and social performance. Instead of focusing on the family as Brodwin does, I focus on responses to somatic pain in the hospital by staff.

24 It was very important to Joan that people within an acceptable reference group acknowledge her. The only members of this reference group Joan interacted with following the death of her husband were doctors she met during hospitalizations.

25 Joan also employed wit and irony as leveling devices, what Scott (1985) has referred to as "weapons of the weak."

26 In some instances Joan resisted alterations in medications because these medications were associated with the idealized memories of good doctors who had helped her in the past. Giving up the medicine meant cutting herself off from these memories of care providers.

27 On the sense of violence that patients feel when doctors produce a medical report out of fragments of historical data, see Poirier and Brauner (1988) who draw on the writings of Derrida.

28 On the means by which time creates and reinforces patterns of control in the hospital see Frankenberg (1988).

29 This care plan was devised in part on the basis of ethnographic data presented in this paper. It was developed by a primary care doctor who was responsive to the growing literature in the 1980s arguing for a biopsychosocial model of medicine (Brody 1980; Engel 1980; Katon and Kleinman 1980; Stoeckle and Barsky 1980). My role as an anthropologist in assisting Joan's medical team to devise a care plan took into consideration the critique of the negotiation model provided by Taussig (1980; 1992).

30 During moments of reflection Joan often shifted from the first to the second person and conceded that loneliness or anger upset her stomach and brought on pain. This was typically followed by a "medical voice" which instantiated her pain as medical not psychological, a medical condition aggravated by stress and worries.

31 Brodwin (1992) following Hughes and Ziman (1978) speaks of a "vocabulary of symptoms" generalized within a family as an idiom of distress. Based upon Joan's description of a good doctor who treated her in the past and "understood," it is possible that such a code influenced her somatization and evaluation of doctors' sensitivity, i.e. ability to understand.

32 Joan found it uncomfortable to eat alone and after her husband's death suffered from anorexia leading her to be tube fed. Following her recovery, she commonly complained of gastric discomfort whenever she ate. Joan lived on a very meager diet at home and conveyed to me that food just didn't "sit right" when she ate alone. When in the company of others, including this researcher, she had a healthy appetite and ate while engaged in conversation. Her appetite constituted a somatic idiom of distress as well as a measure of comfort.

33 At the same time, doctors read Joan's somatization as an inability to come to terms with her feelings leading her to displace them.

34 On the reification of disease as a form of dehumanization see Taussig (1980).

35 "Blaming the victim" (Ryan 1971) has been described as treating the victim as responsible for an occurrence rather than the agents causing or exacerbating misfortune. Joan felt as if she were being blamed for her pain when it was factors beyond her control which provoked her sensitive constitution.

36 Through metonymic as well as metaphoric association individuals become identified by medicines prescribed by doctors or self-administered. Consuming medications is part of the labeling process which often leads to the reification of "the patient."

37 It is not uncommon for the afflicted to take on a positive moral identity following an "impression point" (Stromberg 1985) experience where their life takes on new meaning. Examples include those who are HIV positive who become community activists and drug users who become outreach workers after viewing their affliction as a life lesson or divine calling. See as well the writings of I. M. Lewis (1971) and Victor Turner (1968) on the afflicted (and possessed) becoming healers, once their affliction is interpreted as a calling. On a more general note see the literature on human

response to life disruption and the need to (re)establish some sense of continuity having personal and social meaning (e.g. Luborsky 1987; Becker 1994). I was aware that in as much as coherence and a sense of continuity are often created in the context of (re)telling life narratives (Peacock and Holland 1992), my willingness to listen to Joan may well have contributed to her "working out" a sense of her mission in the hospital.

38 Framing a condition such as this as the weak point in one's body affected by stress has been referred to by Balint (1957) as a "basic fault."

39 Levinas (1969) has pointed out that coping is not just individual, it requires participation. Joan's efforts to express a sense of agency in a world largely viewed as unsupportive may be viewed as a form of coping.

40 Many theorists, e.g., Foucault and Goffman, have described the hospital as a place where constraint is exercised. In the case presented, the hospital is a space where relations of power are contested at the site of the body and agency is expressed.

41 This interplay entails power asserting itself, meeting resistance, and retreating only to invest itself in new ways.

REFERENCES

Abey, S. and Lipowsky, J. P. 1987, "Comprehensive management of persistent somatization: an innovative in-patient program," *Psychother. Psychosom.* 48:110–15.

Alexander, L. 1982, "Illness maintenance and the new American sick role," in Noel Crisman and Tom Maretski (eds.), *Clinically Applied Anthropology*, Boston: Reidel, pp. 351–67.

Bakhtin, M. 1973, *Problems of Dostoevsky's Poetics* (R. W. Rotsel trans.), Ann Arbor: Ardis.

Balint, M. 1957, *The Doctor, His Patient, and the Illness*, London: Pitman Press.

Barsky, A. 1988a, "The paradox of health," *New England Journal of Medicine* 318(7):414–18.

1988b, *The Worried Well*, Boston: Little, Brown and Company.

Bass, C. and Murphy, M. 1995, "Somatoform and personality disorders: syndromal comorbidity and overlapping developmental pathways," *Journal of Psychosomatic Research* 39(4):403–27.

Becker, G. 1994, "Metaphors in disrupted lives: infertility and cultural constructions of continuity," *Medical Anthropology Quarterly* 8(4):383–410.

Bokin, J. A., Reis, R. K. and Katon, W. J. 1981, "Tertiary gain and chronic pain," *Pain* 10:331–5.

Brodwin, P. 1992, "Symptoms and social performances: the case of Diane Reden," in M. J. DelVecchio Good, Paul Brodwin, Byron Good and Arthur Kleinman (eds.), *Pain as Human Experience: An Anthropological Perspective*, Berkeley: University of California Press.

Brody, D. S. 1980, "Physician recognition of behavioral, psychological and social aspects of medical care," *Archives of Internal Medicine* 10:1286–9.

Conrad, P. and Schneider, J. 1980, "The medical control of deviance: contests and consequences," in *Research in the Sociology of Health Care*, Vol. 1, Greenwich, Connecticut: JAI Press, pp. 1–53.

1992, *Deviance and Medicalization: From Badness to Sickness*, Philadelphia: Temple University Press.

Daniels, A. 1969, "The captive professional: bureaucratic limitations in the practice of military psychiatry," *Journal of Health and Social Behavior* 10(4):255–65.

Engel, G. L. 1980, "The clinical application of the biopsychosocial model," *American Journal of Psychiatry* 137(5):535–44.

Foucault, M. 1980a, *The History of Sexuality*, Vol. 1, New York: Vintage.

1980b, *Power/Knowledge: Selected Interviews and Other Writings 1972–1979*, Brighton: Harvester.

Frankenberg, R. 1986, "Sickness as cultural performance: drama, trajectory and pilgrimage. Root metaphors and the making of disease," *International Journal of Health Services* 16(4):603–26.

1988, "'Your time or mine': an anthropological view of the tragic temporal contradictions of biomedical practice," *International Journal of Health Services* 18(1):11–34.

Giddens, A. 1979, *Central Problems in Social Theory*, Berkeley: University of California Press.

Goffman, E. 1974, *Frame Analysis*, New York: Harper and Row.

Hughes, M. and Ziman, R. 1978, "Children with psychogenic abdominal pain and their families," *Clinical Pediatrics* 17:569–73.

Illich, I. 1976, *Medical Nemesis*, New York: Pantheon.

1986, "Body history," *Lancet* December 6:1325–7.

Ingleby, David 1982, "The social construction of mental illness," in P. Wright and A. Treacher (eds.), *The Problem of Medical Knowledge: Examining the Social Construction of Medicine*, Edinburgh: University of Edinburgh Press, pp. 123–43.

1988, "Professionals as socializers: 'the psy complex'", *Research in Law, Deviance and Social Control* 7:79–109.

Katon, W. and Kleinman, A. 1980, "Doctor-patient negotiation and other social science strategies in patient care," in G. L. Eisenberg and A. Kleinman (eds.), *The Relevance of Social Science for Medicine*, Massachusetts: Reidel Publishers, pp. 253–79.

Kleinman, A. 1988, *The Illness Narratives: Suffering, Healing, and the Human Condition*, New York: Basic Books.

Levinas, E. 1969, *Totality and Infinity*, Pittsburgh: Duquesne University Press.

Lewis, I. M. 1971, *Ecstatic Religion: An Anthropological Study of Spirit Possession and Shamanism*, London: Penguin.

Lipowski, Z. J. 1970, "Physical illness, the individual and the coping process," *Psychiatry in Medicine* 1:91–102.

Lipowsky, J. P. 1986, "Somatization: a borderland between medicine and psychiatry," *Canadian Medical Association Journal* 135:609–14.

Luborsky, M. 1987, "Analysis of multiple life history narratives," *Ethos* 15:366–81.

Mayou, R. 1976, "The nature of bodily symptoms," *British Journal of Psychiatry* 124:55–60.

Nadelson, T. 1979, "The Munchausen spectrum: borderline character features," *General Hospital Psychiatry* 1:11–17.

Nelkin, D. and Tancredi, L. 1989, *Dangerous Diagnostics: The Social Power of Biological Information*, New York: Basic Books.

Nichter, M. 1981, "Idioms of distress: alternatives in the expression of psychosocial distress, a south Indian case study," *Culture, Medicine and Psychiatry* 1:9–23.

Nichter, M., Trockman, G. and Grippen, J. 1985, "Clinical anthropologist as therapy facilitator: role development and clinician evaluation in a psychiatric training program," *Human Organization* 44(1):72–9.

Nichter, M. and Vuckovic, N. 1994, "Agenda for an anthropology of pharmaceutical practice," *Social Science and Medicine* 39(11):1509–25.

Parsons, T. 1976, "Definitions of health and illness in the light of American values and social structure," in E. G. Jacco (ed.), *Patients, Physicians and Illness: A Sourcebook of Readings*, New York: Free Press, pp. 107–27.

Peacock, J. and Holland, D. 1992, "The narrated self: life stories in process," *Ethos* 21:367–83.

Poirier, S. and Brauner, D. 1988, "Ethics and the daily language of medical discourse," *Hastings Center Report* August/September:5–9.

Ryan, W. 1971, *Blaming the Victim*, New York: Vintage.

Scheper-Hughes, N. and Lock, M. 1991, "The message in the bottle: illness and the micropolitics of resistance," *The Journal of Psychohistory* 18(4):409–32.

Scott, J. C. 1985, *Weapons of the Weak: Everyday Forms of Peasant Resistance*, New Haven: Yale University Press.

Sonberg, P. and Kema, R. 1986, *Over-the-Counter Drugs: Harmless or Hazardous?*, New York: Chelsea House Publishers.

Stoeckle, J. D. and Barsky, A. J. 1980, "Attributions: uses of social science knowledge in the 'doctoring' of primary care," in L. Eisenberg and A. Kleinman (eds.), *The Relevance of Social Science for Medicine*, Boston: Reidel Publishers, pp. 223–40.

Stromberg, P. 1985, "The impression point: synthesis of symbol and self," *Ethos* 13:56–74.

Taussig, M. 1980, "Reification and the consciousness of the patient," *Social Science and Medicine* 14b:3–13.

1992, *The Nervous System*, New York: Routledge.

Turner, V. 1968, *The Drums of Affliction: A Study of Religious Processes Among the Ndembu of Zambia*, Oxford: Clarendon Press.

Vuckovic, N. and Nichter, M. 1997, "Changing patterns of pharmaceutical practice in the United States," *Social Science and Medicine*, in press.

World Health Organization 1992, "The ICD-10 classifications of mental and behavioural disorders," in *International Classification of Diseases (Tenth Revision)*, Geneva: Division of Mental Health, WHO.

Index